Surgery 1

For Churchill Livingstone

Publisher: Laurence Hunter
Project Editor: Barbara Simmons
Copy Editor: Jane Ward
Project Controller: Nancy Arnott
Design Direction: Erik Bigland, Charles Simpson
Indexer: Anne McCarthy
Page Layout: Gerard Heyburn

Churchill's Mastery of Medicine

Surgery 1

Edited by

Michael Lavelle-Jones

MBChB FRCS (England) FRCS (Edinburgh) MD

Consultant Surgeon, Honorary Senior Lecturer
Ninewells Hospital and Medical School
Dundee

Illustrations by
Peter Cox

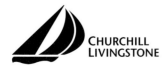
CHURCHILL LIVINGSTONE

NEW YORK, EDINBURGH, LONDON, MADRID, MELBOURNE,
SAN FRANCISCO AND TOKYO 1997

CHURCHILL LIVINGSTONE
Medical Division of Pearson Professional Limited

Distributed in the United States of America by Churchill
Livingstone Inc., 650 Avenue of the Americas, New York,
N.Y. 10011, and by associated companies, branches and
representatives throughout the world.

First published 1997

ISBN 0 443 051720

British Library of Cataloguing in Publication Data
A catalogue record for this book is available from the British
Library.

Library of Congress Cataloging in Publication Data
A catalog record for this book is available from the Library of
Congress.

Medical knowledge is constantly changing. As new information
becomes available, changes in treatment, procedures, equipment
and the use of drugs become necessary. The editors, contributors
and the publishers have, as far as it is possible, taken care to
ensure that the information given in this text is accurate and up
to date. However, readers are strongly advised to confirm that
the information, especially with regard to drug usage, complies
with current legislation and standards of practice.

The
publisher's
policy is to use
**paper manufactured
from sustainable forests**

Produced by Longman Singapore Publishers Pte Ltd
Printed in Singapore

Contributors

Douglas Gentleman BSc MB ChB FRCS (England)
FRCS (Glasgow)
Consultant Neurosurgeon, Dundee Royal Infirmary,
Dundee

C. Goodman MD FRCS (Edinburgh)
Consultant Urologist, Dundee Royal Infirmary,
Dundee

Michael Lavelle-Jones MB ChB FRCS (England)
FRCS (Edinburgh) MD
Consultant Surgeon, Ninewells Hospital and Medical
School, Dundee

Peter T. McCollum MCh FRCS (Ireland)
FRCS (Edinburgh)
Consultant Vascular Surgeon, Ninewells Hospital and
Medical School, Dundee

J. Howard Stevenson MD FRCS (Edinburgh)
Consultant Plastic Surgeon, Dundee Royal Infirmary,
Dundee

W.S. Walker MA MB BChir FRCS (England)
FRCS (Edinburgh)
Consultant Cardiothoracic Surgeon, Royal Infirmary of
Edinburgh, Edinburgh

Contents

Using this book

Philosophy of the book

How much do you know about gallstones? Do you know the right things? Can you answer exam questions on breast cancer? This book aims to help you with these and other similar questions.

In this book essential information is presented in a concise and ordered fashion. Principles are illustrated and mechanisms explained rather than simply giving you lots of facts to memorise. This book does not aim to offer a complete 'syllabus'. It is impossible to draw boundaries around medical knowledge and learning – this is really a continuous process carried out throughout your medical career. With this in mind, you should aim to develop the ability to discern knowledge that *must* be understood, from areas that you *need to know about*, and topics which you should simply *be aware of*.

The aims of this introductory chapter are:

1. to help plan your learning
2. to show you how to use this book to increase your understanding as well as your knowledge
3. to realise how self-assessment can make learning easier and more enjoyable.

Layout and contents

The main part of the text describes important topics in major subject areas. Within each chapter, essential information is presented in a set order with explanations and logical 'links' between topics. Where relevant, key facts about basic sciences/anatomy are outlined. The aetiology, pathological features, clinical features, differential diagnosis and an approach to investigation are then described. Finally, the principles of management and the prognosis are presented. It is recognised that at the level of an undergraduate or newly qualified doctor a detailed understanding is not required; instead the ability to set out principles is all that is expected.

You need to be sure that you are reaching the required standards, so the final section of each chapter is there to help you to check out your knowledge and understanding. The self-assessment is in the form of multiple choice questions, patient management problems, case histories, data interpretation, picture quizzes and viva questions. All of these are centred around common clinical problems that are important in judging your performance as a doctor. Detailed answers are given. These answers will also contain some information and explanations that you will not find elsewhere, so *you have to do the assessment to get the most out of this book*.

How to use this book

I expect you are using this book as part of your exam preparations. Your first task is to map out on a sheet of paper a series of three lists dividing the major subjects (corresponding to the chapter headings) into an assessment of your strong, reasonable and weak areas. This gives you a rough outline of your revision schedule, which you must then fit in with the time available. Clearly, if your exams are looming large you will have to be ruthless in the time allocated to your strong areas. The major subjects should be further classified into individual topics. Encouragement to store information and to test your ongoing improvement is by the use of the self-assessment sections – you must not just read passively. It is important to keep checking your current level of knowledge, both strengths and weaknesses. This should be assessed objectively – self-rating in the absence of testing can be misleading. You may consider yourself strong in a particular area whereas it is more a reflection on how much you enjoy and are stimulated by the subject. Conversely, you may be stronger in a subject than you would expect simply because the topic does not appeal to you.

It is a good idea to discuss topics and problems with colleagues/friends; the areas which you understand least well will soon become apparent when you try to explain them to someone else.

Approaching the examinations

The discipline of learning is closely linked to preparation for examinations. Many of us opt for a process of superficial learning that is directed towards retention of facts and recall under exam conditions because full understanding is often not required. It is much better if you try to acquire a deeper knowledge and understanding, combining the necessity of passing exams with longer term needs.

First, you need to know how you will be examined. Does the examination involve clinical assessment such as history taking and clinical examination? If you are sitting a written examination what are the length and types of questions? How many must you answer and how much choice will you have?

Now you have to choose what sources you are going to use for your learning and revision. Textbooks come in different forms. At one extreme, there is the large reference book. This type of book should be avoided at this stage of revision and only used (if at all) for reference, when answers to questions cannot be found in smaller books. At the other end of the spectrum is the condensed 'lecture note' format, which often relies heavily on lists. Facts of this nature on their own are difficult to remember if they are not supported by understanding. In the middle of the range are the medium-sized textbooks. These are often of the most use whether you are approaching final University examinations or the first part of professional examinations. My advice is to choose one of the several medium-sized books on offer on the basis of which you find the most readable. The best approach is to combine your lecture notes, textbooks (appropriate to the level of study) and past examination papers as a framework for your preparation.

Armed with information about the format of the exams, a rough syllabus, your own lecture notes and some books that you feel comfortable in using, your next step is to map out the time available for preparation. You must be realistic, allow time for breaks and work *steadily*, not cramming. If you do attempt to cram, you have to realise that only a certain amount of information can be retained in your short-term memory, so as the classification of jaundice moves in, the treatment of acute pancreatitis moves out! Cramming simply retains facts. If the examination requires understanding you will be in trouble.

It is often a good idea to begin by outlining the topics to be covered and then attempting to summarise your knowledge about each in note form. In this way your existing knowledge will be activated and any gaps will become apparent. Self-assessment also helps determine the time to be allocated to each subject for exam preparation. If you are consistently scoring excellent marks in a particular subject it is not cost effective to spend a lot of time trying to achieve the 'perfect' mark.

In an essay, it is many times easier to obtain the first mark (try writing your name) than the last. You should also try to decide on the amount of time assigned to each subject based on the likelihood of it appearing in the exam! Commonest things are usually commonest!

The main types of examination

Multiple choice questions

Unless very sophisticated, multiple choice questions test your recall of information. The aim is to gain the maximum marks from the knowledge that you can remember. The stem statement must be read with great care highlighting the 'little' words such as *only, rarely, usually, never* and *always*. Overlooking negatives, such as *not, unusual* and *unsuccessful* often causes marks to be lost. *May occur* has an entirely different connotation to *characteristic*. The latter may mean a feature which should be there and the absence of which would make you question the correctness of the diagnosis.

Remember to check the marking method before starting. Most multiple choice papers employ a negative system in which marks are lost for incorrect answers. The temptation is to adopt a cautious approach, answering a relatively small number of questions. However, this can lead to problems, as we all make simple mistakes or even disagree vehemently with the answer in the computer! Caution may lead you to answer too few questions to obtain a pass after the marks have been deducted for incorrect answers.

Short notes

Short notes are not negatively marked. Predetermined marks are given for each important key fact. Nothing is gained for style or superfluous information. The aim is to set out your knowledge in an ordered *concise* manner. Do not devote too much time to a single question thereby neglecting the rest, and remember to limit your answer to the question that has been set.

Essays

Similar comments apply to essays, but marks may be awarded for logical development of an argument or theme. Conversely, good marks will not be obtained for an essay that is a set of unconnected statements. Always plan your essay answer. Length matters little if there is no cohesion. It is even more important in an examination based on essays to manage your time carefully. *All* questions must be given equal weight. A brilliant answer in one essay will not compensate for not attempting another because time runs out.

Data interpretation

Data interpretation involves the application of knowledge to solve a problem. In your revision you should aim for an understanding of principles; it is impossible to memorise all the different data combinations. In an exam, a helpful approach is to translate numbers into a description; for example, a serum potassium of 2.8 mmol/litre is *low* and the ECG tracing of a heart rate of 120/min shows a *tachy*cardia. This type of question is usually not negatively marked so put down an answer even if you are far from sure that it is right.

Slide/picture quizzes

Recognition is the first step in a picture quiz. This should be coupled with a systematic approach looking for, and listing, abnormalities. For example, breast shadows, bony skeleton, soft tissues, retrocardiac space, etc, can be examined in a chest X-ray. Describe in your mind what you see and try to match it with common problems. Again, even if you are in doubt, put an answer down. Any accompanying statement or data should be used alongside the visual image as it may give a clue as to the answer required; it may also be essential in distinguishing between two conditions that are of the same appearance.

Patient management problems

A more sophisticated form of exam question is an evolving case history, with information being presented sequentially and you being asked to give a response at each stage. They are constructed so that a wrong response in the first part of the question does not mean that no more marks can be obtained from the subsequent parts. Each part should stand on its own. Patient management problems are designed to test the recall and application of knowledge through an understanding of the principles involved.

Vivas

The viva examination can be a nerve-racking experience. You are normally faced with two examiners who may react with irritation, boredom or indifference to what you say. You may feel that the viva has gone well and yet you fail, or more commonly, you think that the exam has gone terribly simply because of the apparent attitude of the examiners.

Your main aim during the viva should be to control the examiners' questioning so they constantly ask you about things you know. Despite what is often said, you can prepare for this form of exam. Questions are liable to take one of a small number of forms centred around subjects that cannot be examined in a traditional clinical exam.

During the viva there are certain techniques which help in making a favourable impression. When dis-cussing patient management, it is better to say 'I would do this' rather than 'the book says this'. You should try and strike a balance between saying too little and too much. It is important to try not to go off the topic. Aim to keep your answers short and to the point. It is worth-while pausing for a few seconds to collect your thoughts before launching into an answer. Do not be afraid to say 'I don't know'; most examiners will want to change tack to see what you do know about.

Conclusions

You should amend the framework for using this book according to your own needs and the examinations you are facing. Whatever approach you adopt your aim should be for an understanding of the principles involved rather than rote learning of a large number of poorly connected facts.

Surgical principles

1.1 Pre- and postoperative management

Preoperative preparation

History and physical examination

A thorough history and physical examination are the key initial steps in the preoperative work-up of any surgical patient. Although the presenting complaint is of prime importance, any previous medical or surgical history, drug history or allergies must be sought as they may influence the choice of operation, anaesthetic or perioperative care.

Laboratory investigations

Biochemical and haematological screening are important in all patients undergoing major surgery and in older patients undergoing minor surgery. These tests can detect an unsuspected metabolic abnormality or anaemia that would require investigation and correction prior to surgery.

Diagnostic radiology

Many patients will have undergone diagnostic radiology prior to surgery and often prior to hospital admission. These films must be available and have been reviewed prior to operation.

Preoperative chest X-ray and ECG

Patients over 50 years of age and younger patients with respiratory or cardiovascular abnormalities detected on history and examination should have a preoperative chest X-ray and/or ECG.

Blood cross-match

Blood samples either for grouping and serum saving or for cross-matching should be taken according to the magnitude of the intended operation.

Informed consent

Obtaining consent should not be delegated to the most junior member of the surgical team. Instead, a careful, logical explanation of the planned operation and any alternatives should be given to the patient, preferably by the surgeon who is to perform the operation.

Medical problems in surgical patients

Many medical disorders can influence the management of the surgical patient. The three most commonly encountered groups of problems are:

- respiratory disease
- cardiovascular disease
- diabetes mellitus.

Respiratory disease

Upper respiratory tract infection

Any patient with evidence of an upper respiratory tract infection should have *elective* surgery postponed until the infection has cleared. Although most of these infections are viral in origin, manipulation during induction and maintenance of anaesthesia render these patients prone to a serious secondary bacterial respiratory tract infection in the postoperative period.

Chronic obstructive airways disease and asthma

Patients known preoperatively to have chronic pulmonary disease must stop smoking 1–2 weeks prior to surgery and should be admitted in advance of their operation to enable the following measures to be undertaken:

- full evaluation of respiratory system: both pulmonary function testing and arterial blood gases
- preoperative physiotherapy
- sputum culture and treatment of any infection
- anaethestic consultation: regional anaesthesia (spinal or epidural) may be more appropriate than general anaesthesia in certain cases.

Cardiovascular disease

Patients with cardiovascular disease are at risk during surgery and in the immediate postoperative period, when fluctuations in blood pressure and fluid balance can compromise a limited cardiac reserve. The decision to operate in this group of patients is a balance of risks which requires close cooperation between surgeon, cardiologist and anaesthetist.

Myocardial infarction and angina

The risks of reinfarction are minimised if surgery can be delayed until at least 6 months after a previous myocardial infarction. Patients with angina should be symptomatically well controlled before undergoing surgery.

Hypertension

Medical therapy and control should be optimised before surgery.

Congestive heart failure

Surgery is likely to aggravate heart failure in these patients when they lie flat on the operating table, particularly if intravenous fluid therapy is needed. Diuretic therapy and cardiac inotropic support should be optimised prior to surgery.

Valvular heart disease

These patients require special precautions to prevent fluid overload as their cardiac reserve may be limited. Many patients will be taking long-term anticoagulation therapy, which will need to be temporarily withdrawn or reduced, and the patient will need to be closely monitored to allow surgery to be undertaken without risk of major bleeding. Antibiotic prophylaxis is essential to prevent endocarditis.

Diabetes mellitus

Glucose, potassium (K⁺) and insulin (GKI) continuous infusion regimens have revolutionised the management of diabetic patients undergoing surgery. The amount of insulin added to the 10% dextrose (glucose) solution is varied depending upon the patient's blood sugar level, which is regularly monitored. An insulin-induced hypokalaemia is prevented by continuous potassium supplementation.

This regimen is established on the morning of surgery for insulin-dependent diabetics and also for those non-insulin-dependent diabetics who usually use oral hypoglycaemic agents. It is continued until patients resume their normal diet after surgery. Special measures are rarely required for diabetics who are normally adequately controlled by dietary measures alone.

Fluid balance and nutrition

Surgery profoundly affects the whole body balance and the distribution of fluids and electrolytes. The principles of fluid management in the surgical patient depend upon an understanding of the baseline daily fluid requirements plus a knowledge of the effects of surgical procedures and disease on normal metabolism.

Fluid and electrolyte balance in the surgical patient

The three most important components are water, sodium and potassium. The normal water and electrolyte turnover in a healthy individual is summarised in Table 1. Fluid and electrolyte therapy depends upon:

- maintenance of daily requirements
- replacement of ongoing fluid losses
- replacement of long-standing fluid deficits.

Maintenance of daily requirements

A healthy 70 kg person needs 2500 ml water plus 100 mmol sodium plus 40 mmol potassium each day. This is equivalent to 2 litres of 5% dextrose with 40 mmol added potassium plus 500 ml 0.9% (normal) saline solution. This fluid regimen will maintain the baseline fluid requirements in most patients.

Replacement of ongoing losses

A daily fluid balance chart has a central role to play in managing each patient's fluid requirements. It is especially important to record fluid losses from:

- nasogastric aspiration
- vomit
- stoma output
- fistula output
- drain output
- urine output.

These volumes shoud be considered together with the daily urine, stool and insensible losses (see Table 1) and should be replaced volume for volume in the following 24 hours with either normal saline or a balanced salt solution (Ringer's solution or Hartmann's solution).

Insensible losses. If a patient is febrile, excess water will be lost through sweating and evaporation and this should be replaced with an extra 500 ml of 5% dextrose solution.

Replacement of long-standing fluid deficits

This is a difficult concept to grasp. In patients who, for example, have had a long-standing bowel obstruction or who have had severe burns, large volumes of fluid will be sequestered either in the intestinal lumen or in the interstitial fluid. This fluid, which has been 'lost' from the circulation and from the intracellular and extracellular fluid spaces, can amount to several litres and if replaced too rapidly would overexpand the circulating plasma volume causing heart failure and gross oedema.

Complex formulae exist that help estimate these losses, which should be replaced slowly over a period of days.

Surgical nutrition

A good nutritional status is vital to ensure repair and healing after surgery. Wherever possible, elective surgery should be postponed until nutritional deficiencies have been corrected.

The key factors that determine a patient's nutritional status are:

- dietary history
- weight loss (> 5 kg is significant)
- anthropomorphic measurements of muscle and fat stores
- serum albumen level.

The optimum diet includes an adequate number of calories, protein, fat, minerals and vitamins to meet the energy and growth and repair demands of daily activi-

Table 1 Normal daily turnover of water and electrolytes

	Intake		Output	
Water (ml)	Food and liquid	2000	Urine	1000
	Internal metabolism	500	Sweat	500–750
			Expired air	250
			Stools	250
Total water (ml)		2500		2500
Sodium (mmol)	Diet 100		Urine 100	
Potassium (mmol)	Diet 100		Urine 60	
			Internal metabolism 40	

Table 2 Essential dietary components

- 2 500 kcal/day caloric intake for a 70 kg human
- 1g/kg protein to supply essential amino acids
- Fat-soluble vitamins: vitamins A, D, K, E
- Water-soluble vitamins: vitamin B group, vitamin C
- Essential fatty acids
- Trace elements: copper, zinc, iron, manganese

ties. These requirements are summarised in Table 2. Calories and nitrogen should be given simultaneously to achieve a positive nitrogen balance (a net synthesis of protein). The optimum ratio is 150 kcal for every gram of nitrogen. At least one half of the calories must be given as glucose (in order to stimulate insulin secretion which in turn facilitates protein synthesis). The remaining calories can be given as fat, which will have the added benefit of providing the essential fatty acids necessary for a balanced diet.

The two main forms of surgical nutrition are:

- enteral nutrition
- parenteral nutrition.

Enteral nutrition, which uses the patient's own gastrointestinal tract for nutrient absorption, is preferable to the parenteral (intravenous route), which is prone to serious complication and is more expensive.

Enteral nutrition

There are three main types of enteral nutrition:

- oral supplementation: using high-calorie/high-protein drinks to supplement oral intake
- nasogastric or nasojejunal tube feeding: using fine-bore silastic tubes to deliver enteral nutrition direct to the small bowel
- feeding gastrostomy or jejunostomy: exteriorising part of the stomach or proximal jejunum as a conduit for feeding.

Enteral nutrition is most useful in patients who have an intact, functioning full-length gastrointestinal tract or at least 300 cm of small bowel. Abdominal cramps, diarrhoea and vomiting are the major side effects and are caused by the delivery of hypertonic enteral feeds directly to the small intestine.

Parenteral nutrition

The composition of parenteral nutrition can be individualised to the nutritional requirements of each patient. Each pharmacy-prepared nutrition bag contains enough nutrients for a 24-hour period and consists of:

- amino acids
- dextrose
- lipids
- vitamins, minerals and trace elements.

This solution is thrombogenic and has to be administered via a large central vein (superior vena cava/right atrium) to avoid thrombosis. The silastic feeding

catheters used are tunnelled subcutaneously from the vein to an exit point usually on the chest wall. Strict aseptic technique must be used when changing the nutrition bag to prevent introducing sepsis.

Parenteral nutrition is best restricted to those patients whose intestinal tract cannot cope with enteral nutrition. Typically this includes:

- patients with Crohn's disease
- patients with high small bowel fistulae
- patients with short gut syndrome following major small bowel resection
- catabolic postoperative patients with septic complications.

Analgesia

Adequate pain control is vital to allay anxiety pre- and postoperatively and to allow patients to rest, recuperate and sleep. Three groups of drugs are used:

- opioids (usually morphine)
- non-steroidal anti-inflammatory agents (NSAIDs)
- mild oral analgesics.

Opioids

These drugs are the most potent analgesics and form the cornerstone of treatment in postoperative analgesia. Newer methods of delivery have supplanted intramuscular and subcutaneous routes, which are prone to unpredictable absorption and may subject patients to overdose, causing respiratory depression, or underdose, causing inadequate pain control.

Patient controlled analgesia. This is the optimum technique for pain management after major surgery. A predetermined bolus of morphine is delivered intravenously from a special pump that is activated by the patient. Overdosage is prevented by a 'lock-out' mechanism that prevents the patient reactivating the pump until a set time has elapsed. In each case, the bolus dose and lock-out time can be adjusted to suit the individual patient's needs.

Epidural opioids. Opioids or local anaesthetic agents (e.g. bupivacaine) can be infused into the epidural space through a suitably postioned catheter. This technique blocks the afferent nerves and effectively controls pain. It is a type of regional anaesthesia. Respiratory depression is less in comparison with opiates which have been administered systemically. Because the vasomotor nerves are also blocked epidural analgesia can cause severe orthostatic hypotension and these patients require careful monitoring of their blood pressure.

Non-steroidal anti-inflammatory drugs

These agents can be administered by intramuscular, rectal or oral routes. They are effective in relieving pain after minor surgery or for patients who have had major surgery and no longer require opioid therapy. They can be used in combination with opioids to reduce the dose of opioid required to relieve pain.

Mild oral analgesics

Many of these are non-opioid analgesics. They occupy the bottom rung of the prescription ladder for pain relief. Paracetamol is the usual starting drug and should be administered on a regular rather than 'as required' basis to provide the maximum benefit. If this is ineffective, weak opioid analgesics such as dihydrocodeine should be used either alone or as a compound analgesic preparation with paracetamol.

Postoperative monitoring

Close observation of a patient's vital signs (pulse/blood pressure/temperature/respiration rate) and careful fluid balance will optimise recovery and enable early detection of impending complications.

In most surgical units there are three levels of postoperative monitoring activity and care:

- general surgical ward
- high dependency unit
- intensive care unit.

The majority of patients undergoing routine elective surgery will be recovered satisfactorily in an ordinary surgical ward. Others with intercurrent medical problems (see p. 6), undergoing epidural anaesthetic techniques (see p. 9) or who have undergone emergency major surgery may require more intensive monitoring. Many of these patients can be effectively managed on a high dependency surgical unit, which provides continuous pulse, blood pressure and oximetry measurements together with hourly fluid balance. The high dependency unit provides a higher nurse/patient ratio than the general surgical ward.

Intensive care is reserved for those patients who require ventilation after surgery or who develop serious respiratory, cardiac or septic complications.

1.2 Postoperative complications

For most patients, postoperative recovery is uneventful and is characterised by a systematic return to normal function. Any deviation from this predicted course is a postoperative complication. Complications are sometimes unavoidable in critically ill patients who undergo urgent surgery. In patients who undergo elective surgery, complications should be rare and may be avoided with careful pre- and perioperative care.

Pulmonary problems

Respiratory complications are the most frequent and are common to all surgical procedures.

Atelectasis and pneumonia

Inadequate ventilation of small pulmonary airways plus retention of respiratory secretions leads to alveolar collapse and atelectasis. If untreated, a secondary bacterial infection will supervene causing lobar or bronchopneumonia. The most important predisposing factors are:

- smoking
- chronic obstructive airways disease (COAD)
- postoperative pain (inhibits respiratory effort) and coughing.

Onset of these complications can be prevented *preoperatively* by:

- stopping smoking before surgery
- preoperative physiotherapy for patients with COAD
- deferring elective surgery for at least 2 weeks in patients with a chest infection.

Important intra operative measures are:

- choice of incision
- deep vein thrombosis prophylaxis (to prevent pulmonary thrombo-embolism).

Important postoperative measures are:

- intensive physiotherapy
- adequate pain relief.

Diagnosis and treatment

An early postoperative fever is caused by a respiratory complication until proved otherwise. It is confirmed on physical examination of the chest or by chest X-ray.

Sputum culture and broad-spectrum antibiotic cover should be instituted in addition to the above measures.

Pulmonary aspiration. Supine posture and the absence of the normal protective reflexes during general anaesthesia predispose surgical patients to pulmonary aspiration. Regurgitated gastric contents usually enter the right main bronchus. Three groups are especially at risk:

- pregnant women
- patients with bowel obstruction
- non-fasted patients requiring urgent surgery.

The most important preventative measures are:

- preoperative nasogastric drainage
- an adequately-fasted patient
- anaesthetic care using cricoid pressure to prevent aspiration during intubation and use of a cuffed endotracheal tube to prevent aspiration while the patient is paralysed and ventilated.

Postoperative respiratory depression

Immediate respiratory depression is caused by the persistent action of opiates or muscular relaxants administered during surgery, or by a massive pulmonary collapse. Respiratory depression later on in the postoperative period is usually caused by oversedation with opioid analgesic agents.

These complications can be prevented by careful prescribing practice and close monitoring of the conscious level and postoperative respiratory effort. A pulse oximeter will give an early indication of arterial desaturation.

Postoperative respiratory failure

Patients with severe intra-abdominal sepsis, fat embolus or those who have had a massive blood transfusion are at risk of developing adult respiratory distress syndrome (ARDS). Untreated, arterial hypoxaemia and carbon dioxide retention will be accompanied by a progressive radiological opacification of the lung fields (Fig. 1). Without treatment these patients will develop irreversible pulmonary failure and will die. Their management is complex and depends upon:

- identifying and eliminating any treatable underlying cause
- intubation and mechanical ventilatory support.

Postoperative shock

Shock is defined as a failure to maintain adequate tissue perfusion. Hypotension, tachycardia, sweating, pallor and peripheral vasoconstriction are the hallmarks of hypovolaemic and cardiogenic shock. Without treatment, oliguria and multisystem organ failure develop and lead to death.

The precise clinical picture will depend on the underlying cause. The three main types of postoperative shock (Table 3) are:

- hypovolaemic
- septic
- cardiogenic.

A

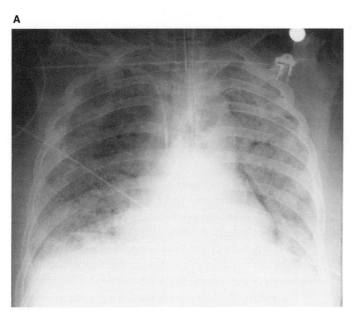

B

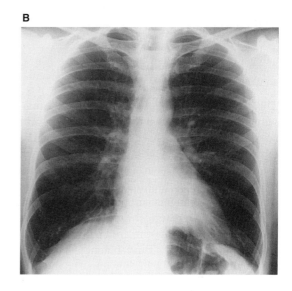

Fig. 1
Adult respiratory distress syndrome (**A**); and a normal chest X-ray (**B**) for comparison.

Table 3 A comparison of the key clinical features in hypovolaemic, cardiogenic and septic shock

	Normal	Hypovolaemic shock	Cardiogenic shock	Septic shock	
				Early	Late
Pulse rate beats/min	72	> 100	40–120, regular or irregular	> 100	> 100
Jugular venous pressure (cm H$_2$O)	5–10	0–5 or negative	> 10	0–5 or negative	0–5 or negative
Skin	—	Cold, clammy	Cold, clammy	Warm	Cold, clammy
Blood pressure mm H$_{(g)}$	120/80	< 100 systolic	< 100 systolic	Normal, or < 100 systolic	< 100 systolic
Urine output (ml/hours)	30	< 30	< 30	30	< 30

Hypovolaemic shock

This is the most common type of postoperative shock. It may be caused by:

- inadequate replacement of pre- or perioperative fluid losses
- continued haemorrhage in the postoperative period.

Treatment
Careful fluid balance will prevent most cases of hypovolaemic shock. Ongoing haemorrhage may be obvious from a chest drain but is less clear after abdominal surgery, when large volumes of blood can collect unnoticed in the abdomen. A careful judgement may be required by the surgeon with regard to the need for re-operation.

The essential management points are:

Replacement. Replace the circulating volume *and* extracellular fluid losses with a combination of whole blood and a balanced salt solution.

Monitor. Monitor the response:

- blood pressure and pulse rate (aim to restore preoperative values)
- urine output (keep at 30ml/hour; 0.5–1ml/kg/hour)
- establish central venous pressure measurement (aim for values between 5–10 cm water).

Appraisal. Think about reoperation if ongoing haemorrhage is suspected.

Septic shock

The most frequent causes of septic shock in the postoperative patient are listed in Table 4. Early septic shock is characterised by a hyperdynamic circulation with fevers, rigors, a warm vasodilated periphery and a bounding pulse. Untreated, late septic shock supervenes with hypotension, peripheral vasoconstriction and anuria.

The essential points of management are:

Assessment. Identify and remedy any underlying cause: this may involve anything from changing an infected central venous line to re-operation for intra-abdominal sepsis.

Antibiotic therapy. Implement broad-spectrum aerobic and anaerobic antibiotic therapy after an infection screen and blood/sputum/urine culture.

Monitor and support. Instigate intensive monitoring plus fluid therapy and respiratory and renal function support to prevent multisystem organ failure.

Cardiogenic shock

This is usually secondary to acute myocardial ischaemia or infarction causing left ventricular failure or a rhythm disturbance. In patients with pre-existing cardiac disease, fluid overload may induce cardiac failure.

In addition to poor peripheral perfusion, these patients will have an elevated jugular venous pressure,

Table 4 Major causes of postoperative fever and sepsis

Day 1	Atelectasis, chest infection
Day 5	Wound infection
Days 7–10	Intra-abdominal sepsis
	Thromboembolism
Any day	Catheter or i.v. line sepsis

basal crepitations and a gallop cardiac rhythm plus acute electrocardiographic changes.

The essential management points are:

Control fluid overload. Establish a diuresis to remove fluid overload.

Monitor. Instigate invasive monitoring of cardiac function (CVP or Swann–Ganz catheter).

Therapy. Use vasoactive or inotropic drugs to optimise myocardial efficiency.

Wound complications

The two most important wound complications are:

- wound infection
- wound dehiscence.

Wound infection

This is one of the most frequent surgical postoperative complications. It is seen least in clean elective surgical wounds (e.g. inguinal hernia repair) and most often in contaminated wounds (e.g. perforated diverticular disease).

The main factors in reducing the risk of wound infection are surgical technique and aseptic care.

Meticulous surgical technique:

- minimise tissue trauma
- preserve wound blood supply
- prevent wound haematoma.

Prevention of wound contamination:

- preoperative bowel preparation
- perioperative antibiotic prophylaxis
- good surgical technique.

Wound infections present with a fever on about the fifth postoperative day. Inspection of the wound site reveals tenderness, erythema and induration. An infected wound should be opened widely to enable release of any contained pus and the wound packed loosely with gauze to ensure adequate drainage. Antibiotics have only a secondary role in wound sepsis and are not a substitute for surgical drainage. After treatment, these wounds should be left to heal by secondary intention.

Wound dehiscence

A wound dehiscence is a failure of wound healing. Although any wound can dehisce, it usually affects abdominal wounds (burst abdomen), which disrupt usually 7–10 days after surgery, leaking serosanguinous fluid and then revealing the viscera.

The two most important groups of factors predisposing to wound dehiscence are poor surgical technique and impaired wound healing.

Iatrogenic (poor surgical technique):

- tight sutures causing wound ischaemia
- suture breakage.

Patient-related (poor wound healing). This occurs more often in patients at increased risk:

- malnourished patients
- septic patients
- patients with inoperable malignancy
- morbidly obese patients
- jaundiced patients.

Treatment. Re-exploration and resuture of the wound under general anaethesia is essential. Dehiscence rarely recurs.

Urinary problems and postoperative renal failure

Acute urinary retention and urinary tract infection are the most common postoperative urinary complications.

Acute urinary retention

There are three major predisposing factors:

- preoperative history of symptoms of bladder outflow obstruction
- postoperative immobility
- postoperative pain.

Retention may be prevented by selective perioperative catheterisation of at-risk patients, e.g. those with symptoms of prostatic outflow obstruction or who are undergoing major abdominal or perineal surgery.

Urinary tract infection

Postcatheterisation urinary tract infection is usually caused by:

- a breakdown in sterile technique during catheter insertion
- contamination of the catheter drainage system.

Infection can be difficult to eradicate. The choice of antibiotics is dictated by the results of urine culture. Prompt removal of the catheter as soon as the patient is ambulant will reduce the frequency of infection.

Postoperative renal failure

Acute renal failure can be:

- prerenal
- renal
- postrenal.

Prerenal failure
Underperfusion of the kidneys is the final common pathway. This is usually caused by inadequate fluid balance during the pre- and perioperative period or by continued haemorrhage and fluid losses that have been overlooked. The management is outlined on page 10.

Renal failure
Uncorrected prerenal failure will eventually cause acute parenchymal renal failure. Other important causes are:

- incompatible blood transfusion
- myoglobinuria from a soft tissue crush injury
- septic shock
- hepatorenal syndrome (renal failure associated with obstructive jaundice).

Treatment. Wherever possible, any underlying cause is treated. Haemodialysis may be necessary until renal function recovers.

Postrenal failure
The two most important causes of postrenal failure are:

- catheter blockage
- ureteric ligation.

Catheter blockage is easily treated. Unilateral ureteric ligation is usually silent and the remaining kidney compensates. Bilateral ligation is rare but may occur in patients who have undergone a difficult surgical dissection in the pelvis.

Thromboembolic disorders

The pathogenesis of venous thrombosis involves stasis, increased blood coagulability and damage to the blood vessel wall (Virchow's triad). Prevention of deep vein thrombosis or early detection of an established thrombosis is essential in order to prevent death from pulmonary embolus. Despite all current measures, 1 in 200 patients undergoing major surgery will die from pulmonary embolus.

Deep vein thrombosis

Most deep vein thromboses start in an area of venous stasis, usually in the calf veins. Local vascular damage and hypercoagulability caused by surgical stress also contribute. The following factors increase the risk of thrombosis:

- **patient-related factors**
  — increasing age, obesity
  — oral contraception
  — prolonged postoperative immobility
  — smoking
  — pregnancy

- **disease-related factors**
  — malignancy
  — recent myocardial infarction

- **procedure-related factors**
  — long operation time
  — limb or hip surgery
  — intra-abdominal pelvic dissection.

Diagnosis

A deep vein thrombosis may be clinically silent or present with a painful, tender swollen calf. It may be a cause of postoperative fever. The diagnosis is confirmed by:

- venography
- Doppler ultrasonography.

Prophylaxis and treatment

Stopping smoking before surgery and losing weight, if appropriate, will help reduce the risk of deep vein thrombosis. A combination of graduated elastic calf compression stockings plus pre- and perioperative cover with low-dose subcutaneous heparin injections effectively reduces the incidence of deep vein thrombosis *and* fatal pulmonary embolus.

An established deep vein thrombosis is treated by immediate full anticoagulation using a continuous intravenous heparin infusion and simultaneous oral anticoagulation with warfarin. Heparin therapy is stopped once the patient is on full oral anticoagulation, which is then continued for 3–6 months.

Pulmonary embolism

Most pulmonary emboli arise from a propagated clot which detaches and embolises from the iliac or femoral veins. The clinical presentation depends on the size of the embolus:

- massive embolus: circulatory collapse, cardiac arrest and death
- small embolus: pleuritic chest pain, haemoptysis, cyanosis, pleural friction rub, tachycardia, tachypnoea, right heart failure
- recurrent embolus: progressive dyspnoea.

Diagnosis

Confirming the diagnosis, particularly if the embolus is small, can be difficult. The following features are usually present either alone or in combination:

- arterial hypoxia
- electrocardiographic changes (S waves, lead 1; Q waves and T wave inversion in lead 3)
- chest X-ray: may be normal or show reduced pulmonary vascular markings
- a mismatched defect on isotope ventilation/ perfusion scanning (this is the most reliable test).

Treatment

The key steps in the treatment of pulmonary emboli are:

- supplemental oxygen therapy
- systemic anticoagulation
  — most pulmonary emboli will be satisfactorily treated by these measures
- surgery: although urgent thoracotomy and open embolectomy for a massive embolus may be life-saving, it is rarely feasible; transvenous embolectomy using a special suction catheter introduced via the femoral vein is sometimes successful. Filters can be placed into the inferior vena cava using radiological techniques to prevent recurrent emboli.

Postoperative intra-abdominal sepsis

Postoperative sepsis is usually caused by anastomotic breakdown or a failure to eradicate infection at the original laparotomy. The infection is either generalised (peritonitis) or localised (intra-abdominal abscess) and can be extremely difficult to diagnose. It should be suspected in any patient who develops signs of sepsis 7–10 days after a laparotomy.

Diagnosis:

Investigations include:

- contrast radiology: to detect any anastomotic leak
- ultrasound or CT scan: to detect any abnormal intra-abdominal fluid collections or abscess
- laparotomy should be undertaken if doubt remains despite negative radiology.

Treatment

Postoperative intra-abdominal abscess can be drained percutaneously using interventional radiology techniques under antibiotic cover. If infection is widespread, causing generalised peritonitis, laparotomy and drainage is usually required with exteriorisation of any disrupted anastomosis. Overall mortality rates are high (30%) for this serious complication.

Self assessment: questions

Multiple choice questions

1. The following are contraindications to major elective surgery requiring general anaesthesia:
   a. A myocardial infarction 12 months ago
   b. A preoperative serum potassium of 2.6 mmol/litre in a patient on diuretic therapy
   c. Previous mitral valve replacement
   d. A resolving upper respiratory tract infection
   e. Unsuspected glycosuria on routine ward urine testing

2. The following statements concerning fluid and electrolyte balance are correct:
   a. Nasogastric aspirates should be replaced volume for volume with 5% dextrose solution
   b. 100 mmol potassium are required each day to replace baseline losses
   c. Long-standing fluid deficits should be replaced within the first 24 hours
   d. Insensible losses are unchanged by fever
   e. A total daily intravenous fluid intake of 1500 ml will maintain baseline fluid requirements in a normal individual

3. Enteral nutrition is:
   a. Highly thrombogenic
   b. Used in patients with the short gut syndrome
   c. A potential cause of abdominal cramps and diarrhoea
   d. More likely to cause septic complications than parenteral nutrition
   e. Contraindicated in patients after a cerebrovascular accident

4. The following features are in keeping with a postoperative opiate overdose:
   a. Hyperventilation
   b. Mydriasis
   c. Hypotension
   d. Tachycardia
   e. Hypoxaemia

5. Venous thromboembolism prophylaxis is required in:
   a. A 24-year-old woman undergoing appendicectomy who uses oral contraception
   b. A 50-year-old woman with rectal cancer requiring anterior resection
   c. An 80-year-old man requiring hip replacement
   d. A 50-year-old woman undergoing palliative bypass for inoperable pancreatic cancer
   e. A 40-year-old man undergoing inguinal hernia repair

6. The following statements concern cardiogenic shock:
   a. It can be distinguished from hypovolaemic shock by central venous blood pressure measurements
   b. It can be distinguished from hypovolaemic shock by systemic blood pressure recordings
   c. It responds to a fluid challenge
   d. It responds to inotropic support
   e. It is a cause of postoperative oliguria

7. The following features are in keeping with a major pulmonary embolus:
   a. A matched defect on isotopic ventilation/perfusion scanning
   b. Pleuritic pain and haemoptysis
   c. Peripheral but not central cyanosis
   d. Tachypnoea
   e. ECG evidence of left ventricular strain

8. An abdominal wound dehiscence:
   a. Usually occurs before the fifth postoperative day
   b. Frequently recurs
   c. Is often fatal
   d. Is more common in jaundiced patients
   e. Is increased in patients on steroid therapy

9. Aspiration pneumonia:
   a. Most commonly affects the left upper lobe
   b. Is more frequent following emergency than elective surgery
   c. Is less likely if cricoid pressure is used during intubation
   d. Is aggravated by gastric acidity
   e. Is less common in patients with reflux oesophagitis

10. Postoperative atelectasis is more common in:
    a. Smokers
    b. Patients undergoing lower abdominal surgery
    c. Obstructed patients
    d. The period between the fifth and tenth postoperative days
    e. Oversedated patients

Case histories

Case history 1

A 61-year-old man develops a fever of 38.4°C 7 days after an anterior resection.

1. What are the most likely causes?
2. What steps would you take to reach the appropriate diagnosis?
3. How would you treat this patient?

Case history 2

You are called to see a patient in the middle of the night. He is a 72-year-old man who had an emergency partial gastrectomy for a bleeding gastric ulcer 6 hours previously. The nursing staff are concerned because he has not passed any urine for 2 hours and has a systolic blood pressure of 95 mmHg.

1. What are the most likely causes?
2. How would you differentiate them?
3. What steps would you take to resuscitate this patient?

Short notes

1. Compare ECG tracing A and B (Fig. 2):
   a. What are the abnormalities on tracing B?
   b. What is the most likely diagnosis?
   c. How would you confirm the diagnosis?
   d. How would you treat this patient?

A

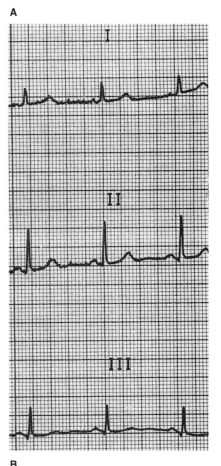

B

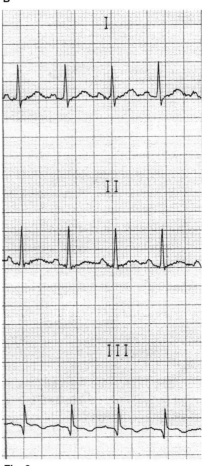

Fig. 2
ECG tracing.

Self-assessment: answers

Multiple choice answers

1. a. **False.** Elective surgery should be postponed for at least 6 months after a myocardial infarction. Thereafter, the risk of reinfarction is about 5%.
   b. **True.** The normal serum potassium ranges from 3.5–5.5 mmol/litre. This patient is hypokalaemic (2.6 mmol/litre) and is at risk of cardiac arrhythmia if anaesthesia is induced. The hypokalaemia should be corrected by slow intravenous potassium infusion over 24–48 hours before proceeding to surgery.
   c. **False.** Patients with previous valvular heart surgery are usually fit enough to undergo surgery. They do require antibiotic prophylaxis to prevent endocarditis, and careful fluid balance to prevent fluid overload together with close monitoring and a temporary reduction of any anticoagulant therapy.
   d. **True.** Patients with evidence of an upper respiratory infection preoperatively who undergo surgery are at risk of developing major respiratory postoperative complications. Elective surgery should be deferred until any infection is completely resolved.
   e. **True.** This may be the first indication of diabetes in an asymptomatic patient. Surgery tends to elevate blood glucose levels and may precipitate a diabetic coma in a previously undiagnosed diabetic. If unsuspected glycosuria is detected surgery should be deferred until the diagnosis of diabetes has been confirmed or excluded.

2. a. **False.** Nasogastric aspirates contain large amounts of sodium, potassium and chloride ions in addition to other elements. Nasogastric losses should be replaced volume for volume by 0.9% saline solution with added potassium or by a balanced salt solution (Hartmann's or Ringer's solution).
   b. **False.** Daily urinary potassium excretion averages 60 mmol/litre.
   c. **False.** Patients with long-standing fluid losses may be deficient of 5 or more litres of extracellular fluid. This should be replaced slowly over the first 48 hours to prevent overexpansion of the circulating plasma volume. It is important to remember while calculating the daily fluid balance that these patients will also need fluid to replace any ongoing losses (nasogastric aspirates, etc.) as well as their baseline daily requirements.
   d. **False.** Insensible losses are increased by fever through sweating and exhalation of warm humidified air. Water is lost in excess of sodium and should be replaced by 5% dextrose solution.

   e. **False.** The daily intravenous fluid requirement is 2500 ml (500 ml 0.9% normal saline, 2000 ml 5% dextrose).

3. a. **False.** Enteral nutrition is delivered via the gastrointestinal tract and is not associated with any thrombogenic risk. Parenteral nutrition is highly thrombogenic hence the need for central venous access where high rates of blood flow reduce the risk of thrombosis.
   b. **False.** Patients with a short gut have limited absorptive capacity. They are best fed via the parenteral route.
   c. **True.** Enteral nutrition is hyperosmolar and can stimulate gastrointestinal motility producing diarrhoea and cramps.
   d. **False.** Parenteral nutrition requires strict asepsis to prevent catheter sepsis, thrombosis and septicaemia. Enteral nutrition using the gut is less prone to septic complication.
   e. **False.** Provided these patients have an intact gag and cough reflex they can be fed enterally without a significant risk of aspiration.

4. a. **False.** Opiate overdosage causes respiratory depression.
   b. **False.** Opiates cause pupillary constriction rather than dilatation.
   c. **True.**
   d. **False.** Opiate overdosage causes circulatory collapse producing hypotension and a bradycardia.
   e. **True.** Hypoxaemia is a secondary effect of respiratory depression.

5. a. **True.** The risk of thrombosis is increased even in a relatively short operation in a patient using oral contraception.
   b. **True.** Patients of any age group undergoing surgery that involves a pelvic dissection are at increased risk of thromboembolism.
   c. **True.** Hip surgery is one of the operations with the highest incidence of thromboembolism, up to 50% of patients being affected.
   d. **True.** Patients with malignancy are at increased risk. Prophylaxis should be given even for a short palliative operative procedure.
   e. **False.** Short operations in young patients that are followed by early ambulation do not require prophylaxis.

6. a. **True.** CVP measurements are usually elevated in patients with cardiogenic shock because of right heart failure or fluid overload. CVP measurements are reduced in hypovolaemic shock as a result of diminished venous return.

b. **False.** Both types of shock are associated with systemic hypotension.

c. **False.** Hypovolaemic shock will respond to a fluid challenge. Cardiogenic shock may be aggravated by a fluid challenge, which will expand the circulating volume, increase the venous return and aggravate any cardiac failure.

d. **True.** Inotropic support will improve myocardial efficiency and cardiac output.

e. **True.** Cardiogenic shock will lead to renal hypoperfusion and oliguria.

7. a. **False.** The defect following a pulmonary embolus is usually mismatched, i.e. there is a defect on the perfusion scan in an area of normal ventilation.

b. **True.** These features are often the hallmark of a major pulmonary embolus.

c. **False.** A major pulmonary embolus will cause arterial hypoxaemia. Cyanosis will be central and peripheral.

d. **True.** Shallow, fast respiration is a frequent finding.

e. **False.** A major pulmonary embolus causes right ventricular strain caused by a sudden increase in pulmonary artery resistance.

8. a. **False.** Dehiscence usually presents around 7–10 days after surgery.

b. **False.** Recurrence is uncommon.

c. **False.** Most patients make an uneventful recovery after abdominal resuture.

d. **True.** Wound healing is impaired in patients with jaundice.

e. **True.** Steroid therapy impairs wound healing.

9. a. **False.** The right lung is most often affected because the right main bronchus is wider and has a more vertical course. The middle and lower lobe segments are most frequently affected.

b. **True.** These patients are frequently obstructed or require urgent surgery with limited opportunity for preoperative fasting. The risks of aspiration are increased.

c. **False.** Cricoid pressure during induction of anaesthesia is an essential manoeuvre which protects the airway immediately prior to endotracheal intubation.

d. **True.** Gastric acid can cause an intense chemical pneumonitis that after secondary bacterial infection leads to a severe aspiration pneumonia.

e. **False.** Patients with severe gastro-oesophageal reflux are more likely to regurgitate gastric contents once consciousness is depressed during anaesthesia.

10. a. **True.** Smoking impairs the ciliary clearance mechanism and makes bronchial mucus more viscid.

b. **False.** Upper abdominal incisions inhibit abdominal respiration more than lower abdominal incisions and thus contribute to shallow breathing, a factor linked to postoperative atelectasis and pneumonia.

c. **True.** Bowel obstruction and abdominal distension can lead to diaphragmatic splinting and basal atelectasis.

d. **False.** Atelectasis begins early often within the first 24 postoperative hours.

e. **True.** Oversedation can cause respiratory depression and hypoventilation, which predispose to collapse of the small airways and absorption of alveolar air causing atelectasis. Major airway obstruction may develop because of suppression of the cough reflex.

Case history answers

Case history 1

1. There are many causes of postoperative fever. In a patient who is 7 days postcolectomy the most likely causes are:
a. wound infection
b. anastomotic leak
c. chest infection
d. DVT
e. i.v. line or catheter sepsis.

2. The patient should be examined to see if there are any respiratory symptoms, any new abdominal aches or pains or any calf tenderness. Look for:
- signs of collapse or consolidation in the chest
- evidence of a wound infection or peritonitis
- evidence of a DVT
- any signs of cellulitis around any remaining i.v. lines.

There are several key investigations:
- chest X-ray
- blood cultures
- wound swab
- urine and sputum culture
- contrast X-rays or CT scan if anastamotic leakage is suspected.

The choice of investigation will depend on the physical findings.

3. Specific treatment is also related to the underlying cause, for example:
- wound infection: lay open wound to allow drainage
- anastomotic leakage: requires reoperation and exteriorisation or drainage under broad-spectrum antibiotic cover
- chest infection: intensive physiotherapy, broad-spectrum antibiotic cover
- an infected i.v. line will require resiting.

Case history 2

1. The most likely cause of hypotension and oliguria in an elderly patient soon after major surgery is hypovolaemic shock. Other possible causes are:
   - opiate overdose
   - cardiogenic shock
   - septic shock (less likely).

2. Look for signs of hypovolaemia: collapsed jugular veins or low central venous pressure (CVP), peripheral shut down or excessive blood loss from drains. Pin-point pupils and a depressed respiration rate would suggest an opiate overdose. If the jugular veins were engorged or the CVP raised and there were signs of cardiac failure, a cardiac cause would have to be considered. Warm peripheries with a fast bounding pulse would suggest a septic cause for the patient's hypotension.

3. Treatment would depend on the underlying cause. Hypotensive shock should respond to resuscitation with blood or plasma, aiming to restore the systolic blood pressure to above 100 mmHg and to achieve a urine output of 30 ml/hour. Continued blood loss from the drain or failure to respond to fluid resuscitation may be an indication of internal bleeding requiring reoperation. If narcotic overdose is suspected, opiate analgesics should be withdrawn or counteracted with a specific antagonist such as naloxone. Cardiogenic shock should respond to intravenous fluid restriction plus diuretic therapy or inotropic support. If a septic cause is suspected, a full sepsis screen should be instituted.

Short notes answers

1. a. ECG B shows S waves in lead I and Q waves in lead III and inverted T waves in lead III.
   b. These changes are in keeping with a right heart strain secondary to a pulmonary embolus.
   c. The diagnosis would be supported by a history of pleuritic chest pain, haemoptysis and a pleural rub on examination with or without evidence of a deep vein thrombosis (DVT). The diagnosis would be confirmed by demonstrating a mismatched ventilation/perfusion defect on V/Q scanning.
   d. Full systemic anticoagulation is required initially with intravenous heparin by continuous infusion, to be followed by 3–6 months of oral anticoagulation with warfarin.

Surgical gastroenterology

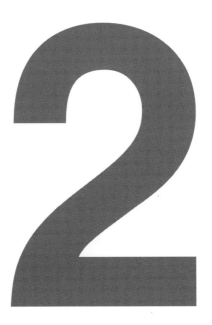

2.1 Diseases of the oesophagus

The oesophagus is a muscular tube that extends from the pharynx to the gastric cardia. Its prime function is to act as a conduit for the passage of food. Muscular sphincters control entry and exit of food into the oesophagus. In health, the lower 2 inches (5 cm) of the oesophagus and the gastro-oesophageal junction lie below the oesophageal hiatus of the diaphragm.

The most important oesophageal diseases are:

- hiatus hernia with or without reflux oesophagitis
- carcinoma of the oesophagus
- achalasia
- oesophageal strictures and perforation.

Hiatus hernia with or without reflux oesophagitis

These are separate but related conditions and together are the most common oesophageal disorder. There are two types of hernia: a sliding hernia (Fig. 3A) and a paraoesophageal or rolling hernia (Fig. 3B). Reflux oesophagitis is caused by acid or bile regurgitation into the oesophagus and is more common in patients with a sliding hiatus hernia. Reflux oesophagitis can occur in patients without a hiatus hernia.

Sliding hiatus hernia

Aetiology
Ageing and obesity slacken the oesophageal hiatus and allow the gastro-oesophageal junction to slide upwards into the chest. In this position, the lower oesophageal sphincter is less effective and allows reflux of gastric contents. Acid, bile and pepsin all contribute to the erosive oesophagitis and oesophageal ulceration.

Clinical features
Heartburn, regurgitation and waterbrash are the primary symptoms. They are worse at night when the patient is recumbent.

Complications
There are two main complications:

- reflux-induced oesophageal 'peptic' stricture which may require dilatation
- Barrett's oesophagitis.

Chronic irritation of the lower oesophagus by reflux can promote replacement of the normal squamous epithelium with columnar (Barrett's) epithelium. Long-standing Barrett's oesophagitis that does not respond to anti-reflux treatment is unstable and an adenocarcinoma may develop.

Diagnosis
A sliding hiatus hernia can be detected on a barium

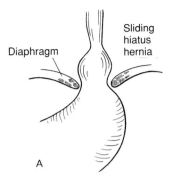

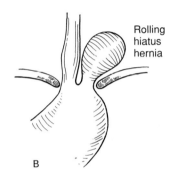

Fig. 3
A. Sliding hiatus hernia. **B**. Rolling, paraoesophageal hiatus hernia.

swallow and meal examination or at endoscopy. Biopsy is necessary to assess the severity of any associated oesophagitis.

Specialised oesophageal function studies, which include manometry, 24-hour ambulatory pH monitoring and radioisotope transit tests, are mandatory prior to surgical treatment.

Treatment
Antacids regimens and weight reduction form the cornerstone of medical treatment. Elevation of the bed head may relieve night-time symptoms. Patients should also be encouraged to cut down alcohol intake and stop smoking. These measures are effective in 90% of patients; the remainder require surgery. The aim of surgery is to *prevent* gastro-oesophageal reflux by restoring the gastro-oesophageal junction and lower oesophagus to its normal position below the oesophageal hiatus and to strengthen the lower oesophageal sphincter by some form of fundal wrap. The operation can be performed through the chest (Belsey repair) or through the abdomen (Nissen fundoplication). The oesophageal hiatus is also tightened.

Paraoesophageal or rolling hiatus hernia

All or part of the stomach herniates through the oesophageal hiatus adjacent to the gastro-oesophageal junction, which remains in its normal anatomical position (Fig. 3B)

Clinical features

Usually asymptomatic, the rolling hiatus hernia only presents when complications develop. Incarceration of the hernia causes:

- gastric outlet obstruction
- strangulation
- gastric stasis and ulceration.

Diagnosis

A rolling hiatus hernia is detected by a chest X–ray, barium swallow and meal examination or by gastroscopy.

Treatment

Because the complications are dangerous, early surgery is required. The herniated stomach is reduced through an abdominal incision and the defect in the oesophageal hiatus repaired.

Carcinoma of the oesophagus

True primary oesophageal cancers are of squamous cell origin. Adenocarcinomas in the lower third of the oesophagus are usually gastric in origin or have developed in a Barrett's oesophagus. Both types of tumour spread by direct invasion of local structures, via the bloodstream to liver, lungs and bone, and by lymphatics to the regional lymph glands.

Aetiology

The causes of carcinoma of the oesophagus are:

- high alcohol and tobacco consumption
- malnutrition
- certain chemicals, e.g. nitrosamines
- stasis of food caused by an oesophageal web, achalasia or stricture.

Clinical features

Progressive dysphagia of solids then liquids with severe weight loss are the hallmark of oesophageal cancer. Chest pain and hoarseness are grave symptoms and indicate local spread within the chest to involve the recurrent laryngeal nerve. Some patients will present with recurrent chest infections or an aspiration pneumonia caused by regurgitation of food from the obstructed oesophagus.

Complications

These include:

- aspiration pneumonia
- inability to swallow saliva
- tracheo-oesophageal fistula.

Diagnosis

A barium swallow will demonstrate an irregular stricture. The diagnosis must be confirmed by endoscopy and biopsy. A computerised tomography (CT) scan of the chest will help 'stage' the disease and assess resectability.

Treatment

As in all patients with cancer the choice of treatment lies between aggressive surgery/radiotherapy/chemotherapy in an attempt to cure the patient, or a lesser procedure aimed at relieving (palliating) the patient's symptoms. The decision taken will be based on many factors including the stage or extent of the disease, the age and fitness of the patient and also the patient's wishes.

Surgical resection should be attempted whenever possible as this provides the best symptom palliation. However, many patients are unfit or have advanced disease and only 10% will undergo a successful resection. Most *squamous* cell cancers and some adenocarcinomas are sensitive to radiotherapy, which can be used as an alternative to surgery either as primary treatment in an attempt to 'cure' the disease or simply in a palliative dose to relieve dysphagia. Swallowing can also be restored by intubation using pulsion tubes (e.g. the Nottingham tube) which are pushed through the tumour from above (through the mouth) or by traction tubes (e.g. the Celestin tube) which are pulled into place through a gastrotomy at open operation.

Prognosis

Survival is poor. The operative death rate is 5–10% and less than 10% of patients will survive 5 years even after apparently successful treatment.

Achalasia

Achalasia is a functional not a mechanical obstruction of the oesophagus. It is the most important of all the oesophageal motility disorders.

Aetiology

Achalasia is caused by an idiopathic degeneration of the ganglion cells of Auerbach's myenteric plexus. As a result, primary peristalsis is absent and the lower oesophageal sphincter fails to relax on swallowing.

Young adults + elderly

Clinical features

↳ may be central not local neuro defect

Dysphagia without weight loss is the cardinal symptom. Pain is uncommon.

More probs c fluids ∵ overspill → trachea

Complications

Solids sink to lower end of oes.

These include:

- night-time regurgitation — aspiration pneumonia
- oesophageal stasis — ulceration.

Diagnosis

A barium swallow is the primary investigation. The proximal oesophagus is dilated and tortuous and merges into a smooth cone-shaped narrowed segment above the gastro-oesophageal junction.

Oesophageal manometry (pressure studies) will confirm absent primary peristalsis and failure of the lower oesophageal sphincter to relax on swallowing.

During endoscopy, the narrow lower oesophageal sphincter offers no mechanical resistance to the passage of the gastroscope. A mucosal biopsy should be taken to exclude a cancer.

CxR: ↑ed mediastinum + fluid level in oes behind heart

[handwritten notes in top margin: Oesophageal web / circumferential mucosal fold / upper oesophagus + severe Fe def anaemia / Plummer Vinson's Dysphagia / Anaemia glossitis / Atrophic glossitis]

Differential diagnosis. It is important to differentiate achalasia from other major causes of dysphagia, e.g. benign strictures, oesophageal carcinoma.

Treatment

Achalasia can be relieved by forceful disruption of the lower oesophageal sphincter using endoscopically guided balloon dilatation or by open surgical division of the sphincter (Heller's cardiomyotomy). The risk of oesophageal perforation and recurrent achalasia are higher with balloon dilatation, which is usually reserved for patients unfit for surgery.

*[handwritten: * Abdo approach. longitudinal incision of lower oes + upper gastric wall but not of mucosa]*

Oesophageal strictures and perforation

Strictures

Most oesophageal strictures present with dysphagia. The diagnosis is confirmed by barium swallow and endoscopy. Usually they are the result of long-standing oesophageal reflux. Other important causes are:

- oesophageal cancer
- corrosive ingestion
- collagen diseases, e.g. scleroderma.

The majority of benign strictures can be managed by endoscopic dilatation and treatment of the underlying condition.

Perforation

Perforation of the oesophagus is a recognised complication of forceful dilatation of an oesophageal stricture. It can also complicate diagnostic endoscopy as a result of either a technical error or tearing of the oesophagus by the endoscope against the cervical spine.

Spontaneous oesophageal perforation (Boerhaave's syndrome) is the sequel to a violent bout of vomiting or retching, often precipitated by a bout of heavy eating or drinking. The tear usually occurs just above the gastro-oesophageal junction on the left side.

Clinical features
These include:

- agonising pain in the chest, neck or upper abdomen
- cervical crepitus and subcutaneous emphysema
- hydropneumothorax on a chest X-ray caused by air leaking from the oesophageal lumen into the pleural cavity.

Diagnosis
A water-soluble contrast swallow will demonstrate the site of the leak.

Treatment
Most instrumental cervical perforations and some minor intrathoracic perforations can be treated conservatively with systemic antibiotics and oral fluid restriction. All others require thoracotomy, closure of the perforation and

chest drainage. If surgery is delayed beyond 24 hours in these cases, the survival rate will be less than 50%.

2.2 Diseases of the stomach and duodenum

The two most important conditions that affect the stomach and duodenum are:

- peptic ulcer disease
- carcinoma of the stomach.

Peptic ulcer disease

This is the most common disorder of the stomach and duodenum. Peptic ulceration occurs at any site where gastrointestinal mucosa is subject to the corrosive action of acid gastric juices. The most frequent sites are:

- duodenum: causing a duodenal ulcer
- oesophagus: causing a peptic stricture
- stomach: causing a gastric ulcer
- following gastroenterostomy: causing a stomal ulcer.

Aetiology
The causes of the disease are:

- high gastric acid output
- alcohol and tobacco consumption
- salicylates, steroids, non-steroidal anti-inflammatory drugs
- antral helicobacter infection.

Clinical features
Cyclical epigastric pain relieved by food, milk or antacids characterises uncomplicated peptic ulcer disease. Epigastric tenderness is usual.

Diagnosis
Gastroscopy is the most valuable investigation. It will detect small superficial ulcers and any inflammation, which may be overlooked on a barium meal.

Treatment
Most uncomplicated peptic ulcers respond to medical therapy. Surgery is only occasionally needed.

Medical treatment. Histamine H_2 receptor antagonists, which reduce gastric acid secretion, are the mainstay of treatment. Peptic ulcers are characterised by a rapid symptomatic response to these drugs and to the withdrawal of any causative agents. Resistant ulcers usually respond to proton pump inhibitors such as omeprazole, which is a more potent inhibitor of acid secretion. Some ulcers respond to chealating agents such as bismuth compounds or sucralfate. Less than 1% of patients with peptic ulcer disease will have a persistent ulcer that will require surgery.

Helicobacter infection. In patients with a biopsy-proven gastric helicobacter infection and a duodenal

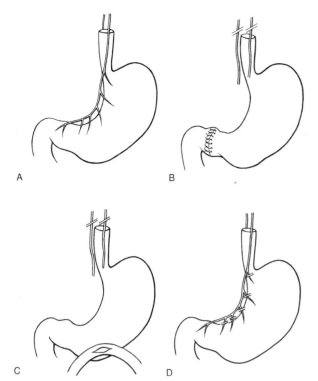

Fig. 4
The principal surgical operations for peptic ulcer disease.
A. Normal anatomy. **B.** Truncal vagotomy and pyloroplasty.
C. Truncal vagotomy and gastroenterostomy. **D.** Highly selective
vagotomy.

ulcer there is increasing evidence to show that eradicating the infection using a combination of antibiotics together with a histamine H_2 receptor antagonist or proton pump inhibitor is the most effective method, inducing permanent healing.

Elective surgery for peptic ulcer disease

The primary goal of operative management is to cut down gastric acid secretion. There are three commonly used operations (Fig. 4).

- truncal vagotomy plus a drainage procedure
- highly selective vagotomy
- vagotomy and antrectomy (a type of partial gastrectomy).

Division of the main vagal nerve trunks inhibits gastric acid output production but it also impairs gastric emptying. A drainage procedure, either pyloroplasty or gastroenterostomy, is essential to prevent gastric stasis.

Highly selective vagotomy is technically a more difficult operation but has the advantage of denervating the acid-producing parietal cell mass in the body of the stomach while preserving the vagal motor function of the pylorus. As gastric emptying is not affected, a drainage procedure is not required. Truncal vagotomy and antrectomy completely denervates the stomach and removes the gastrin-secreting gastric antrum. This procedure eliminates the two major stimuli to gastric acid secretion and is a most effective antiulcer operation.

Because it is a more extensive operation, the morbidity and mortality are higher and the procedure is reserved for patients with severe ulcer disease or ulcers that have recurred after less complex surgery.

Complications of gastric surgery
The complications seen are:

- recurrent ulceration
- postgastrectomy syndromes
- nutritional deficiencies.

Recurrent ulceration. Ulcers that recur after surgery usually develop because the original operation was inadequate or incomplete. They present with ulcer pain or bleeding or both. Reoperation can be complex and difficult. Wherever possible histamine H_2 receptor antagonists should be tried first to promote healing.

Postgastrectomy syndromes. There are two postgastrectomy syndromes:

Postvagotomy diarrhoea. After truncal vagotomy, 1% of patients develop incapacitating explosive diarrhoea. The mechanism is poorly understood but may be caused by rapid gastric emptying and fast small bowel transit.

Dumping syndrome. Two types are recognised:

- Early dumping syndrome (vasomotor dumping). This occurs shortly after eating and patients experience sweating, palpitations, lightheadedness and abdominal cramps and feel compelled to lie down. The cause is uncertain but appears related to the uncontrolled entry of hypertonic food boluses from the stomach into the small bowel. Treatment is difficult. Some patients relieve their symptoms by taking small frequent dry meals.
- Late dumping syndrome or reactive hypoglycaemia. In these patients, rapid absorption of a large glucose load from the small bowel is followed by a 'rebound' hypoglycaemia caused by prolonged insulin action.

Nutritional deficiencies. Iron deficient anaemia is common and is caused by a failure to absorb dietary iron. A macrocytic anaemia can also develop because of Vitamin B_{12} malabsorption. This can be prevented by 3-monthly Vitamin B_{12} injections.

Complications of peptic ulcer disease

There are three major complications:

- haemorrhage
- perforation
- pyloric stenosis.

Haemorrhage
Bleeding is the most frequent and most lethal complication of peptic ulcer disease. Sudden, massive haemorrhage presents with haematemesis, melena and shock. Less often, chronic blood loss can cause anaemia with or without melena. The principles of management of a

bleeding peptic ulcer are fully outlined in section 4.3. The most important points are:

- resuscitate with blood products
- confirm diagnosis by endoscopy within 24 hours
- urgent surgery if no response to resuscitation.

Endoscopic treatment. Bleeding can be arrested by injecting sclerosing agents into the bleeding site or by laser coagulation. Both procedures can be performed at the same time as the diagnostic gastroscopy.

Surgical treatment. Three-quarters of all patients will stop bleeding after resuscitation alone or following endoscopic treatment. Continuing haemorrhage or rebleeding is an indication for emergency surgery. Simple oversew of the bleeding ulcer is effective in combination with histamine H_2 receptor antagonists or with vagotomy and pyloroplasty to reduce gastric acid output. Major surgery such as a gastrectomy should be avoided if possible because the surgical mortality is high.

Prognosis. Up to 10% of patients with bleeding ulcers will die. Elderly patients or those who have rebled are at greatest risk.

Perforation

Most ulcers that perforate are sited on the anterior wall of the duodenum or stomach. The release of food and digestive enzymes into the peritoneal cavity initially causes a chemical peritonitis. Secondary bacterial peritonitis evolves later.

Clinical features:

- agonising central epigastric pain, shoulder tip radiation
- rigid, silent abdomen
- subdiaphragmatic gas on an *erect* chest X-ray.

Treatment. Nasogastric decompression is essential to minimise further intraperitoneal contamination. After intravenous fluid resuscitation, urgent laparotomy and simple oversew of the perforation with an omental 'patch' is required. Thorough peritoneal lavage will minimise the risks of postoperative abscess formation.

Prognosis. As with haemorrhage, 10% of these patients also will die. At special risk are the elderly and patients in whom a late diagnosis is made.

Pyloric stenosis

This is the result of fibrotic scarring from a long-standing duodenal or pyloric channel ulcer. It can also result from spasm or oedema caused by an acute ulcer. Pyloric stenosis is the least common complication of peptic ulcer disease.

Clinical features:

- a long history of peptic ulcer symptoms
- vomiting unaltered foodstuffs
- weight loss and dehydration
- a succussion splash on examination.

Diagnosis. Barium meal and gastroscopy are complementary in the evaluation of gastric outlet obstruction. Barium meal will demonstrate delayed gastric emptying while gastroscopy will help distinguish spasm from fibrosis and exclude a gastric outlet cancer. Before either investigation is attempted, the stomach should be decompressed by nasogastric suction and lavaged to remove food debris.

Treatment. Some patients with an acute ulcer and spasm will respond to intravenous histamine H_2 receptor blockade and a period of nasogastric decompression. Most require a gastric drainage procedure (either pyloroplasty or gastroenterostomy) combined with a truncal vagotomy to cut down acid secretion.

Prognosis. In contrast to haemorrhage and perforation, the outlook for patients with pyloric stenosis is excellent.

Benign gastric ulcers

These are less common than duodenal ulcers and occur in an older age group. It is *essential* to differentiate them from an ulcerating gastric cancer.

Aetiology:
The causes are:

- high acid output
- non-steroidal anti-inflammatory drugs
- *Helicobacter pylorii* infection
- duodenogastric bile reflux.

Clinical features
Epigastric pain, vomiting, weight loss and anaemia are the chief symptoms. They are common to patients with a gastric ulcer or a *gastric cancer*.

Diagnosis
Gastroscopy and biopsy is essential in order to confirm the diagnosis, exclude gastric cancer and to detect helicobacter infection. Classically a punched out ulcer crater is in keeping with a benign gastric ulcer whereas a rolled everted ulcer edge is suspicious of malignancy. Repeated biopsy may be necessary to rule out a gastric cancer.

Treatment
Histamine H_2 receptor antagonists form the mainstay of treatment. Some ulcers, especially those associated with helicobacter infection respond to chelating compounds such as bismuth or sucralfate or to combinations of antibiotic therapy plus histamine H_2 receptor antagonists. Repeat endoscopy after 6–8 weeks of treatment is mandatory to ensure the ulcer heals. Non-response or relapse after treatment is more common in gastric than in duodenal ulceration. It may also indicate that the ulcer is malignant.

A recurring or non-healing gastric ulcer in the body of the stomach is best treated by partial gastrectomy (Fig. 5). Local excision plus vagotomy and drainage is

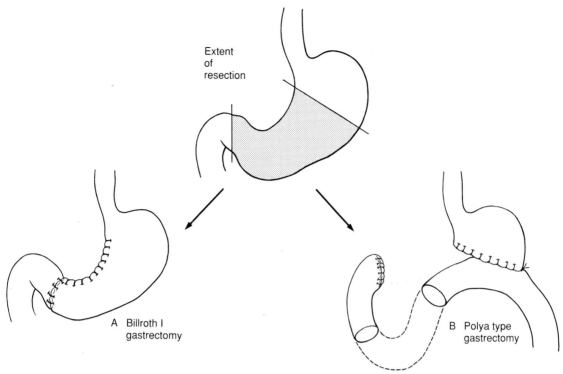

Fig. 5
Billroth I (**A**) and Polya type (**B**) gastrectomies for peptic ulcers (**A** or **B**) or gastric cancer (**B**).

also effective, particularly in elderly patients. Ulcers in the gastric antrum are treated like duodenal ulcers.

Carcinoma of the stomach

Nearly all gastric cancers are adenocarcinomatous in origin. The disease is twice as common in men as in women and has a peak incidence in the sixth decade. Spread occurs by direct invasion of local structures, e.g. the pancreas; via the bloodstream to the liver; by lymphatics to regional lymph glands; and across the peritoneal cavity (transcoelomic) to form peritoneal deposits or metastases in the ovaries (Krukenberg tumours).

Aetiology
Gastric cancer is more common in patients with:

- pernicious anaemia and achlorhydria
- type A blood group
- previous partial gastrectomy
- positive family history
- smoking and spicy foods
- a history of gastric adenomatous polyps.

There are four main pathological types:

- ulcerative
- polypoid
- linitis plastica ('leather bottle stomach'): a diffuse infiltrating cancer affecting all layers of the stomach wall
- superficial spreading cancer: an uncommon variant restricted to the mucosa and submucosa and associated with a better prognosis.

Clinical features
Gastric cancer often presents late. Patients may present with symptoms and signs of the *primary tumour* (dyspeptic symptoms, vomiting, epigastric mass), signs of *secondary disease* (left supraclavicular lymphadenopathy from spread via the thoracic duct) or *systemic symptoms* such as weight loss, poor appetite, anaemia. Usually patients have a long history often of initially rather vague symptoms. A few tumours that block the cardia and cause dysphagia or those that obstruct the pylorus and cause vomiting present earlier.

Patients with unremitting, gnawing epigastric pain and a palpable epigastric mass or a hard liver edge usually have advanced, inoperable disease.

Diagnosis
Gastroscopy and biopsy is the key investigation. It provides a tissue diagnosis and detects those cancers that because of size or site may be missed on a barium meal examination.

Abdominal ultrasound and CT scanning can be used independently or in combination to look for liver metastases.

Treatment
Once the diagnosis is confirmed, a barium meal is a useful aid in planning the surgical treatment. Radical surgical resection provides the only hope of cure. It is also the best way to palliate the patient's symptoms. Cancer of the body of the stomach requires en-bloc removal of the entire stomach together with the adjacent omentum, regional lymph nodes and spleen. Continuity of the

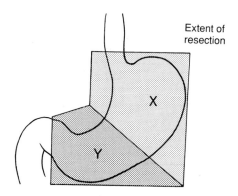

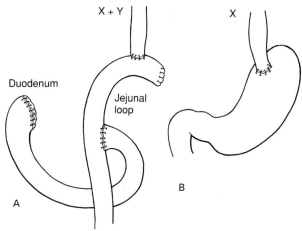

Fig. 6
A. Total abdominal gastrectomy for gastric cancer (resection of X and Y). **B.** Proximal gastrectomy for cancer of the gastric cardia (removal of X only).

gastrointestinal tract is restored using the jejunum (Fig. 6A). For cancers involving the fundus or cardia, the distal stomach can be preserved and used to restore continuity to the oesophagus (Fig. 6B). For a cancer of the antrum or pylorus, the spleen and proximal stomach are preserved and gastrointestinal continuity restored with a Polya type gastrectomy (Fig. 5).

Radical gastric resection is contraindicated if liver metastases are present. These patients cannot be cured. A lesser gastric resection may be chosen to simply remove the bulk of the tumour. A palliative by-pass (gastroenterostomy) may help relieve symptoms caused by an obstructing cancer that cannot be removed.

Prognosis
Because this disease presents late, is locally invasive and disseminates widely, only 10% of patients will survive 5 years. A few patients with superficial spreading cancers that are diagnosed early are the only exception. They can expect a 90% 5-year survival.

2.3 Biliary and pancreatic disease

There are four important biliary disorders:

- common
  — gallstone disease
  — obstructive jaundice
- uncommon
  — cholangiocarcinoma
  — carcinoma of the gallbladder.

The three most important diseases affecting the pancreas are:

- acute pancreatitis
- chronic pancreatitis
- carcinoma of the pancreas.

Biliary disease

Gallstone disease: biliary colic and acute cholecystitis

Gallstones are common. Up to 20% of all individuals over the age of 60 have gallstones. Although the vast majority of gallstones are asymptomatic, cholecystectomy for gallstone disease is the most frequent major elective operation carried out in Britain and the USA today.

There is a considerable overlap beween biliary colic and acute cholecystitis. Biliary colic is caused by the transient impaction of a gallstone in the neck of the gallbladder (Hartmann's pouch). Acute cholecystitis implies the development of bacterial infection in the gallbladder wall, which may or may not be preceded by biliary colic.

Clinical features
Biliary colic has the following characteristics:

- sudden of onset of right subcostal pain which subsides gradually *over a few hours*
- radiation around costal margin and shoulder tip
- nausea and vomiting
- symptoms that may not be severe enough for the patient to urgently attend hospital
- fever (uncommon).

Acute cholecystitis is the sequel to secondary bacterial infection caused by gut-derived Gram-negative bacteria (e.g. *Escherichia coli*), which spread to the gall-bladder via the bile or bloodstream.

Additional clinical features are:

- signs of systemic sepsis
- subcostal tenderness (Murphy's sign)
- jaundice
- fever (common).

Acute cholecystitis can also occur without gallstones (acalculous cholecystitis). This condition, which is rare, occurs in debilitated, septic patients, burn victims or patients on long-term parenteral nutrition.

Diagnosis
This diagnosis is established primarily by history and physical examination. It is confirmed by:

- ultrasound scan: will detect 95% of all gallstones
- radionuclide biliary excretion scan (HIDA): used when ultrasound scanning is unsuccessful and will detect a blocked cystic duct
- oral cholecystogram: *this is of no value* in acute cholecystitis as it requires a functioning gallbladder to produce a result: the test is used electively to detect gallstones in patients with biliary colic.

Medical treatment

The key steps in the initial management of acute chole-cystitis are:

1. establish i.v. fluid regimen, restrict oral intake
2. broad-spectrum intravenous antibiotic cover
3. parenteral opioid analgesia.

About 90% of all attacks will resolve using this conservative regimen. Those that do not respond within 24–48 hours have usually developed a septic complication of gallstone disease that will require urgent surgery.

Surgical treatment for acute cholecystitis

For the majority of cases that settle with conservative treatment, there are two choices:

- early cholecystectomy: performed during the same hospital admission within 5–7 days of the acute attack
- elective cholecystectomy: 4–6 weeks after the acute attack following convalescence at home.

Currently, most patients with gallstones will have their gallbladder removed using laparoscopic surgical techniques. Open cholecystectomy is reserved for those patients in whom technical difficulties are encountered or for patients undergoing urgent surgery for the complications of biliary disease. Some surgeons routinely perform an operative cholangiography during cholecystectomy to check the biliary anatomy and to look for common bile duct stones (see below for management of common bile duct stones).

Urgent surgery and the complications of acute cholecystitis

Urgent surgery is required for those patients with acute cholecystitis who do not respond quickly to medical treatment, usually because of the onset of complications. These can be classified according to the site of the gallstones in the biliary tree (see Fig. 7):

Stones remaining in the gallbladder:

- common complications
  — pericholecystic abscess
  — empyema
  — mucocoele
- uncommon complications
  — gangrene
  — free perforation
  — gallstone ileus.

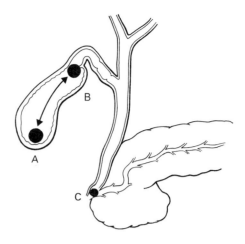

A – Acute cholecystitis
B – Biliary colic
  – Empyema
  – Pericholecystic abscess
  – Perforation
  – Gangrene
C – Ascending cholangitis
  – Obstructive jaundice
  – Gallstone pancreatitis

Fig. 7
Complications of gallstones.

Stones that migrate to the common bile duct:

- obstructive jaundice
- ascending cholangitis
- gallstone pancreatitis.

Surgery for gallstones remaining in the gallbladder

There are two surgical options for complicated gallstone disease where the gallstones have remained in the gallbladder.

Emergency cholecyst*ectomy*. Removing the diseased gallbladder and stones plus draining the associated sepsis.

Emergency cholecyst*ostomy*. Using a tube to drain the gallbladder after removing the stones. This is a safer option in frail, septic patients. The gallbladder can be removed at a later date when the patient's condition allows.

Surgery for gallstones in the common bile duct

Gallstones are found in the common bile duct in 5% of all patients with gallstone disease (choledocholithiasis). Most migrate from the gallbladder. Occasionally stones form primarily in the common bile duct. In addition to the three main clinical presentations outlined above, common duct stones can also be silent and present unexpectedly during routine elective or emergency cholecystectomy.

Obstructive jaundice. This is caused by common duct stones and may be painless or associated with biliary colic or cholecystitis. The diagnosis is confirmed by ultrasound demonstration of a dilated biliary tree. There are two options for treatment.

Open common bile duct exploration plus cholecystectomy.

In this procedure, the bile duct is opened and any stones removed. The bile duct is closed over a T-tube and a cholecystectomy is usually performed.

Endoscopic retrograde cholangiopancreatogram (ERCP), sphincterotomy and stone removal. This technique has the advantage of avoiding a laparotomy. It is especially suitable for frail elderly patients whose main symptoms relate to the common bile duct stones and who do not have acute cholecystitis, and also for those patients with common bile duct stones who have previously had a cholecystectomy.

Ascending cholangitis. Rigors, jaundice and fever are the hallmark of ascending cholangitis; these are caused by a combination of obstruction and infection in the biliary tree. Untreated, this lethal combination will lead to death from septicaemia and liver abscess. Treatment involves urgent decompression of the biliary tree under antibiotic cover, by either ERCP or open exploration; this is a life-saving measure.

Gallstone pancreatitis (see acute pancreatitis, p. 29). Elective biliary surgery is characterised by a low morbidity and mortality. Patients at highest risk are those undergoing urgent or emergency surgery for the complications of gallstone disease.

Obstructive jaundice

The main *surgical* causes of jaundice are:

- common causes
  - common bile duct stones
  - pancreatic cancer
- uncommon causes
  - cholangiocarcinoma
  - extrinsic compression by malignant hilar lymph glands
  - metastatic liver disease.

These conditions have to be differentiated from the many medical causes, the most common being:

- hepatitis A, B, and C
- drug-induced jaundice
- primary biliary cirrhosis
- alcoholic liver disease.

Clinical features

Most patients will be obviously jaundiced. Some will have hepatomegaly which may be smooth or irregular. A palpable gallbladder is suspicious of malignant biliary obstruction with passive massive distension of an obstructed gallbladder. There may be stigmata of cirrhotic liver disease (see section 2.4). Usually diagnostic tests will be essential to determine the cause.

Diagnosis

The key tests are:

- liver function tests
  - serum bilirubin
  - alkaline phosphatase
  - liver transaminases

Massive elevation in the liver transaminases is in keeping with a hepatocellular cause for jaundice. Major elevations in the serum alkaline phosphatase with normal liver transaminase levels suggest an obstructive jaundice. These tests are not infallible.

- hepatitis screen, A, B, C
- biliary ultrasound scan: the identification of a dilated biliary tree will confirm the diagnosis of an obstructive jaundice; liver metastases may also be detected
- ERCP examination: frequently an essential diagnostic and therapeutic step once biliary tree dilatation is detected; the cause of obstruction can be identified and endoscopic treatment may be possible.

Treatment

This depends on the underlying cause. Treatment of the various surgical causes of obstructive jaundice is discussed in detail in the relevant sections of this chapter. Any jaundiced patient faced with surgery has three additional problems to surmount:

- coagulopathy
- hepatorenal failure
- increased risk of infection.

Any coagulopathy must be corrected before surgery by vitamin K injection plus fresh frozen plasma infusion (contains a high concentration of clotting factors). The risk of hepatorenal failure is minimised by keeping jaundiced patients well hydrated before, during and after surgery. All these patients require antibiotic prophylaxis.

Cholangiocarcinoma

This cancer can arise anywhere in the biliary tree; usually it will eventually cause obstructive jaundice.

Treatment

Cure is infrequent; most patients present with advanced disease and require endoscopic (ERCP) intraluminal stenting to relieve the jaundice and intense pruritus that often accompanies the disease. Occasionally surgical resection of the tumour is possible.

Carcinoma of the gallbladder

Gallbladder cancer is rare. Sometimes it is identified as an unexpected finding in a gallbladder removed and submitted for histopathological examination. More often the disease will present with a painful biliary mass and the diagnosis will be made unexpectedly at operation for 'gallstone disease'. Usually these cancers cannot be removed and the survival is poor.

Diseases of the pancreas

Acute pancreatitis

Aetiology

Gallstone disease or alcohol excess account for 70% of all episodes of acute pancreatitis. A transient obstruction of the ampulla of Vater during passage of a common duct stone is the most likely mechanism in biliary pancreatitis. Alcohol may act as a pancreatic toxin or may damage the pancreas by simultaneously inducing pancreatic hypersecretion and spasm of the sphincter of Oddi. Less common causes of acute pancreatitis include:

Pancreas divisum. This is a congenital abnormality where the body of the pancreas drains via the accessory and not the main pancreatic duct.

Metabolic abnormalities. These include hyperlipidaemia or hypercalcaemia.

Trauma. This can occur either after a blunt abdominal injury or following a peroperative injury, or after ERCP.

Mumps.

Despite thorough evaluation, 10–20% of all cases of pancreatitis will prove to be idiopathic.

The clinical course and outcome depend on the severity of the attack. In a mild attack, the pancreas becomes oedematous. If the injury continues, oedema will progress to haemorrhage and ultimately pancreatic necrosis. All attacks of pancreatitis are aseptic initially. Secondary infection develops in areas of pancreatic necrosis and can cause a pancreatic abscess. Fluid and blood loss into the pancreas and retroperitoneum are caused by an increase in capillary permeability and produce shock. Fluid and pancreatic enzymes may become sequestered in the lesser sac and produce a pseudocyst.

Clinical features

Acute pancreatitis is characterised by a rapid onset of agonising epigastric pain that spreads to the back and flanks. Patients are usually nauseated and will vomit. Early in the attack, abdominal tenderness is maximal in the epigastrium and later becomes more generalised. Some but not all patients will be shocked. The degree of shock will depend on the severity of the attack.

Diagnosis

Almost invariably the diagnosis is confirmed by an elevated serum amylase level. Plain abdominal X-rays may be normal or may show an isolated dilated loop of bowel (a sentinel loop) caused by a local ileus. A swollen oedematous pancreas can be demonstrated on ultrasound or CT examination, which may also detect any gallstones.

Differential diagnosis. The two most important conditions that mimic acute pancreatitis and can be associated with an elevated serum amylase are:

- perforated peptic ulcer
- mesenteric vascular occlusion.

Treatment

Surgery has no role to play in the early management of acute pancreatitis. Aggressive supportive medical therapy forms the cornerstone of treatment. The key features are:

1. withdraw all oral intake, institute nasogastric suction
2. establish intravenous fluid support and resuscitation
3. monitor response
   - catheterise, measure hourly urine volumes
   - record vital signs
   - record central venous pressure
4. draw blood for
   - serum amylase
   - calcium
   - blood glucose
   - arterial blood gases
   - liver and serum biochemistry
5. obtain a baseline chest X-ray
6. provide adequate opioid analgesia.

Most patients respond rapidly to this regimen. A few will progressively deteriorate and develop respiratory and renal failure. Failure to respond indicates a severe (necrotising) attack, development of a complication or an incorrect diagnosis.

Necrotising pancreatitis can be detected on a CT scan; radical surgical debridement of the dead tissue is sometimes the only option.

Complications

The two most important complications of acute pancreatitis are:

- pancreatic pseudocyst
- pancreatic abscess.

Two less common complications of pancreatitis are:

- pancreatic ascites
- pancreatic pleural effusion.

Pancreatic pseudocyst. A pseudocyst consists of a fluid collection rich in pancreatic secretions that usually develops in the lesser sac. Pseudocysts present as an epigastric mass about 1 week after the onset of pancreatitis. The diagnosis is confirmed on ultrasound or CT scan. Most resolve spontaneously. Large cysts that persist or cause pain or jaundice can be drained either percutaneously under ultrasound/CT-guided control or internally at laparotomy into the back wall of the stomach (an operation known as a marsupialisation). Occasionally pseudocysts can become infected and form an abscess or may erode a major blood vessel causing haemorrhage and collapse. Both complications need emergency surgical intervention.

Pancreatic abscess. This is the sequel to secondary

bacterial infection in an area of pancreatic necrosis, usually with a mixed growth of aerobic and anaerobic organisms. This diagnosis should be suspected in patients with pancreatitis who become severely septic with a tender abdominal mass. The diagnosis is confirmed on ultrasound/CT scanning and urgent surgical drainage is mandatory.

Pancreatic ascites and pleural effusion. This develops as a result of disruption of the main pancreatic duct by the acute inflamatory process. Leakage of pancreatic secretion into the peritoneal cavity may lead to a pseudocyst (localised leak) or pancreatic ascites (generalised leak) or a pleural effusion if fluid leaks via the diaphragm and mediastinum into the chest. Surgical treatment is complex and the overall outcome is poor.

Prognosis
Of all patients with acute pancreatitis 10–15% will die of their disease. Death is more likely in the elderly with fulminant, severe attack or in patients with septic complications and multisystem organ failure.

Chronic pancreatitis

Chronic pancreatitis is usually the sequel to repeated attacks of alcohol-induced acute pancreatitis. Rarely, it follows an injury to the pancreas caused by surgery or external trauma.

Clinical features
Chronic pancreatitis is characterised by recurrent severe abdominal pain, or signs of pancreatic insufficiency (malabsorption and diabetes mellitus). Most patients give a history of alcohol abuse. Occasionally patients will present with a complication of chronic pancreatitis, e.g. abscess or pseudocyst.

Diagnosis
Plain abdominal film shows pancreatic calcification and endoscopic retrograde cholangiopancreatography (ERCP) shows pancreatic duct strictures and dilatation. It is extremely important to exclude pancreatic cancer as the presentation is similar.

Medical treatment
Malabsorption and steatorrhoea can be reduced by oral pancreatic enzyme supplements, which may also reduce narcotic analgesic requirements. Diabetic patients require insulin therapy. Chronic pain is a major clinical problem and narcotic addiction is commonplace.

Surgical treatment
The main indication for surgical intervention is relief of pain. Operative treatment is complex and should be reserved for the few well-motivated patients who have a clear structural abnormality in the pancreas detected on CT scan or ERCP. Unreformed alcoholics who are

addicted to narcotics are unlikely to benefit from surgery.

There are two main options:

- pancreatic ductal drainage
- major pancreatic resection.

Drainage of a dilated ductal system either by an ampullary sphincteroplasty (Fig. 8) or by anastomosing the pancreatic duct to a loop of jejunum using various techniques (Fig. 9) will relieve pain. If the pancreatic duct is not dilated, resection of the diseased gland is the only other option. Resection should be tailored to the extent of the disease. Unlike pancreatic resection for cancer, the pylorus and duodenum are preserved whenever possible.

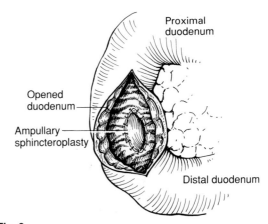

Fig. 8
Ampullary sphincteroplasty for chronic pancreatitis.

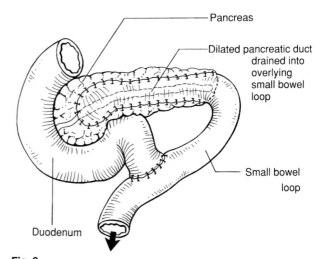

Fig. 9
Pancreatic ductal drainage procedure for chronic pancreatitis.

Carcinoma of the pancreas

Pancreatic ductal adenocarcinoma accounts for 90% of all cancers arising from the pancreas. The remainder, which are derived from the ampulla of Vater or the adjacent duodenal mucosa, are termed periampullary cancers. These cancers present early with obstructive

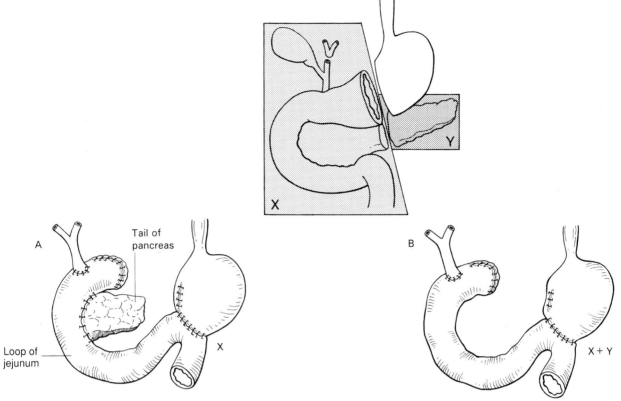

Fig. 10
A. Pancreaticoduodenectomy. **B.** Total pancreatectomy.

jaundice, are biologically less aggressive and are associated with a better prognosis.

Pancreatic cancer is becoming increasingly common in both men and women. Many have advanced disease at presentation and symptom palliation is often all that can be offered.

Clinical features

Weight loss, abdominal pain, back pain and jaundice are the cardinal features of pancreatic cancer. Jaundice is most common in cancers of the pancreatic head (caused by early obstruction of the common bile duct) and is less frequent in a cancer of the body and tail of the gland, where malignant obstruction of the common bile duct occurs later. A mass may be palpable in the epigastrium together with an enlarged liver. In patients with jaundice and pancreatic cancer, the gallbladder may be painlessly distended (Courvoisier's law).

Diagnosis

Abdominal ultrasound and CT scan. These are the key investigations. A dilated common bile duct plus a soft tissue mass in the pancreas is virtually diagnostic of pancreatic cancer. Liver metastases may also be detected.

Endoscopic retrograde cholangiopancreatography. ERCP can distinguish pancreatic ductal carcinoma from the various periampullary cancers. ERCP techniques can be used to insert a stent through a malignant biliary stricture caused by cancer of the pancreas or ampulla and will relieve obstructive jaundice.

Surgical treatment

Cancer of the body and tail of the pancreas is inevitably inoperable. Only one in 10 patients with cancer of the pancreatic head is resectable and of these very few will be long-term survivors. Resection is prevented either by direct invasion of vital local structures (e.g. portal vein, hepatic or mesenteric vessels) or because of coexistent hepatic metastases.

There are two surgical options for the few patients with early resectable cancer of the pancreatic head. They are:

Pancreaticoduodenectomy (Whipple's operation). En-bloc resection of the pancreatic head bearing the tumour, duodenum, pylorus and distal bile duct (see Fig. 10A).

Total pancreatectomy. Complete removal of pancreas, duodenum, pylorus and distal common bile duct (see Fig. 10B).

There is considerable debate as to the relative merits of these two operations. Periampullary cancers are usually treated by Whipple's operation.

Symptom palliation

The three predominant symptoms are:

- obstructive jaundice: this can be relieved by palliative open surgical by-pass (cholecyst-jejunostomy) or by ERCP and stenting

- pain: high doses of oral or subcutaneously infused opioids may be required
- pruritus: this requires operative or endoscopic relief of obstructive jaundice.

Prognosis

There are few long-term survivors even after apparently successful pancreatic resection for pancreatic ductal adenocarcinoma. Most die of local recurrence. In contrast one in three patients with periampullary cancer can expect to live 5 years after resection.

2.4 Diseases of the liver and spleen

Surgery has a role to play in two important groups of liver diseases:

- primary and secondary liver cancer
- portal hypertension and cirrhosis.

Primary and secondary liver cancer

Worldwide, primary liver cancer is common. It is only in Europe, North America and Australasia that secondary metastatic liver cancer is seen more often.

Primary hepatocellular carcinoma

Aetiology

Chronic *hepatitis B infection* is the primary aetiological factor. In Africa, for example, 80% of all patients with hepatocellular carcinoma are seropositive. In the USA, *alcoholic cirrhosis* is the major predisposing factor, whereas in the Orient infestation with *liver flukes* is linked to the increased incidence of the disease. Elsewhere, a high dietary intake of *aflatoxins* (products of the mould aspergillus found in wheat and soyabean) coincides with an increased incidence of primary hepatocellular cancer.

Pathology

Usually, the cancer develops as a single mass and later develops satellite nodules. In a fibrous cirrhotic liver, the cancer may be nodular and surrounded by a pseudocapsule. Less often a young adult (usually without any aetiological risk factors) will develop a fibrolamellar carcinoma characterised by multiple nodules separated by fibrous septae. This variant of the disease has a better prognosis. Primary hepatocellular carcinoma spreads to the coeliac and hilar lymph glands and can invade the portal and hepatic veins giving rise to pulmonary metastases.

Clinical features

Patients frequently present late with weight loss, abdominal pain and an upper abdominal mass. Less than one half will be jaundiced. Some will have stigmata of underlying liver disease.

Diagnosis

Most patients will have an elevated oncofetoprotein and α-fetoprotein (AFP) level. Ultrasound or CT evaluation of the liver is the key diagnostic test. Tissue diagnosis is confirmed either by ultrasound or CT-guided percutaneous biopsy or by laparoscopy and biopsy.

Treatment

Liver resection offers the only hope of long-term survival. Extensive disease or poor residual liver function resulting from coexisting cirrhosis precludes resection in all but a few patients. Attempts to devascularise the tumour by hepatic artery ligation or to destroy the tumour by direct infusion of cytoxic agents via the hepatic artery have limited success.

Prognosis

Long-term survival is poor; most patients are dead within 1 year of diagnosis. Less than 20% of the few patients undergoing resection will survive 5 years.

Secondary liver cancer

Almost all primary cancers can metastasise to the liver. The most common primary sites are:

- lung
- breast
- stomach
- pancreas
- colorectum.

The deposits, which may be single or multiple, are caused by spread of primary tumour cells to the liver via the portal or systemic circulation and less often via the lymphatics.

Clinical features

Metastatic liver disease may be detected during the preoperative work-up of a patient with cancer or is discovered unexpectedly during elective or urgent surgery for cancer. Less often, patients will present primarily with pain, ascites, jaundice or hepatomegaly caused by metastatic disease with a 'silent' underlying primary cancer.

Diagnosis

Diagnosis is by CT, ultrasound or hepatic radioisotope scan. Any of these tests will confirm the presence of hepatic metastases. Ultrasound or CT can be combined with percutaneous needle biopsy to provide a tissue diagnosis. An alternative is a laparoscopically guided biopsy, which provides the opportunity to inspect the rest of the peritoneal cavity in cases where no primary site is obvious.

Treatment

The detection of liver metastases often alters the surgical management of patients with cancer. Since most of these patients will have incurable disease, the primary goal of surgical intervention is to palliate distressing symptoms rather than undertake radical surgical resection. The management of colorectal and renal cell cancer metastases is an exception to this rule.

Hepatic lobectomy in patients with metastases from colorectal cancer can give a 25% 5-year survival, whereas some renal secondaries will regress after resection of the primary tumour.

Some gastrointestinal metastases will respond to chemotherapy using 5-fluorouracil, by either systemic or direct intrahepatic arterial perfusion. An alternative treatment currently under investigation is hepatic cryotherapy, a technique that causes necrosis of the tumour deposits by freezing.

Prognosis
Overall, less than 10% of patients will survive more than 1 year after diagnosis. The outlook is slightly better for patients with hepatic colorectal metastases.

Portal hypertension and cirrhosis

Increased resistance to intrahepatic blood flow or extrahepatic portal vein obstruction causes portal hypertension. This leads to the diversion of portal venous blood to the systemic circulation through the collateral circulation, which exists between the portal and systemic circulations. The most important plexus of veins lies around the gastro-oesophageal junction. These veins become progressively dilated and varicose forming oesophageal varices which lie just beneath the oesophageal mucosa. These fragile veins can rupture causing an exsanguinating haemorrhage and death. Surgical treatment is aimed either at mechanically obliterating the varices or at creating a venous shunt between the portal and systemic circulations which decompresses the portal circulation and thus reduces the pressure and risk of bleeding from the oesophageal varices.

Aetiology
Most cases of portal hypertension are caused by cirrhosis, which is usually the sequel to alcohol abuse or viral hepatitis. Infrequently, portal hypertension can result from isolated thrombosis of the portal or splenic vein (prehepatic causes) or by restriction of blood flow through the hepatic veins (posthepatic causes).

Clinical features
Cirrhotic patients may present with the classic triad of ascites, hepatomegaly and spider naevi. Palmar erythema, gynaecomastia and testicular atrophy are other key physical signs. Some patients will present with a catastrophic haematemesis following oesophageal variceal rupture.

Diagnosis
Gastroscopy is the key investigation that will detect any

oesophageal or gastric fundal varices: suspect this diagnosis in every cirrhotic patient.

Treatment of the acutely bleeding patient
All patients require immediate resuscitation as outlined on page 76. Many patients will have a coagulopathy because of their underlying liver disease coupled with the massive blood losses. This requires correction with fresh frozen plasma, clotting factors and vitamin K.

The following steps should be taken to arrest the haemorrhage:

Injection sclerotherapy. This is performed at the same time as the diagnostic gastroscopy. A sclerosant (e.g. ethanolamine oleate) is injected into or around the bleeding varix.

Splanchnic vasoconstriction. Vasopressin, somatostatin or propranolol may reduce splanchnic blood flow and portal venous pressure and hence stop bleeding.

Balloon tamponade. A Sengestaken–Blakemore tube (Fig. 11) can be used to control bleeding by applying direct pressure to the varices. It can be particularly useful in controlling gastric fundal varices, which may be difficult to control with sclerotherapy. Occasionally, in patients who are exsanguinating, immediate placement of a Sengestaken–Blakemore tube will be a life-saving manoeuvre carried out in advance of sclerotherapy or endoscopy.

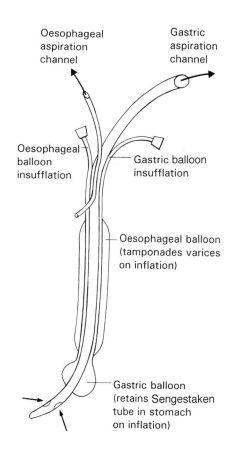

Fig. 11
Sengestaken–Blakemore tube.

Emergency surgery. Patients who do not respond to these measures require emergency surgery.

Oesophageal transection. Direct obliteration of the bleeding varices using a staple gun to completely transect and reanastomose the oesophagus.

A porto-systemic shunt procedure. See below.

Treatment of patients who are not bleeding acutely

Patients with varices who have bled but are no longer acutely bleeding can be treated by two main options:

- injection sclerotherapy
- elective surgery.

Varices can be obliterated by a programme of repeated sclerosant injections, which produces fibrosis and thrombosis. This reduces the death rate from bleeding, but these patients will still die from their underlying cirrhotic liver disease.

Operative diversion of blood from the portal to the systemic circulation (porta-systemic shunt) will decompress the varices and prevent further bleeding. Its use is restricted to a selected group of patients who have previously bled, are at a high risk of rebleeding and who are fit enough to undergo the procedure. Overall, the operative death rate is 10%. Diversion of blood away from the liver by the procedure can lead to an increased risk of liver failure and hepatic encephalopathy. Patient selection is difficult and is aided by Child's criteria, which use hepatic function and patient nutritional status to identify those patients suitable for surgery.

There are many types of shunt operation, but the three most commonly used are:

- end-to-end porta-caval (Fig. 12)
- side-to-side porta-caval (Fig. 13)
- distal spleno-renal shunt (Fig. 14).

Both porta-caval shunts decompress high-pressure portal venous blood into the low-pressure inferior vena cava. A major advantage of the distal spleno-renal shunt

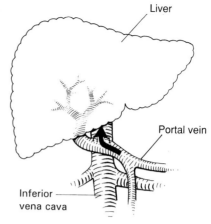

Fig. 13
Side-to-side porta-caval shunt.

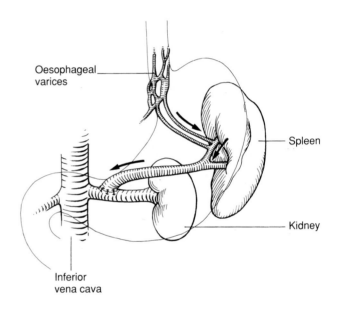

→ Flow of blood decompressing portal venous blood into systemic circulation

Fig. 14
Distal spleno-renal shunt.

is that it selectively decompresses the oesophageal varices and preserves the liver perfusion. It is a more difficult operation.

Surgery and the spleen

Despite its protected position behind the left costal margin, the spleen remains vulnerable to trauma, particularly after a violent acceleration or deceleration injury. In the adult, the spleen produces plasma cells, monocytes and lymphocytes and functions as a filter to remove defunct circulating red blood cells. It also functions as a store for platelets and has a pivotal role in antibody production.

There are three main indications for splenectomy:

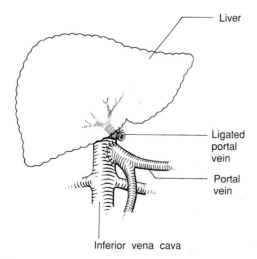

Fig. 12
End-to-end porta-caval shunt.

- trauma
- incidental splenectomy during elective intra-abdominal surgery
- symptomatic splenomegaly or hypersplenism.

Trauma

Splenic rupture should be considered in any blunt or penetrating injury to the upper abdomen or lower chest. Patients may show signs of hypovolaemic shock, although this may be absent in the early stages after injury. Rib fractures or a complaint of left shoulder tip pain caused by the subdiaphragmatic collection of blood should also raise suspicion of injury. In patients with multiple trauma, the diagnosis may be overlooked unless a diagnostic peritoneal lavage is performed.

Occasionally a delayed splenic rupture may occur several weeks following the initial injury after the late rupture of a slowly expanding subcapsular haematoma.

Diagnosis

In a shocked patient following major trauma with no other overt sign of blood loss, it may be necessary to proceed immediately to a life-saving diagnostic laparotomy. Here, the diagnosis may be made at operation.

In less urgent circumstances, the diagnosis may be suspected by a positive diagnostic peritoneal lavage and confirmed by CT or ultrasound abdominal scan.

Treatment

Total splenectomy is usually the only operative option. Occasionally it may be possible to conserve the spleen by repair of any isolated tears (splenorrhaphy) or by tamponade (wrapping the organ in an absorbable woven mesh).

Splenectomy during intra-abdominal surgery

The spleen may be removed as part of a radical surgical procedure for cancer of the oesophagus or stomach in an attempt to ensure complete removal of the lymphatic drainage bed. Splenectomy may also be necessary as a result of inadvertent injury during surgery of the stomach and gastro-oesophageal junction or during mobilisation of the splenic flexure during colonic surgery.

Symptomatic splenomegaly or hypersplenism

Congenital haemolytic anaemias. Splenectomy will prevent haemolysis in congenital haemolytic anaemias (e.g. hereditary spherocytosis, thalassaemia) or in autoimmune haemolytic anaemia.

Idiopathic thrombocytopenic purpura. This condition, characterised by a shortened platelet lifespan causing a bruising and bleeding tendency, can be effectively treated by splenectomy if patients fail to respond to steroid therapy. In this disease, the spleen may function as a source of circulating antiplatelet antibodies as well as the site of their extraction from the circulation.

Hodgkin's disease. Splenectomy is now rarely performed in staging Hodgkin's disease.

The consequences of splenectomy

After splenectomy, there is often a massive rise in the circulating platelet level (up to 0.5–1.0 million cells per μl). This can persist for up to 12 months, but the risks of thrombosis are slight and patients do not need anticoagulation.

All patients after splenectomy are at risk of a severe postsplenectomy infection. The infection starts as a flu-like illness and rapidly progresses to a septicaemia causing multiple organ failure and death. The increased risk is greatest in the first 2 years after surgery but persists throughout life. The most common pathogen is *Streptococcus pneumoniae*. All patients undergoing splenectomy should be immunised preoperatively, when possible, with a pneumococcal vaccine, followed by lifelong antibiotic prophylaxis with a low-dose penicillin.

2.5 Diseases of the small bowel and appendix

Small bowel disease falls into three major categories:

- small bowel obstruction
- inflammatory disease of the small bowel
- mesenteric ischaemia.

Acute appendicitis is the most important surgical condition that affects the appendix.

Small bowel obstruction

Aetiology
The two main causes of small bowel obstruction are:

- postoperative adhesions
- irreducible external hernias, e.g. inguinal, femoral or umbilical.

Less frequent but important causes are:

- caecal carcinoma obstructing the ileocaecal valve
- Crohn's disease
- ischaemic stricture from radiation enteritis or mesenteric ischaemia
- gallstone ileus
- food bolus or foreign body
- congenital adhesions
- intussusception
- small bowel volvulus.

Clinical features

Colicky abdominal pain is the most constant feature of small bowel obstruction. Other symptoms and signs depend upon the level of obstruction.

Distal small bowel obstruction is associated with progressive abdominal distension and dehydration.

Mid small bowel obstruction is characterised by severe colic.

High small bowel obstruction can be deceptively pain free with profuse vomiting and rapid dehydration.

Physical examination classically reveals a tympanitic distended abdomen with tinkling bowel sounds together with clues as to the likely underlying cause of the obstruction, e.g an irreducible hernia or a previous laparotomy scar.

Diagnosis

This is usually established on clinical grounds and confirmed by plain abdominal X-ray. Distended small bowel loops on a supine film and multiple fluid levels on an erect film are the hallmark of small bowel obstruction (Fig. 15).

Strangulation. This is a life-threatening complication and implies obstruction of the blood supply to the affected segment of small bowel by either venous congestion or arterial occlusion. It is more common in:

- a closed loop obstruction (where a single loop of bowel becomes obstructed between two fixed points and rapidly distends)
- small bowel volvulus

- irreducible incarcerated external hernias.

Differential diagnosis. Clinical and biochemical indices differentiate poorly between strangulating and 'simple' small bowel obstruction, but strangulation should be suspected in patients with:

- localised abdominal tenderness
- fever, leucocytosis, tachycardia
- constant rather than colicky pain.

Treatment

Urgent surgery is only indicated if there is a suspicion of strangulation. At least one half of episodes of simple adhesive obstruction will settle with conservative treatment and will not need surgery. Those patients who do not settle after 2–3 days or who have an obvious underlying cause, e.g. an external hernia, all require surgery after appropriate preoperative preparation.

The key preoperative steps are:

- stop oral intake
- apply nasogastric suction
- provide intravenous fluid replacement and resuscitation
- correct any fluid and electrolyte imbalance.

Surgery

Most cases of small bowel obstruction needing operation are the result of adhesions. The surgery involves meticulously unravelling the entire small intestine by careful division of all adhesive bands. Any non-viable

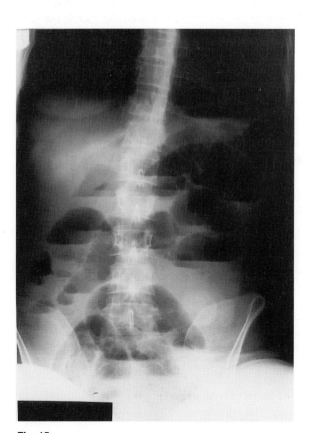
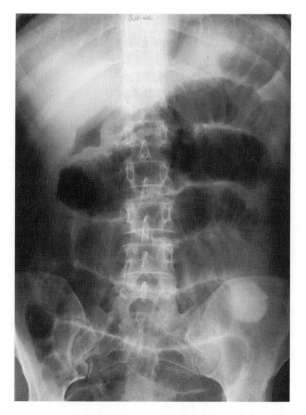

Fig. 15
X-ray appearances of a small bowel obstruction—erect abdominal film (left); supine abdominal film (right).

segments of bowel (as a result of strangulation) should be resected. Any associated disease (e.g. hernia or colon cancer) should be dealt with at the same time.

Prognosis

Surgery for simple small bowel obstruction is a low-risk procedure. If strangulation supervenes, death rates may reach 10%, especially in the elderly. This emphasises the need for careful appraisal and prompt management of patients in whom strangulation is suspected.

Inflammatory diseases of the small bowel

Crohn's disease is the most important condition in this category. In addition, there are many infective causes of small bowel inflammation:

- *Campylobacter coli*
- *Yersinia enterocolitica*
- *Salmonella typhii*
- Tuberculous enteritis.

Crohn's disease

Aetiology and pathology

Crohn's disease is an idiopathic transmural inflammatory disease of the intestinal wall. It can affect any part of the gastrointestinal tract from the mouth to the anus. The disease is characterised by focal areas of lymphocytic infiltration and the presence of non-caseating epithelioid granulomas. Mucosal ulceration, skip lesions (segments of normal bowel interspersed between grossly diseased bowel) and deep fissures, which sometimes connect with adjacent viscera causing fistulation, are the hallmark of Crohn's disease.

The most frequent distribution of the disease is:

- terminal ileum and caecum
- perineum
- colon.

Clinical features

Most patients will present with one or a combination of the following symptoms:

- gastrointestinal
  — colicky abdominal pains
  — diarrhoea
  — perianal sepsis, abscesses and fistulae
- chronic systemic disease
  — weight loss, malnutrition, anaemia
  — failure to thrive.

Occasionally the disease presents acutely and mimics appendicitis.

Although some patients will exhibit no gross abnormal physical signs in the early stages of the disease, others will exhibit a range of physical findings:

- evidence of recent weight loss
- small bowel obstruction
- abdominal mass caused by matted intestinal loops
- entero-cutaneous fistula
- chronic perianal sepsis.

Diagnosis

Depending on the symptom pattern, confirmation of Crohn's disease can be obtained by two main methods.

Sigmoidoscopy/colonoscopy. This provides direct visualisation of Crohn's ulceration and biopsy evidence of pathognomonic granulomata if the large intestine is involved.

Barium studies. A barium follow through is the single most useful examination for small bowel Crohn's disease. Cobblestone mucosa, rose thorn fissures, multiple small bowel strictures, interloop fistulae and 'skip lesions', appearing in any combination, are classic features of small bowel Crohn's disease (Fig. 16).

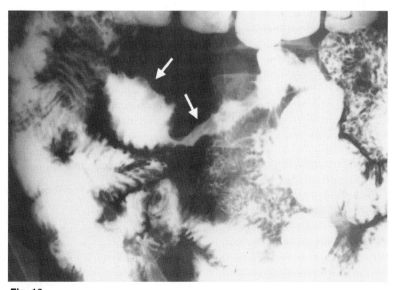

Fig. 16
X-ray appearances of small bowel Crohn's disease showing strictured and dilated segments.

Differential diagnosis. The differential diagnosis of Crohn's disease is extremely wide, encompassing almost all intra-abdominal pathologies. Two important conditions in the differential diagnosis of small bowel Crohn's disease which should not be overlooked are:

- tuberculous enteritis
- small bowel lymphoma.

Both these conditions may present with weight loss and a right iliac fossa mass, with similar radiological findings on a small bowel follow through. Often the diagnosis is only realised after surgical resection and histopathology examination.

Complications. The two most important groups of complications are:

- fistula and abscess formation
  — entero-cutaneous
  — entero-enteric
  — entero-vesical
  — interloop abscess
- small bowel obstruction.

Treatment

The natural history of Crohn's disease is of spontaneous relapses and remissions. This makes evaluation of any therapy difficult. Generally, the first-line management is medical, with surgery reserved for the management of complications.

Medical therapy. Steroids and/or immunosuppressive therapy combined with nutritional support form the cornerstone of medical treatment.

Steroids. Intermittent high-dose courses are used alone or in combination with low-dose steroid maintenence therapy.

Azathioprine or cyclosporin. These immunosuppressive agents suppress the chronic inflammatory reaction associated with Crohn's disease.

Metronidazole or sulphasalazine. These agents are most effective in colonic Crohn's disease (see p. 46).

Nutritional support. Total parenteral or enteral nutrition can effectively treat malnutrition caused by malabsorption, although it is unlikely to influence the course of the disease.

Surgery in Crohn's disease. Conservative surgery is the keynote of operative management in Crohn's disease. Abscesses and fistulae are the main indications for surgery in small bowel Crohn's disease. Wherever possible, the affected segments of bowel should be resected and gastrointestinal continuity restored rather than performing a by-pass operation that short circuits but leaves behind the affected Crohn's disease segment. Surgery is sometimes required for chronic small bowel obstruction caused by a strictured segment of Crohn's disease. The same surgical principles apply.

Prognosis

Management of patients with Crohn's disease is a life-long task best provided by a dedicated team of gastroenterologists and surgeons with a special interest in the disease. Surgery does not cure the disease and some patients will require repeated surgical procedures. Overall, the death rate of Crohn's disease patients is tow to three times higher than that of the general population.

Mesenteric ischaemia

Lack of blood supply to the small intestine can be acute or chronic. Whereas the blood supply to the foregut (from the coeliac axis) or to the hindgut (from the inferior mesenteric artery) can be sustained by collateral blood flow immediately after an acute occlusion, the blood supply to the midgut cannot, hence the catastrophic consequences of an acute occlusion of the superior mesenteric artery.

The three most important types of occlusion are:

- acute superior mesenteric artery occlusion
- acute mesenteric venous occlusion
- chronic superior mesenteric artery occlusion.

Acute superior mesenteric artery occlusion

Acute occlusion is caused by arterial embolisation, usually from a mural thrombus in the heart or great vessels or by thrombosis of an atherosclerotic superior mesenteric artery.

Clinical features

Agonising abdominal pain, vomiting and diarrhoea, and gastrointestinal blood loss are the hallmarks of an acute occlusion. Typically, the patient is elderly, has atrial fibrillation and may have a previous history of peripheral vascular disease.

Generalised tenderness is evident on abdominal examination. Without treatment, sepsis and irreversible shock rapidly supervene.

Diagnosis

Making the diagnosis can be difficult as there are few specific signs. The following features suggest a diagnosis of acute mesenteric ischaemia:

- massive leucocytosis
- a mild hyperamylasaemia, which can cause diagnostic confusion with acute pancreatitis
- lack of intestinal gas on plain abdominal X-ray.

Treatment

There is rarely time for sophisticated investigation and in many cases a suspected diagnosis will only be confirmed at an urgent laparotomy after resuscitation.

In elderly patients with total small bowel infarction, surgery has no role to play. Laparotomy merely confirms the diagnosis and inevitably there is a fatal outcome. Less extensive infarction is amenable to resection. In other patients, revascularisation by either embolectomy or by-pass grafting may revive an ischaemic but not an infarcted bowel.

Mesenteric venous thrombosis

Venous infarction is much less common than arterial occlusion. It is usually idiopathic but may be the result of sepsis, liver disease or other hypercoagulable states. The presentation and management are essentially the same as for an acute mesenteric arterial occlusion.

Chronic superior mesenteric vascular occlusion

Incomplete occlusion of the superior mesenteric artery causes chronic small bowel ischaemia. This manifests as post-prandial pain coupled with weight loss and diarrhoea caused by malabsorption. The clinical picture may mimic advanced malignancy and requires a superior mesenteric angiogram to clinch the diagnosis.

Endarterectomy or the use of a vein graft to by-pass the occlusion can produce a dramatic resolution of the symptoms.

Prognosis. The overall prognosis for patients with mesenteric ischaemia is poor. Over 50% of patients will die of the acute event.

Acute appendicitis

Appendicectomy for acute appendicitis is one of the most common surgical emergencies. The disease can occur at any age and overall mortality rates are less than 1%. Those at greatest risk of dying of the disease are the very young and the very old.

Aetiology

There is no single satisfactory explanation for the cause of appendicitis. A combination of luminal obstruction by faecoliths or lymphoid follicular hyperplasia with secondary bacterial invasion of the appendicular wall by enteric organisms have been implicated.

Clinical features

The initial symptoms are vague. Patients complain of nausea, anorexia and a poorly localised abdominal discomfort. Later, as serosal inflammation of the appendix develops, pain localises in the right iliac fossa and becomes aggravated by movement. A low-grade fever with tenderness and guarding over McBurney's point (one third of the way along a line drawn from the anterior superior iliac spine to the umbilicus) are classical physical signs. Rectal examination is essential to detect pelvic appendicitis.

The history and physical signs will differ depending on the site of the appendix (Fig. 17) and in patients at the extremes of life.

Retrocaecal appendicitis. Pain remains poorly localised as the appendix is not in contact with the parietal peritoneum. It can mimic renal colic or pyelonephritis.

Pelvic appendicitis. There are no abdominal signs; patients may have diarrhoea or urinary frequency because of irritation of the rectum or bladder by the

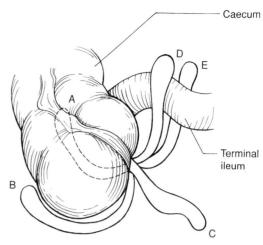

Fig. 17
Anatomical positions of the appendix in relation to the caecum and ileum. A. retrocaecal; B. paracaecal; C. pelvic; D. preileal; E. postileal

inflamed appendix. It can mimic gastroenteritis, cystitis or acute salpingitis.

Appendicitis and an abnormally sited caecum. In patients with a high caecum or those with a malrotation, appendicitis may mimic cholecystitis or diverticulitis.

Diagnosis

In the majority of cases, the diagnosis of acute appendicitis is based on the case history and physical examination. Special investigations have little role to play except in young women, in whom the diagnosis may be difficult to distinguish from gynaecological disease. In these patients ultrasound examination or diagnostic laparoscopy is useful.

Diagnosing appendicitis in children can be difficult as the history may not be clear. Appendicitis may also be overlooked in the elderly patient with a lax abdominal wall where guarding cannot be elicited.

Differential diagnosis. The differential diagnosis in acute appendicitis is wide and is summarised in Table 5.

Complications

Perforation. This is more common in the young and the elderly or where there is a delay in diagnosis.

Appendix mass. The acutely inflamed appendix, which may have perforated, becomes 'walled off' from the peritoneal cavity by adjacent loops of intestine and

Table 5 Differential diagnosis of acute appendicitis

Common
Mesenteric lymphadenitis
Gastroenteritis
Salpingitis
Ruptured ovarian follicle
Pyelonephritis/ureteric colic

Uncommon
Ectopic pregnancy
Torted ovarian cyst
Acute Crohn's disease
Cholecystitis

omentum that prevent a generalised peritonitis. A tender mass is palpable in the right iliac fossa.

Treatment

Appendicectomy is mandatory once the diagnosis has been made and the patient made fit for surgery; the only exception being an appendix mass that can be treated conservatively with antibiotics, intravenous fluids and bed rest until the mass resolves. In these cases, appendicectomy is undertaken at a later date unless an appendix abscess develops that requires incision and drainage.

Tumours of the appendix

These are rare and of two types:

- benign and malignant carcinoid tumours
- adenocarcinoma of the appendix.

Benign and malignant carcinoid tumours

The appendix is the most common primary site for these tumours. They develop from specialised cells, namely the argentaffin cells, which have an endocrine function. These tumours are usually found by chance at the tip of the appendix during appendicectomy and they have a characteristic yellow-brown colour. Although microscopically they have many of the features of an invasive carcinoma, their biological behaviour is benign and only a few will metastasise.

A carcinoid tumour of the tip of the appendix can be treated by appendicectomy. Carcinoid tumours of the base of the appendix are more likely to invade adjacent structures and are best treated by right hemicolectomy. Appendicular carcinoids are usually incidental findings during laparotomy or appendicectomy. Occasionally they present late when metastatic liver deposits give rise to the carcinoid syndrome (flushing, diarrhoea, borborygmi) caused by the release of vasoactive amines, C_5 hydroxytryptamine, into the systemic circulation.

Adenocarcinoma of the appendix

This diagnosis is rarely made preoperatively and may be difficult to distinguish from a caecal carcinoma. A right hemicolectomy is the treatment of choice.

Uncommon small bowel diseases

Radiation enteritis and small bowel lymphoma are two uncommon but important small bowel diseases.

Radiation enteritis

Irradiation injury to the small bowel is usually the sequel to pelvic radiotherapy for gynaecological cancer. The early mucosal injury presents with bloody diarrhoea and abdominal cramps. Injury to the blood vessels can present up to 20 years later with chronic ischaemia causing formation of fibrotic strictures and symptoms of chronic small bowel obstruction.

Treatment.

Early symptoms resulting from the mucosal injury are treated conservatively and usually settle spontaneously. Major small bowel resection is required to relieve the late obstructive symptoms.

Small bowel lymphoma (non Hodgkin's and T-cell lymphoma)

The presenting symptoms are similar to small bowel Crohn's disease. Sometimes the diagnosis is only confirmed after resection of the affected segment of small intestine. Radiotherapy and chemotherapy are usually used in conjunction with surgery.

2.6 Diseases of the large intestine

The most important surgical diseases affecting the large bowel are:

- carcinoma of the colon
- colonic polyps
- Crohn's colitis and ulcerative colitis
- diverticular disease.

All of these conditions usually present with an alteration in bowel habit often associated with the passage of blood, mucus and slime. The principles of investigation are common to all; namely, a careful contrast radiological evaluation of the colon coupled with endoscopy and biopsy using sigmoidoscopy or colonoscopy as appropriate. Some affected patients will present acutely with a large bowel obstruction.

Large bowel obstruction

The obstructed colon distends progressively as the small bowel continues to pour its contents through the ileocaecal valve. As the distended colon contracts and attempts to overcome the obstruction, the peristaltic waves are perceived as colic. If the ileocaecal valve is competent (Fig. 18B) and prevents reflux of the intestinal contents back into the small intestine, a closed-loop obstruction develops with massive and rapid distension of the colon. Left untreated, the thin-walled highly distensible caecum will perforate. If the ileocaecal valve is incompetent (Fig. 18C), intestinal contents will flow back into the small bowel, which will in turn distend and eventually cause vomiting.

Aetiology

Cancer of the colon is by far the most common cause of large bowel obstruction (see p. 42).

Less frequent causes are sigmoid or caecal volvulus, 'pseudo-obstruction', chronic constipation and faecal impaction, and finally a diverticular stricture or acute diverticulitis.

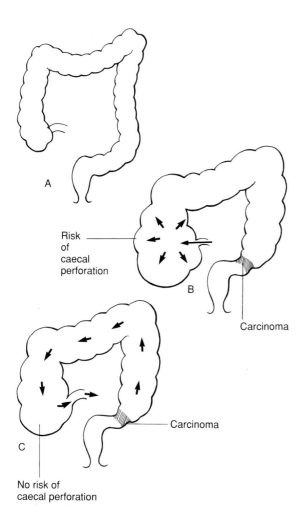

Fig. 18
Large bowel obstruction. **A.** Normal anatomy. **B.** Closed-loop
large bowel obstruction. **C.** 'Open' loop obstruction with
retrograde decompression of the colon into the small bowel.

Clinical features

Large bowel obstruction is characterised by colicky
lower abdominal pains, abdominal distension and an
alteration in bowel habit. As the obstruction progresses,
constipation becomes absolute and the passage of flatus
ceases. Unlike small bowel obstruction, vomiting is a
late feature.

Physical examination often reveals a tense tympanitic distended abdomen in a dehydrated patient. The
bowel sounds are high-pitched and tinkling. Localised
tenderness, particularly over the caecum, suggests
imminent caecal perforation.

Diagnosis

Large bowel obstruction is investigated by two main
methods.

Plain abdominal X-ray. Gross colonic dilatation on a
supine abdominal film with large bowel fluid levels on
an erect film are the classical features. The extent of any
caecal dilatation in a closed-loop obstruction will also
be evident.

**Sigmoidoscopy and/or gentle contrast enema exam-
ination.** If the patient's condition permits, the level of
the obstruction must be assessed prior to surgery. These
tests are important in order to help plan the most appropriate operation and to rule out a pseudo-obstruction or
faecal impaction, which can be treated without operation.

Treatment

Once the patient has been adequately resuscitated,
rapid surgical relief of the mechanical obstruction is
the primary aim of treatment in order to prevent
colonic perforation and a potentially lethal faecal
peritonitis. Treatment depends on the cause of the
obstruction.

Carcinoma of the colon. An obstructing cancer of the
caecum or ascending colon can usually be treated by
right hemicolectomy with an immediate reanastomosis
(Fig. 19). Left-sided cancers that obstruct are more difficult to manage. Primary reanastomosis after resection is
rarely feasible as the obstructed bowel heals poorly and
the risks of anastomotic leakage are high. In frail, ill
patients, a defunctioning transverse colon loop
colostomy may be life-saving. Primary resection without reanastomosis (Hartmann's operation, Fig. 20) is a
good alternative in a fitter patient.

Sigmoid or caecal volvulus. Decompression of a sigmoid volvulus (Fig. 21) using a flatus tube introduced

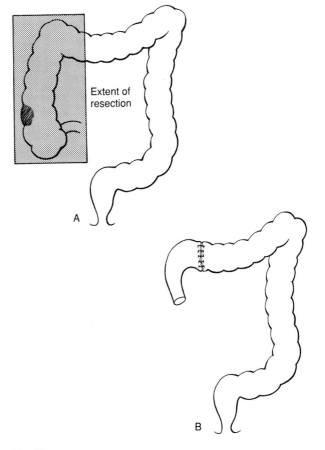

Fig. 19
Right hemicolectomy.

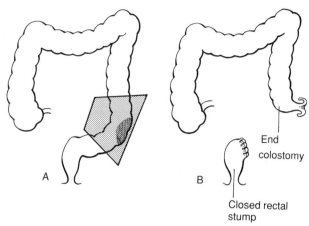

Fig. 20
Hartmann's operation.

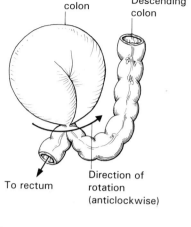

Fig. 21
Sigmoid volvulus.

per rectum can be a life-saving manoeuvre. The volvulus is likely to recur and wherever possible resection either with or without primary reanastomosis should be attempted. A caecal volvulus is less common. Here the caecum is abnormally mobile and may twist, compromising its own blood supply and causing an intestinal obstruction. A right hemicolectomy is the operation of choice.

Pseudo-obstruction. This condition mimics a true mechanical bowel obstruction. It is caused by abnormal gut motility and the diagnosis is confirmed by a contrast enema examination, which will fail to show any evidence of a mechanical obstruction despite the plain abdominal X-ray findings. A pseudo-obstruction often responds to correction of any electrolyte imbalance, rehydration and supplemental oxygen. Occasionally, massive caecal distension will occur and it will be necessary to decompress the colon by caecostomy.

Faecal impaction. Faecal impaction, often in elderly bed-ridden patients, can present as a large bowel obstruction that can be relieved by either manual disimpaction or a series of enemas. These patients should be investigated by sigmoidoscopy and barium enema to exclude an underlying cause for their impaction.

Prognosis
This depends on the cause. The mortality rates after laparotomy for large bowel obstruction are about 15% and are doubled in patients with faecal peritonitis from an associated perforation.

Carcinoma of the colon (and rectum)

Carcinoma of the colon and rectum are closely related and are considered together. Colorectal cancer is a common malignancy and is second only to lung cancer in incidence. It develops slowly and has usually been present for several years before becoming clinically apparent. The distribution of colorectal cancer is shown in Figure 22. Primary cancers in the caecum and ascending

colon develop into a large fungating mass that rarely obstructs the intestinal lumen. Elsewhere, colonic cancer slowly encircles the bowel and will eventually produce obstruction. The disease spreads via the lymphatics to regional and distant lymph node groups and by haematogenous routes to liver and lungs. Spread also occurs across the peritoneal cavity to form multiple metastatic serosal seedlings.

Survival is closely linked to the pathological stage (Duke's staging) at the time of resection (Table 6).

Aetiology
The most important aetiological factors predisposing to carcinoma of the large intestine are:

- diet: a high ratio of animal protein to fat, low-fibre diet
- strong family history of colon cancer
- adenomatous colonic polyps
- familial polyposis coli
- chronic ulcerative colitis.

Clinical features
The presentation depends on the site of the cancer:

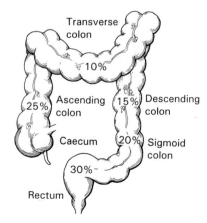

Fig. 22
Distribution of colorectal cancer.

Table 6 Duke's staging for colorectal cancer

Stage	Extent	5-Year survival (%)
A	Limited to bowel wall	80
B	Extends through bowel wall; no lymph node metastases	60
C	Lymph node metastases	30
D	Distant metastases	10

Right hemicolon: anaemia, tiredness, abdominal mass and vague abdominal pain.

Left hemicolon: altered bowel habit, blood mixed with stools and large bowel obstruction.

Rectum: altered bowel habit, rectal bleeding and a mucous rectal discharge, tenesmus. The cancer may be palpable on rectal examination.

Carcinoma of the rectum and right-sided large bowel cancer rarely present with obstruction.

Diagnosis

Investigations must visualise the entire colon, using a combination of three tests.

Rigid or flexible sigmoidoscopy. Up to 50% of all colonic cancers can be reached by these simple endoscopic tests and a diagnostic biopsy obtained.

Double-contrast barium enema. This will outline the entire colon and detect the majority of cancers and colonic polyps.

Colonoscopy. With an experienced endoscopist, the entire colon can be directly visualised. It has the advantage that diagnostic biopsy can be obtained and the disadvantage that the caecum may not always be reached. In the UK, it is reserved for those patients for whom a barium enema raises suspicion of cancer but is not diagnostic.

Abdominal ultrasound. The liver should be carefully examined for metastases.

Surgical treatment: colonic carcinoma

The goal of surgery is to remove the tumour-bearing areas of the colon together with a wide margin of normal bowel and the adjacent regional lymphatic drainage. Gastrointestinal continuity is restored by an end-to-end anastomosis. Liver metastases are not a contraindication to resection. Solitary metastases can be resected.

The precise operation depends on the site of the tumour.

Cancer in the right colon requires a right hemicolectomy (Fig. 19).

Cancer in the transverse colon requires a transverse colectomy or an extended right hemicolectomy (Fig. 23).

Cancer in the left colon requires a left hemicolectomy (Fig. 24A).

Cancer in the sigmoid colon requires a sigmoid colectomy (Fig. 24B).

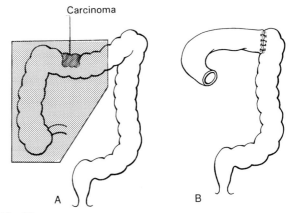

Fig. 23
Surgery for cancer of the transverse colon: extended right hemicolectomy.

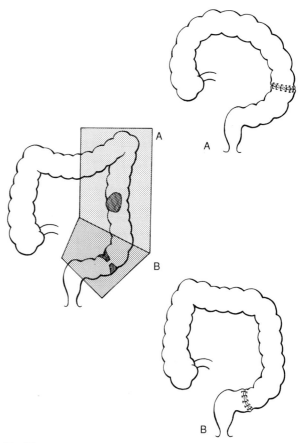

Fig. 24
A. Left hemicolectomy. **B.** Sigmoid colectomy.

Surgical treatment: rectal carcinoma

Treatment of rectal carcinoma is more complex. The surgical options depend upon the size and site of the tumour, together with the build of the patient. Carcinoma of the upper rectum can be dealt with by an extended sigmoid resection and reanastomosis (anterior resection, Fig. 25A). Cancers of the lower rectum, usually those that can be felt on rectal examination, require excision of the entire rectum and anal canal with the formation of a permanent end colostomy in the left iliac

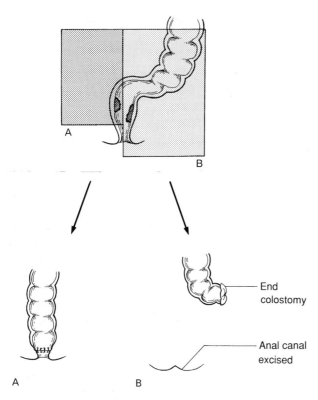

Fig. 25
A. Anterior resection. **B.** Abdomino-perineal resection.

fossa (abdomino-perineal resection, Fig. 25B). Cancers in the mid rectum are the most difficult to manage. A large tumour in a small male pelvis may require an abdomino-perineal resection, whereas a small tumour in a wide female pelvis may be manageable by a low anterior resection.

Radiotherapy and chemotherapy in colon and rectal cancer

These are complex issues and their precise roles have not yet been defined. Radiotherapy seems to reduce the likelihood of local recurrence and is especially useful in rectal cancer. It may be administered pre- or postoperatively. Currently the role of the chemotherapeutic agent 5–fluorouracil in colorectal cancer is being evaluated.

Prognosis

Outcome is closely linked to the pathological staging at the time of resection (see Table 6). It is worse for patients who undergo urgent surgery for obstructed or perforated cancers.

Colonic polyps

Colonic polyps are of great importance because they may be the precursor to colon cancer:

- up to 50% of polyps 2 cm or greater in size are malignant
- one third of patients with colon cancer also have colonic polyps

- colonic polyps can recur or develop at new sites
- malignant potential is also related to the histological type of the polyp (villous > tubulo-villous > tubular adenoma).

Clinical features
Most polyps will be asymptomatic and may not present until the patient develops symptoms of colonic cancer. Rectal bleeding is the most frequent symptom.

Diagnosis
Diagnosis is by air-contrast barium enema or by sigmoidoscopy or colonoscopy plus biopsy.

Treatment
Single polyps. Most polyps are on a stalk and can be snared and removed during sigmoidoscopy or colonoscopy. Sessile polyps, which cannot be safely snared, may require colonic resection. All polyps must be subject to a careful histological examination. Pedunculated polyps bearing a focus of malignancy but no evidence of any invasion of the stalk require no further treatment. Other polyps with malignant invasion of the stalk require resection of the segment of colon bearing the polyp.

Multiple polyps. Colonic polyps are often multiple and the detection of a single polyp demands evaluation of the entire colon and complete clearance of any additional polyps.

Familial polyposis coli. Occasionally, this rare autosomal dominant condition will be encountered. It is characterised by the development of hundreds of polyps throughout the colon after the age of puberty and the development of cancer in at least one of these polyps by the age of 40. There are two treatment options.

Panproctocolectomy. Total removal of the colon, rectum and anus with formation of a permanent ileostomy (see Fig. 26C).

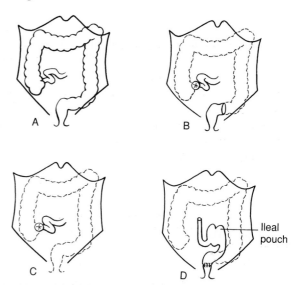

Fig. 26
Surgery of the large bowel and rectum. **A.** Normal anatomy. **B.** Subtotal colectomy. **C.** Panproctocolectomy. **D.** Total colectomy, ileo-anal anastomosis with ileal pouch.

Near total colectomy. As above, with preservation of the anal canal to allow either an ileo-anal anastomosis or construction of an ileal pouch or reservoir (see Fig. 26D).

Prognosis

Regular endoscopic follow-up is essential in patients who have had colonic polyps. In this way, recurrent or new polyps can be removed before malignancy supervenes.

Diverticular disease

Multiple colonic diverticulae (mucosal herniation through the large bowel circular muscle layers) are a common finding. Although they can develop in any part of the colon, they are most frequent in the sigmoid colon. Diverticular disease is a condition of Western society and is linked to a low dietary intake of fibre.

Clinical features

Diverticular disease may be an incidental finding on a barium enema or sigmoidoscopy. Colonic symptoms should not be attributed to it until full colonic investigations have ruled out any coexisting pathology.

Acute diverticulitis is caused by infection of one or more diverticulae and inflammation of the adjacent colon. Patients present with left iliac fossa pain of variable severity, systemic signs of sepsis and an altered bowel habit (either diarrhoea or constipation). On examination, there may be tenderness in the left iliac fossa or signs of local peritonitis or an abdominal mass.

Diagnosis

Acute diverticulitis is a clinical diagnosis and the immediate treatment is based on the history and physical findings. Once the patient's condition has responded to treatment, the diagnosis is confirmed by flexible sigmoidoscopy or barium enema examination.

Treatment

Intravenous antibiotic therapy, bowel rest and analgesia are the cornerstone of medical management. Most patients will settle on this regimen. Those who do not or who develop complications require resection of the diseased segment of bowel. Because of the surrounding inflammation and infection, it is usually necessary to perform a Hartmann's procedure (Fig. 20).

Complications. There are five major complications:

- pericolic abscess
- perforation
- fistula formation: usually to the bladder or vagina causing a vesico-colic or a vagino-colic fistula
- major haemorrhage
- diverticular stricture.

Some patients will present primarily with these complications, which usually require urgent surgery after resuscitation. Again, a Hartmann's procedure is the most useful operation.

Large bowel inflammatory disease

Ulcerative colitis and Crohn's colitis are two of the most common causes of large bowel inflammatory disease. The clinical picture may vary from a chronic low-grade colitis that may persist for many years to an acute fulminant attack of colitis. Infective colitis and ischaemic colitis are two other important causes of acute colitis.

Clinical features

Bloody diarrhoea is the key presenting symptom in acute colitis. In a severe attack, patients may be septic with abdominal pain and tenderness. Patients may also present with chronic colitis causing loose stools, weight loss and anaemia.

Diagnosis

A plain abdominal film is essential in all patients presenting acutely with colitis in order to detect toxic dilatation or colonic perforation (see p. 40).

The three most important elective investigations are:

- stool cultures: to detect any infective causes of colitis
- sigmoidoscopy and biopsy: to obtain a tissue diagnosis
- barium enema: to assess the extent and severity of the disease.

Treatment

The key steps in managing an acute severe attack of colitis are:

- intravenous fluid resuscitation
- restrict oral intake
- intravenous steroid therapy once infective or ischaemic colitis ruled out
- consider subtotal or panproctocolectomy if no remission after 5 days of intensive medical therapy or if complications supervene.

Ulcerative colitis

This idiopathic condition is characterised by mucosal and submucosal inflammation. In contrast to Crohn's disease, the muscular and serosal layers are spared. During active phases of the disease, the mucosa is densely infiltrated with leucocytes and plasma cells, and crypt abscesses form at the base of the villae. Mucosal ulceration develops as the disease progresses. The disease only affects the colon and rectum.

Exacerbations and remissions of the disease, which causes diarrhoea and rectal bleeding, are typical. In addition there are a variety of extracolonic disorders that affect some but not all patients (Table 7).

Diagnosis

Diagnosis is by barium enema, where the classical features are a shortened colon (lead pipe appearance) in chronic ulcerative colitis with mucosal ulceration

Table 7 Extracolonic manifestations of ulcerative colitis

Eye disorders	Iritis
	Conjunctivitis
Joint disorders	Arthralgia
	Ankylosing spondylitis
	Sacroiliitis
Skin disorders	Erythema nodosum
	Pyoderma gangrenosum
Liver disorders	Sclerosing cholangitis

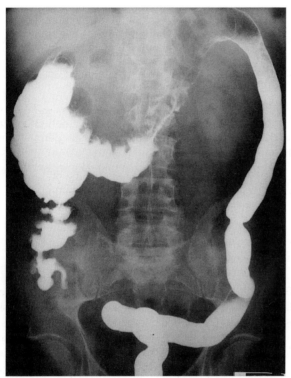

Fig. 27
Radiological appearance of ulcerative colitis.

(Fig. 27) and pseudopolyps in acute colitis and by sigmoidoscopy/colonoscopy and biopsy to provide a tissue diagnosis.

Medical treatment
Most mild attacks will respond to treatment with:

- oral or topical (enema or suppository) steroids
- oral or rectal administration of sulfasalazine compounds.

Low doses of these agents either alone or in combination are used to maintain disease remission.

Surgical treatment
There are four main indications for surgical intervention:

- failure of medical therapy
- acute, fulminant disease
- onset of complications
- malignant change.

Excision of the colon, rectum and anus (panproctocolectomy) will cure the disease (Fig. 26C). A panprocto-

colectomy will leave the patient with a permanent ileostomy. This operation is a major undertaking in an ill, toxic patient with complications of the disease. A subtotal colectomy (excision of the colon with preservation of the rectum and anus (Fig. 26B)) is less extensive and better tolerated by these patients.

Total colectomy with an ileo-anal anastomosis and an ileal pouch (Fig. 26D) is an alternative to these procedures. It is a technically complex operation which has the advantage of avoiding the need for an ileostomy.

Complications
There are four major complications of ulcerative colitis:

Toxic dilatation. Gross dilatation of the transverse colon in a severely ill patient. This is an indication for urgent colectomy before perforation occurs.

Massive haemorrhage.

Perforation. This may occur without dilatation in acute fulminant colitis.

Malignant change. Dysplasia and eventually malignancy will develop in 10–20% of patients who have poorly controlled total colitis of 10 or more years in duration.

Crohn's colitis

Unlike ulcerative colitis, acute colitis caused by Crohn's disease is a transmural inflammation with classic microscopic Crohn's features (see p. 37). Macroscopically, the inflammation may be patchy with areas of normal colon interspersed between areas of disease. Sometimes the rectum is spared. There is often severe perianal disease with multiple fistulae and abscesses.

Treatment
Medical treatment is with steroids (systemic or topical) and for rectal metronidazole.

When medical treatment fails colectomy is the only option, sometimes if only a seqment of colon is diseased a limitedf reseltion can be undertaken e.g. a right hemi colectomy. If the entire colon is involved the patient will require a panproctocolectomy or if the rectum is spared a subtotal colectomy with an ileorectal anastomosis. Ileal pouches are avoided because of the risk of developing crohn's disease in the pouch itself.

Infective colitis

Acute colitis may also be caused by various infections (Table 8). Usually these infections are self-limiting or respond to an appropriate course of antibiotics. Surgical intervention is rarely required.

Table 8 Infective causes of acute colitis

Shigella sonnei
Salmonella typhimurium
Escherichiae coli
Staphylococcus aureus
Clostridium welchii
Entamoeba histolytica (amoebic dysentery)
Schistosoma mansoni (schistosomiasis)

Antibiotic-associated colitis

Overgrowth of *Clostridium difficile*, a normal component of the intestinal flora, can follow ampicillin, clindamycin or cephalosporin therapy. Endoscopic examination of the colon will reveal a pseudomembrane made up of necrotic epithelium and leucocytes. The diagnosis is confirmed by stool culture. The causative antibiotic should be withdrawn and oral vancomycin therapy instituted occasionally colectomy is required.

Ischaemic colitis

This condition usually affects elderly arteriopaths. It is caused by acute or chronic occlusion of the inferior mesenteric artery. The left side of the colon is mainly affected. Clinically, the condition can be difficult to differentiate from other causes of colitis. The diagnosis is usually made on the barium enema appearances: either oedematous mucosa and 'thumb-printing' or a diseased strictured segment of colon in the region of the splenic flexure. Most patients settle on conservative management, otherwise resection is necessary.

Colonic angiodysplasia

This is the most common cause of an obscure gastro-intestinal haemorrhage (i.e. when routine investigation has failed to find an obvious cause). The caecum and ascending colon are the most frequent sites for these submucosal capillary blood lakes to develop. They can cause a chronic anaemia or a torrential haemorrhage.

Diagnosis

Diagnosis is by angiography during active haemorrhage or by colonoscopy, which allows direct visualisation of the angiomata.

Barium enema examination will not detect these vascular lesions.

Treatment

Frequently the bleeding will cease spontaneously and often the precise site of blood loss is never determined. A right hemicolectomy is the operation of choice for patients who continue to bleed.

2.7 Diseases of the rectum and anus

Anorectal problems are a frequent presenting complaint for patients with surgical diseases. The most important are:

- carcinoma of the rectum (see p. 42)
- anorectal sepsis
- haemorrhoids and anal fissures
- pilonidal sinus
- carcinoma of the anal canal

- rectal prolapse and faecal incontinence
- faecal impaction.

Anorectal sepsis

Most episodes of acute anorectal sepsis start with an infection in the intersphincteric space, usually in an anal gland. A primary infection of the anal gland will produce an intersphincteric abscess. Infection from here will spread in several directions (Fig. 28) and lead to:

- perianal abscess
- ischio-rectal abscess
- supralevator abscess or pelvic abscess.

Spontaneous or surgical external drainage will produce a fistula if the connection between the underlying anal gland and the anal canal remains patent. Occasionally, a deep abscess will rupture and drain into the rectum to produce a high fistula (Fig. 28).

Chronic anorectal sepsis results from:

- incomplete treatment of the acute infection
- a persisting anorectal fistula
- underlying chronic inflammation, e.g. Crohn's disease, tuberculosis
- carcinoma of the rectum or anus.

Clinical features

Perianal pain, swelling and erythema are the hallmarks of anorectal sepsis. Pain is maximal in those lesions nearest the anal verge. Swelling and tenderness may be less apparent in deep seated ischio-rectal or supralevator abscesses and may be only detected on rectal examination. These patients will show signs of systemic sepsis.

Treatment

An acute abscess needs prompt incision and drainage under general anaesthetic. A deep ischio-rectal abscess may contain multiple loculi and may extend behind the anal canal into the opposite ischio-rectal fossa (a horseshoe abscess). A careful sigmoidoscopic examination

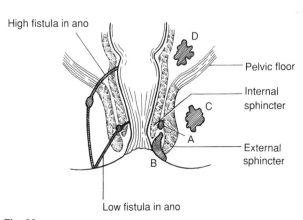

Fig. 28
Perianal sepsis and fistulae: **A.** intersphincteric abscess; **B.** perianal abscess; **C.** ischio-rectal abscess; **D.** pelvic abscess.

plus biopsy of the abscess wall is important to rule out any associated serious pathology.

An anorectal fistula (fistula in ano) may present as an abscess or as a spontaneously discharging opening on the perineum (Fig. 28). The principle of surgery is to lay open the fistula between its internal and external openings and to allow healing by secondary intention. A careful examination under anaesthetic is essential in order to assess the relationship of the fistula to the underlying sphincters. Most fistulae are 'low' and can be safely laid open without complete division of the sphincters, which would cause incontinence. A few fistulae will be found to be 'high', opening into the rectum above the anal sphincters and requiring complex surgical management.

Haemorrhoids and anal fissures

More than 50% of the population have symptoms caused by haemorrhoids at some stage of their lives. The condition should be considered a variant of normal.

Haemorrhoids develop when the normal prolapse of the anal mucosa and its underlying venous plexus becomes exaggerated and leads to symptoms.

Clinical features
Rectal bleeding with or without pain is the hallmark of haemorrhoids. Because these symptoms can also be caused by many other colorectal diseases, in particular *colorectal cancer*, all patients should be carefully evaluated to exclude other more serious causes for their rectal bleeding.

Haemorrhoids are classified according to their severity:

First degree: rectal bleeding
Second degree: prolapse with spontaneous reduction
Third degree: prolapse requiring manual reduction
Fourth degree: permanent prolapse with or without thrombosis.

Diagnosis
Diagnosis is by proctoscopy and sigmoidoscopy. Co-existing colorectal pathology should be excluded using a barium enema in all patients over 40 years of age.

Treatment
Dietary measures. Promoting increased stool softness and bulk by increasing intake of fibre will 'cure' most first- and second-degree haemorrhoids.

Band ligation or injection sclerotherapy. These simple measures are effective for persistent bleeding and mild prolapse.

Haemorrhoidectomy. This is reserved for major prolapse (third and fourth degree) or where other measures fail to control the symptoms.

Acutely prolapsed thrombosed piles
This painful condition should be treated by bed-rest and analgesia. An elective haemorrhoidectomy is carried out at a later date.

Anal fissure

An anal fissure is an ulcer at the mucocutaneous junction between the anal canal and the rectum. It usually lies in the posterior or anterior midline. Often, the underlying cause is unknown. Sometimes it is are associated with underlying inflammatory bowel disease.

Clinical features
Patients present with fissures that cause excruciating anal pain during defecation. The discomfort, which lasts for several hours after each bowel movement, is prolonged by a reflex spasm of the anal sphincters. Patients with fissures frequently defer defecation in order to avoid pain. The constipation that results aggravates the symptoms. Bleeding is usually slight but bright red in colour.

Inspection of the perineum sometimes reveals a sentinel pile at the site of the fissure caused by oedema and inflammation of the adjacent perianal skin. Rectal examination and proctoscopy is usually impossible because of pain and intense spasm of the anal sphincters.

Differential diagnosis.

- carcinoma of the anal canal
- perianal Crohn's disease.

Treatment
Healing of the fissure occurs rapidly once spasm of the anal sphincters is reduced. This is achieved in two ways:

Anal dilatation. A controlled forceful manual partial disruption of the anal sphincters under general anaesthetic.

Lateral sphincterotomy. Surgical division of the *internal* anal sphincter under general anaesthetic.

Prognosis
Most fissures rapidly resolve after surgery. Incontinence as a result of treatment is rare.

Pilonidal sinus

Aetiology
A pilonidal sinus is the result of an ingrowth of dead hairs through small pits usually in the midline of the natal cleft between the buttocks. It occurs in hirsute men and women and usually only presents when infection supervenes, often around puberty when hair growth and sebaceous gland activity peaks.

Clinical features
Most patients present with pain, swelling and discharge or with an acute abscess between the buttocks that sometimes ruptures spontaneously before treatment to produce a chronically discharging sinus. Inspection usually reveals the sinus opening, often stuffed with protruding hairs some distance from the abscess itself, although both are connected by a subcutaneous tunnel.

Treatment

As with any abscess, incision and drainage is the key treatment. All underlying granulation tissue and ingrown hairs should be removed and the underlying cavity deroofed. Postoperative care is particularly important if recurrence is to be avoided. The area must be kept clean and shaved and allowed to heal by *secondary intention*.

Prognosis

Despite meticulous attention, as many as one in 10 patients will develop a recurrence.

Carcinoma of the anal canal

This disease is rare in comparison with carcinoma of the rectum. In the early stages, it may present as a small nodule that eventually will ulcerate and become fixed to the underlying sphincters. As well as local invasion, the cancer will spread to the pelvic lymph glands and to the *inguinal* lymph glands. The disease is confirmed by proctoscopy and biopsy.

Treatment

Radiotherapy and chemotherapy are the first-line treatment. Surgical excision by abdomino-perineal resection (Fig. 25B) is reserved for patients who do not respond or have recurrent disease.

Rectal prolapse and faecal incontinence

Rectal prolapse

Rectal prolapse is most common at the extremes of life. In a complete rectal prolapse, the entire rectal wall including its coverings turns inside out and slides out of the anus. Thus it is anatomically different from a simple rectal mucosal prolapse, which is associated with haemorrhoids.

Adult rectal prolapse predominates in the elderly and is more common in women. The underlying problem does not appear to be muscular damage caused by previous childbirth but instead is a reduction in tone of the anal sphincters.

Clinical features

The rectum prolapses as a conical mass outside the anal canal. Initially this follows defecation and spontaneous reduction occurs. Eventually with progressive muscular laxity, a permanent prolapse develops which causes soiling and excoriation and may eventually ulcerate.

Treatment

Most prolapses can be easily reduced manually only to recur as soon as the patient strains or becomes ambulant. The most effective surgical procedure is a transabdominal rectopexy, hitching the rectum to the sacrum either with sutures or with a non-absorbable mesh.

An alternative procedure in a frail patient unfit to withstand an abdominal operation is to encircle the anal canal with a non-absorbable submucosal suture (Thiersch wire technique) which constricts the anus and prevents prolapse.

Faecal incontinence

This implies the loss of voluntary control of defecation. It often accompanies rectal prolapse but may occur independently. Incontinence may be secondary to birth trauma or surgical injury or organic disease of the ano rectum, such as Crohn's disease or cancer. Many cases are idiopathic and these patients have a combination of defects of the anal sphincters, pelvic floor and their innervation.

Treatment

Some mild cases respond to pelvic floor exercises. Iatrogenic sphincter damage (e.g. during haemorrhoidectomy) is amenable to surgical repair or sphincteroplasty. A general tightening of the pelvic floor muscles and anal sphincters *behind* the anal canal (postanal repair, Fig. 29) is the most frequently used operation for idiopathic faecal incontinence.

Faecal impaction

Faecal impaction can occur at any age. It is especially frequent in the elderly bed-ridden patient who may be recovering from an operation. Constipation-inducing analgesic agents, which contain codeine, may cause constipation that progresses to faecal impaction. Paradoxically, the initial presentation may be a spurious diarrhoea caused by overflow of liquid faeces and mucus from the proximal colon around the impacted faecal bolus. The diagnosis is confirmed by rectal examination.

Treatment

Sometimes the faecal bolus can be broken up by enemas and stool softeners. More often, digital breakdown followed by a manual evacuation is required. Oral laxatives are important to prevent recurrence, and a sigmoidoscopy should be undertaken to make sure an underlying carcinoma has not precipitated the impaction.

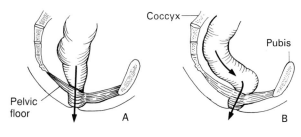

Fig. 29
Postanal repair for faecal incontinence.

Self-assessment: questions

Multiple choice questions

1. Barrett's oesophagus is:
   a. Unrelated to gastro-oesophageal reflux
   b. Best diagnosed using contrast radiology
   c. Best treated by surgical resection
   d. A premalignant condition
   e. Associated with stricture formation

2. A paraoesophageal hiatus hernia:
   a. Is a common cause of gastro-oesophageal reflux
   b. Is less common than a sliding hiatus hernia
   c. Is usually repaired through the chest
   d. Is lined by Barrett's epithelium
   e. Can cause gastric outlet obstruction

3. The following statements are true regarding instrumental oesophageal perforation:
   a. It may cause a pneumothorax
   b. A mediastinal crunch can be detected on auscultation
   c. It always requires operative intervention
   d. It follows a prolonged bout of vomiting
   e. It is infrequently detected using contrast radiology

4. The following statements relate to peptic ulcer disease:
   a. Ulcers are most reliably detected by a barium meal
   b. Pyloric stenosis is the least frequent complication
   c. Elective surgery is rarely required
   d. A drainage procedure is always required after truncal vagotomy
   e. Radiological evidence of subdiaphragmatic gas is always present after peptic ulcer perforation

5. Malignant gastric ulcers:
   a. Can be reliably diagnosed on barium meal examination
   b. Can be differentiated from benign peptic ulcers on history alone
   c. Respond to histamine H_2 receptor antagonists
   d. Can cause pyloric stenosis
   e. Are usually cured by partial gastrectomy

6. The following are classical features of a perforated peptic ulcer:
   a. Succussion splash on examination
   b. A long antecedent history
   c. Shoulder tip pain
   d. Rebound tenderness
   e. Absent bowel sounds

7. The following statements are true concerning gastric carcinoma:
   a. It is twice as common in females as in males
   b. It is linked to patients with type O blood group
   c. It often presents with a major gastrointestinal haemorrhage
   d. It is sited mainly on the lesser curvature of the stomach
   e. It can metastasise to the ovaries

8. Ascending cholangitis:
   a. Can cause collapse in the elderly
   b. Is caused by stone impaction in Hartmann's pouch
   c. Can be treated endoscopically
   d. Is cured by cholecystectomy
   e. Is usually caused by Gram-positive organisms

9. In patients with acute cholecystitis:
   a. Gallstones are always present
   b. Diagnosis is usually confirmed by an oral cholecystogram
   c. A pericholecystic abscess is the most common complication
   d. The presence of icterus invariably implies a coexisting common bile duct stone
   e. Complications are more likely if the patient is a diabetic

10. The following statements relate to common bile duct stones:
    a. Most are formed primarily in the common bile duct
    b. Most are associated with an elevated serum alkaline phosphatase
    c. About 50% are asymptomatic
    d. They are often associated with a palpable gallbladder
    e. They cause at least one third of all episodes of pancreatitis

11. An elevated serum amylase is seen in:
    a. Mesenteric ischaemia
    b. Acute cholecystitis
    c. Idiopathic pancreatitis
    d. Perforated peptic ulcer
    e. Acute hepatitis

12. Necrotising pancreatitis:
    a. Complicates one half of all episodes of acute pancreatitis
    b. Is associated with a poor outcome
    c. Can be diagnosed on ultrasound scanning
    d. Responds to radical surgical debridement
    e. Is usually sterile

13. In patients with pancreatic cancer:
    a. Cancer of the tail of the gland can often be treated by distal pancreatectomy

b. Maturity onset diabetes is not uncommon
c. Obstructive jaundice is infrequent
d. Periampullary cancers have a better prognosis
e. They can present with a deep vein thrombosis

14. Injection sclerotherapy:
   a. Is particularly useful in controlling gastric fundal varices
   b. Can cause an oesophageal stricture
   c. Reduces blood flow through the varices through vasopressin release
   d. Can be used in conjunction with balloon tamponade
   e. Causes variceal thrombosis

15. The following statements relate to surgery and the spleen:
   a. After splenectomy the circulating platelet count falls
   b. It is the first-line management for patients with idiopathic thrombocytopenic purpura
   c. Isolated tears in the spleen can be repaired
   d. A delayed splenic rupture usually occurs within 48 hours
   e. Postsplenectomy pneumococcal infection is more common in young patients

16. Strangulating small bowel obstruction is more common in:
   a. Small bowel volvulus
   b. High small bowel obstruction
   c. An incarcerated external hernia
   d. Obstructed patients with constant not colicky abdominal pain
   e. A closed-loop obstruction

17. Crohn's disease:
   a. Rarely fistulates
   b. May present as a recurrent perianal abscess
   c. Can involve the mouth
   d. Is characterised by caseating epithelioid granulomas
   e. Occasionally causes a fulminant colitis

18. In small bowel mesenteric ischaemia:
   a. An absence of intestinal gas is a common finding
   b. A history of atrial fibrillation is common
   c. The coeliac axis is usually occluded
   d. Venous infarction is more common than arterial occlusion
   e. About 50% of patients die of the acute event

19. The following statements relate to large bowel obstruction:
   a. Caecal perforation is more likely if the ileocaecal valve is incompetent
   b. It is usually caused by carcinoma of the colon
   c. Vomiting is an early feature

d. Distension is usually marked
e. The rectum is usually dilated and empty

20. In colorectal cancer:
   a. At least 50% of all cancers are in the rectum and sigmoid colon
   b. Low anterior resection is easier in males than in females
   c. 60% of patients with lymph gland involvement will survive 5 years
   d. Most 1 cm polyps contain a focus of cancer
   e. Alteration in bowel habit is uncommon in right-sided cancers

21. With regard to diverticular disease:
   a. This is the most common cause of a colovesical fistula
   b. It can present with massive rectal haemorrhage
   c. Colonic resection and primary reanastomosis is the treatment of choice for severe acute diverticulitis
   d. Diverticulae are a common incidental finding on a barium enema examination
   e. Colorectal cancer is rare in patients with diverticular disease

22. Ulcerative colitis is characterised by:
   a. Mucosal skip lesions
   b. Rectal sparing
   c. Crypt abscesses
   d. Transmural inflammation
   e. A lead pipe appearance on barium enema examination

23. Carcinoma of the anal canal:
   a. Is usually treated by abdomino-perineal resection
   b. Can present with an inguinal lymphadenopathy
   c. Is less common than rectal cancer
   d. Is usually painless
   e. Is radiosensitive

24. The following are characteristic of ischio-rectal abscesses:
   a. They are usually situated above levator ani
   b. They can be multilocular
   c. They cause severe perianal tenderness
   d. They are common in patients with ulcerative colitis
   e. Recurrence is often related to an underlying fistula

25. A pilonidal sinus:
   a. Is usually congenital
   b. Is best treated by primary excision and closure
   c. Affects men more than women
   d. Often presents as an acute abscess
   e. Frequently presents at puberty

Case histories

Case history 1

A 47-year-old previously healthy man presents with an eighteen month history of dysphagia for solids. Recently he has had several prolonged chest infections. A barium swallow has been arranged by his general practitioner (Fig. 30).

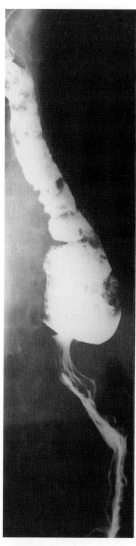

Fig. 30
Barium swallow.

1. What is the most likely diagnosis?
2. How would you confirm the diagnosis?
3. What is the cause of the recurrent chest infections?
4. What treatment would you advise?

Case history 2

A 59-year-old man presents with a 6-week history of jaundice and pruritus. He had a cholecystectomy for acute cholecystitis 12 years ago.

1. What is the most likely differential diagnosis?
2. How would you investigate this patient?
3. If this patient required surgery, what points would be important in his pre- and perioperative management?

Case history 3

A 70-year-old woman presents with a 2-week history of cystitis and pneumaturia. On examination, she has a mass in the left iliac fossa.

1. What is the most likely diagnosis?
2. What is the differential diagnosis?
3. How would you confirm the diagnosis?
4. How should this patient be treated?

Case history 4

A 40-year-old alcoholic man who has been on a drinking binge is admitted collapsed after a haematemesis. He has a pulse rate of 120 and a systolic blood pressure of 80 mmHg.

1. What are the key steps in his resuscitation?
2. What are the possible causes of his haematemesis?
3. How would you establish the diagnosis?

Case history 5

A 70-year-old woman who some years ago had a laparotomy for perforated appendicitis was admitted with a 3-day history of colicky abdominal pains and vomiting. On examination, the patient was dehydrated with a soft, slightly distended abdomen.

1. What is the most likely diagnosis?
2. How would you confirm the diagnosis?
3. How would you manage this patient?
4. When would you operate on this patient?

Essays

1. Discuss the steps you would take to reach a diagnosis in a 45-year-old woman who presents with a 2-week history of right iliac fossa pain. On examination she is afebrile and has a slightly tender mass in the right iliac fossa.
2. During an open cholecystectomy, routine cholangiography is carried out. This demonstrates a stone at the lower end of the common bile duct. Discuss the management from this point.
3. Write short notes on Boerhaave's syndrome.

Photograph questions

Photograph 1

1. What is this X-ray examination (Photograph 1A)?
2. What abnormality can you see?
3. What are the treatment options?

A

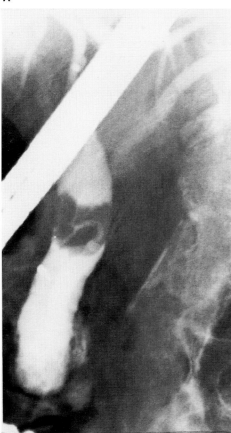

B 'Normal' x-ray for comparison

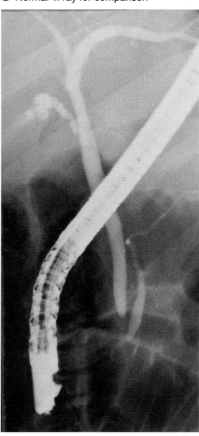

Photograph 1

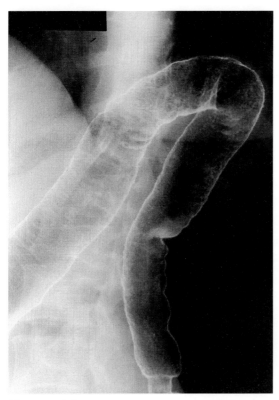

Photograph 2

Photograph 2

1. What abnormal features are shown on this X-ray?
2. What is the diagnosis?
3. What complications can develop?

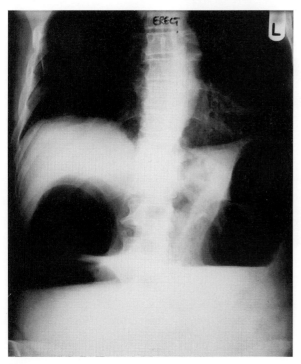

Photograph 3

Photograph 3

1. What is the diagnosis?
2. How would you confirm the cause?
3. What is the risk if treatment is delayed?

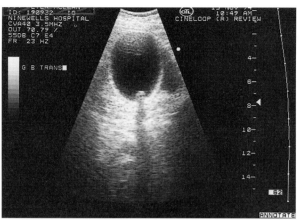

Photograph 4

Photograph 4

1. What examination is this an example of?
2. What abnormality is shown?
3. How else can this diagnosis be confirmed?

Self-assessment: answers

Multiple choice answers

1. a. **False.** Barrett's oesophagus is caused by gastro-oesophageal reflux.
    b. **False.** It is a tissue diagnosis usually confirmed by endoscopic biopsy — there may be no evidence on a barium swallow.
    c. **False.** Barrett's oesophagus usually responds to standard antireflux treatment. Surgery is restricted to patients with the complications of Barrett's oesophagus such as a stricture or malignant change.
    d. **True.** Severe dysplasia or in situ carcinoma may develop in an area of Barrett's oesophagitis that does not respond to medical therapy.
    e. **True.** Stricture formation is a complication of long-standing Barrett's oesophagitis.

2. a. **False.** The gastro-oesophageal junction lies in its anatomically correct position; the lower oesophageal sphincter continues to function normally; reflux does not occur.
    b. **True.** This type of hiatus hernia is relatively uncommon.
    c. **False.** This type of hiatus hernia is most easily repaired through the abdomen. The hernia usually contains stomach lined by normal gastric mucosa.
    d. **False.** Barrett's epithelium is an abnormal columnar epithelium lining the lower oesophagus in association with a sliding hiatus hernia.
    e. **True.** Large portions of the stomach can slip into the chest causing acute angulation of the gastric outlet and obstruction.

3. a. **True.** Rupture of the intrathoracic part of the oesophagus may cause a pneumothorax; air enters the pleural space through the oesophageal perforation.
    b. **True.** A mediastinal crunch is caused by the heart beating against air-filled tissues.
    c. **False.** Cervical perforations are usually treated conservatively with antibiotics and fluid restriction as are many minor perforations of the thoracic oesophagus.
    d. **False.** Perforation following instrumentation is usually a direct result of damage during diagnostic endoscopy or forceful dilatation of an oesophageal stricture.
    e. **False.** Water-soluble contrast studies are the best way of identifying the site of perforation.

4. a. **False.** Ulcers are best detected by gastroscopy. Small ulcers and erosions can be missed by barium studies.

    b. **True.** The complications of peptic ulcer disease in order of decreasing frequency are: haemorrhage, perforation and pyloric stenosis.
    c. **True.** Most ulcers will heal by medical means using histamine H_2 receptor blocking drugs or proton pump inhibitors.
    d. **True.** Truncal vagotomy denervates the pylorus and the antral mill. Either a pyloroplasty or gastroenterostomy is needed to prevent gastric stasis.
    e. **False.** Subdiaphragmatic gas will be absent in at least 10% of patients; if the rest of the history and examination fits, the diagnosis must still be considered.

5. a. **False.** Gastroscopy is the key investigation as it allows direct visualisation of the ulcer plus a biopsy for tissue diagnosis.
    b. **False.** Peptic ulcer and gastric cancer symptoms have a considerable overlap. The diagnosis must be confirmed by gastroscopy and biopsy.
    c. **True.** Histamine H_2-blocking drugs can partly heal malignant ulcers and provide symptomatic relief. This underlines the importance of establishing a firm diagnosis in gastric ulceration before starting treatment.
    d. **True.** A malignant ulcer in the gastric antrum or pyloric ring can cause gastric outlet obstruction.
    e. **False.** Most gastrectomies for gastric cancer are palliative. Overall 5-year survival is around 20%.

6. a. **False.** A succussion splash is pathognomonic of gastric outlet obstruction usually caused by pyloric stenosis.
    b. **False.** Perforation is usually unexpected, with no antecedent history.
    c. **True.** Shoulder tip pain is caused by diaphragmatic irritation from gastric contents released into the peritoneal cavity, which track upwards between the liver and diaphragm.
    d. **False.** Rebound tenderness is unusual. Most patients exhibit a board-like abdominal rigidity caused by spasm of the rectii muscles.
    e. **True.** The severe peritonitis after perforation induces a generalised ileus.

7. a. **False.** Gastric cancer is twice as likely in males as in females.
    b. **False.** Gastric cancer is more common in patients with blood group A. Peptic ulceration has been linked to blood group O patients.
    c. **False.** Blood loss from a gastric ulcer is usually occult. Patients may present with an undiagnosed anaemia.
    d. **True.** Approximately one half are found in this location.
    e. **True.** These are known as Krukenberg deposits.

8. a. **True.** Although rigors, jaundice and fever are the classical triad of symptoms, septicaemia caused by cholangitis can cause collapse in the elderly and must be considered in the differential diagnosis.
   b. **False.** This is more likely to cause empyema or acute cholecystitis. Cholangitis is caused by a combination of infection and obstruction in the common bile duct.
   c. **True.** Cholangitis caused by common bile duct stones or a stricture can be relieved by ERCP coupled with sphincterotomy and stone extraction or endoscopic stenting techniques.
   d. **False.** The bile duct obstruction must be relieved. Cholecystectomy will cure cholecystitis or other gallbladder-related complications of gallstones.
   e. **False.** Most cases of cholangitis are caused by Gram-negative organisms such as *Escherichia coli* or *Klebsiella* spp.

9. a. **False.** Acalculous cholecystitis can occur in immunocompromised patients or critically ill patients in an intensive care setting. It can also affect patients who have been on prolonged parenteral nutrition.
   b. **False.** Oral cholecystography is completely unreliable in acute cholecystitis as it requires a functioning gallbladder to concentrate and reveal the contrast medium. The diagnosis is confirmed by ultrasound or biliary scintiscanning.
   c. **True.** A pericholecystic abscess is the most common cause of a palpable gallbladder mass.
   d. **False.** The presence of an acutely inflamed gallbladder lying adjacent to the common bile duct is enough to cause cholestasis and jaundice in some patients.
   e. **True.** Diabetic patients are at special risk. They are more likely to develop the complications of acute cholecystitis.

10. a. **False.** Most common duct stones are formed in the gallbladder and migrate to the common bile duct.
    b. **True.** Major elevations in the serum alkaline phosphatase with lesser elevations in the liver transaminases are the hallmark of obstructive jaundice.
    c. **True.** At least 50% of common duct stones are silent.
    d. **False.** A palpable gallbladder is associated with malignant biliary obstruction caused by pancreatic cancer or a primary cholangiocarcinoma. In patients with gallstone disease, the gallbladder is usually shrunken from chronic inflammation.
    e. **True.** 'Gallstone' pancreatitis is one of the most common causes of acute pancreatitis. The other is alcohol abuse.

11. a. **True.** Mesenteric ischaemia causes severe abdominal pain. It can often only be differentiated from acute pancreatitis by laparotomy.
    b. **False.** Acute cholecystitis alone rarely elevates the serum amylase. Gallstone pancreatitis is associated with the passage of a gallstone through the ampulla of Vater.
    c. **True.** Idiopathic pancreatitis accounting for 10% of all episodes is associated with hyperamylasaemia.
    d. **True.** The elevation in amylase is usually small.
    e. **False.** The amylase level is normal. Liver transaminases are massively raised.

12. a. **False.** Necrotising pancreatitis complicates less than 10% of all episodes of pancreatitis.
    b. **True.** Mortality rates exceed 30%.
    c. **False.** CT scanning with intravenous contrast enhancement will delineate the necrotic (non-enhancing) from the viable (enhancing) pancreatic tissue.
    d. **True.** Pancreatic debridement (necrosectomy) is sometimes the only treatment option for pancreatic necrosis that becomes secondarily infected.
    e. **False.** Secondary bacterial infection with a mixture of aerobic and anaerobic organisms is common.

13. a. **False.** Cancer of the pancreatic tail is inevitably inoperable by the time it presents.
    b. **True.** Diabetes often predates pancreatic cancer by several months or years.
    c. **False.** Obstructive jaundice is the most common presenting symptom in pancreatic cancer.
    d. **True.** They present early with jaundice and biologically are less aggressive.
    e. **True.** Pancreatic and gastric cancer can present with a DVT. The reason is unknown.

14. a. **False.** Gastric fundal varices are difficult to treat endoscopically. Often they can only be controlled by tamponade (using a Sengestaken–Blakemore balloon) or by surgery.
    b. **True.** Repeated sclerotherapy induces fibrosis, which can cause an oesophageal stricture.
    c. **False.** Vasopressin has to be exogenously infused. It reduces variceal blood flow by decreasing the splanchnic blood flow.
    d. **True.** A combination of sclerotherapy followed by tamponade is often effective in stopping variceal bleeding.
    e. **True.** Sclerotherapy obliterates varices by thrombosis and fibrosis.

15. a. **False.** The platelet count rises following splenectomy.
    b. **False.** Splenectomy is reserved for patients who do not respond to steroid therapy.

c. **True.** The spleen can be conserved following minor injuries.

d. **False.** Delayed rupture of a subcapsular haematoma usually follows 1–2 weeks after the initial injury.

e. **True.** Children and young adults are especially at risk. Pneumococcal vaccine should be given prior to splenectomy followed by at least a 2-year course of low-dose penicillin V.

16. a. **True.** A small bowel volvulus rotates around the axis of its mesentery rapidly occluding the mesenteric blood supply and causing strangulation.

b. **False.** Strangulating obstruction can occur at any level of small bowel obstruction. It is perhaps less common in high obstruction.

c. **True.** An incarcerated hernia often has a tight neck that interferes with the blood supply to the trapped small bowel loops.

d. **True.** Constant severe pain is one of the hallmarks of strangulation.

e. **True.** A closed-loop small bowel obstruction rapidly distends. This increase in internal pressure within the loop compromises the blood supply and predisposes to strangulation.

17. a. **False.** Fistulae are common in Crohn's disease and reflect the transmural inflammatory process.

b. **True.** Recurrent perianal sepsis is one of the commonest presentations of Crohn's disease.

c. **True.** Crohn's disease can affect the entire gastrointestinal tract from the mouth to the anus.

d. **False.** Crohn's granulomas are non-caseating. Caseating granulomas are usually tuberculous.

e. **True.** Fulminant Crohn's colitis is less common than fulminant ulcerative colitis.

18. a. **True.** The radiological features are often non-specific: absent gas shadows or, alternatively, gaseous small bowel distension.

b. **True.** Most patients are arteriopaths. A recent myocardial infarction or a history of atrial fibrillation is common.

c. **False.** The superior mesenteric artery is occluded.

d. **False.** Arterial occlusion is more common than venous infarction.

e. **True.** Many patients are elderly with extensive or total small bowel infarction.

19. a. **False.** An incompetent ileocaecal valve will allow reflux of colonic contents back into the small bowel preventing overdistension of the colon and reducing the risk of perforation.

b. **True.** Pseudo-obstruction, volvulus and constipation are infrequent causes.

c. **False.** Vomiting occurs late, once small bowel obstruction develops secondary to the large bowel obstruction.

d. **True.** The abdomen is usually massively distended and tympanitic with tinkling bowel sounds.

e. **True.** Unless the obstruction is caused by constipation, the rectum is often dilated and empty.

20. a. **True.** The caecum is the second most common site for a colorectal cancer.

b. **False.** The wide female pelvis often facilitates this operation.

c. **False.** Patients with a Duke's grade C tumour have a 30% 5-year survival rate.

d. **False.** Polyps of 1 cm are rarely malignant. Cancer is associated with polyps greater than 2 cm in size.

e. **False.** Right-sided cancers present with anaemia, malaise or a right iliac fossa mass.

21. a. **True.** Crohn's disease and colorectal cancer are less frequent causes of a colovesical fistula.

b. **True.** Haemorrhage can be life-threatening and an indication for urgent colectomy.

c. **False.** This operation carries a high risk of anastomotic dehiscence. A Hartmann's resection is the procedure of choice.

d. **True.** However, they should not be assumed to be the source of a patient's symptoms.

e. **False.** Patients with diverticular disease are as likely as any to have a bowel cancer. The two conditions frequently coexist.

22. a. **False.** Skip lesions are a characteristic of Crohn's disease.

b. **False.** Rectal sparing is a feature of Crohn's disease. In ulcerative colitis the rectum is frequently the most diseased segment of the colon.

c. **True.** Crypt abscesses on biopsy are a hallmark of ulcerative colitis.

d. **False.** Inflammatory changes in ulcerative colitis are confined to the mucosa and submucosa. Transmural inflammation typifies Crohn's disease.

e. **True.** This is caused by chronic inflammation and a generalised shortening of the bowel.

23. a. **False.** Radiotherapy is the first-line treatment for anal cancer.

b. **True.** Anal cancers drain to the inguinal lymph glands.

c. **True.** Anal cancer is comparatively rare.

d. **False.** A painful ulcer is a common presentation.

e. **True.** Anal cancers are highly sensitive to irradiation.

24.
a. **False.** They are centred in the ischio-rectal fossae below levator ani.
b. **True.** An ischio-rectal abscess is usually multilocular. All loculi must be broken down to provide satisfactory surgical drainage.
c. **False.** Severe perianal tenderness is characteristic of a perianal abscess. An ischio-rectal abscess is deep seated and may only be detected on rectal examination.
d. **False.** Underlying Crohn's disease is more likely.
e. **True.** An undetected fistula at the primary operation is the most common cause of recurrence.

25.
a. **False.** Most are acquired by the ingress of hair and faecal matter into the natal cleft caused by movement and friction.
b. **False.** Most pilonidal sinuses are infected. After excision the wounds are best left open to heal by secondary intention.
c. **False.** Recurrence is not uncommon.
d. **True.** The condition is particularly common in hirsute males.
e. **True.** During this period hair growth and sebaceous gland activity increases.

Case history answers

Case history 1

1. Achalasia. The proximal oesophagus is dilated and contains food debris. There is a smooth cone-shaped area of narrowing in the distal oesophagus.
2. A gastroscopy would help rule out other causes of dysphagia such as carcinoma or a peptic stricture. The diagnosis could be confirmed using oesophageal manometry to demonstrate absent primary peristalsis and a failure of the lower oesophageal sphincter to relax on swallowing.
3. Aspiration pneumonia caused by night-time regurgitation of food debris retained in the oesophagus.
4. In a young fit patient, a Heller's cardiomyotomy would be the procedure of choice rather than balloon dilatation.

Case history 2

1. The most likely causes of jaundice in this patient are:
   a. a common bile duct stone
   b. carcinoma of the pancreas
   c. cholangiocarcinoma
   d. acute hepatitis
   e. hepatic metastases.

2. Liver function tests would be important. The pattern of these would suggest whether the jaundice was hepatocellular (elevated transaminases) or obstructive (elevated alkaline phosphatase) in origin. A specimen for serology to exclude hepatitis A, B and C should also be obtained. An ultrasound scan would be the most important non-invasive test. This might show:
   - biliary tree dilatation
   - evidence of a pancreatic mass
   - evidence of liver metastases.

ERCP or CT scanning would be the next step. An ERCP would be most useful if there was ultrasound evidence of biliary tree obstruction. Common bile duct stones could be treated definitively by endoscopic sphincterotomy or a stent could be passed through a malignant stricture caused by a cholangiocarcinoma or pancreatic cancer.

If a pancreatic cancer is suspected, a CT scan would be useful in determining the extent of the disease if surgical resection is to be considered.

3. Jaundiced patients undergoing surgery are prone to the following problems:
   - coagulopathy
   - hepatorenal failure
   - infection.

The patient's coagulation profile should be checked preoperatively and prophylactic vitamin K administered. Fresh frozen plasma might be necessary in the immediate perioperative period.

Postoperative renal failure is a major problem in patients with jaundice. It can be prevented by ensuring the patient is well hydrated before surgery, using intravenous fluids. Mannitol or dopamine can be used to maintain the diuresis perioperatively.

Jaundiced patients are at special risk of infection.

Appropriate broad-spectrum antibiotic prophylaxis should be used.

Case history 3

1. The presence of pneumaturia indicates that this patient has an enterovesical fistula. The cystitic symptoms are secondary to the resultant infection. Most vesical fistulae are colonic in origin (vesicocolic) and this would be in keeping with the patient's left iliac fossa mass.
2. The most likely causes of a colovesical fistula are:
   - diverticular disease
   - Crohn's disease
   - carcinoma of the sigmoid colon.

3. A barium enema and a cystoscopy would be the most useful diagnostic tests.
4. A vesicocolic fistula is unlikely to heal spontaneously. The patient will require a laparotomy and resection of the affected segment of bowel together with an oversew of the bladder fistula. Preoperative bowel preparation would be important. There are two main surgical options:
   - primary reanastomosis

- resection and exteriorisation (Hartmann's procedure).

  The choice will depend on the degree of inflammation and infection present at operation. A primary anastomosis is unsafe in the presence of severe infection and localised peritonitis.

Case history 4

1. The patient's vital signs indicate that he has had a major gastrointestinal bleed. The key steps to his resuscitation are:
   a. establish intravenous access; use multiple sites if necessary
   b. draw blood for urgent cross-match, baseline haematology, biochemistry and coagulation screen
   c. give supplemental oxygen
   d. restore the circulating volume by infusion of colloid (plasma protein substitute) or a plasma expander (such as Haemacel) together with normal saline while waiting for cross-matched blood to arrive
   e. catheterise the patient
   f. monitor the response to treatment in terms of pulse rate, blood pressure and urine output.

   Most patients will respond to this initial regimen once 1–2 litres of crystalloid/colloid have been infused. A failure to respond suggests ongoing haemorrhage. These patients may require:
   - urgent transfusion of uncross-matched blood (O negative)
   - central venous pressure monitoring
   - consideration for urgent diagnostic investigation and possibly surgical treatment.

2. The possible causes of his haematemesis are:
   - oesophageal varices
   - peptic ulcer
   - acute gastritis
   - Mallory–Weiss tear.

3. An urgent gastroscopy would be the key investigation. The examination would also provide a therapeutic option for injection sclerotherapy for varices or a bleeding ulcer.

Case history 5

1. With the history of a previous laparotomy for a septic intra-abdominal condition plus colicky pains and distension, a bowel obstruction secondary to adhesions would be the most likely diagnosis.

2. The presence of tinkling bowel sounds on auscultation would support this diagnosis. It would also be important to rule out any other causes of obstruction, e.g. an irreducible inguinal hernia during the physical examination. The diagnosis would be confirmed by a plain abdominal X-ray. In a small bowel obstruction (the most usual finding in

adhesive obstruction), It is usual to find a ladder pattern of distended small bowel loops. In this patient where the distension is not marked, only a few loops may be present, in keeping with a more proximal obstruction.

3. The initial treatment would be conservative. The key steps are:
   a. establish i.v. access for fluid resuscitation and maintenance
   b. obtain baseline blood for biochemical and haematological indices
   c. restrict oral intake
   d. pass a nasogastric tube, keep the stomach empty
   e. catheterise the patient
   f. correct any dehydration with normal (N) saline or a balanced salt solution
   g. maintain a careful fluid balance.

4. Non-response to 24–48 hours' conservative management would be an indication for surgical intervention. This could be assessed on clinical grounds (decreasing distension; passage of flatus, etc. indicates improvement) and by repeated radiology looking for resolution of the small bowel distension. Earlier surgery would be indicated if the patient developed signs of strangulation, such as:
   - abdominal tenderness
   - continuous not colicky pain
   - fever.

Essay answers

1. The differential diagnosis here is wide. The possibilities are:
   - Crohn's disease
   - an appendix mass
   - an ovarian cyst
   - caecal carcinoma
   - small bowel lymphoma.

   Evaluation would begin with a full history and physical examination. Key points would be:
   - a history in keeping with acute appendicitis several weeks ago
   - small bowel colic suggesting a subacute obstruction in Crohn's disease; a previous or family history of inflammatory bowel disease
   - weight loss or general malaise, non-specific symptoms suggesting a serious pathology such as caecal cancer, Crohn's disease or a lymphoma.

   Important points on physical examination would be fixity, degree of tenderness or whether or not the mass appeared to arise from the pelvis. A rectal and vaginal examination would be important as would signs of anaemia and weight loss.

   An ultrasound scan would be a key investigation. This would confirm or refute the diagnosis of an ovarian cyst or may show features in keeping with an appendix mass or abscess. Contrast barium studies would be the next step using a barium enema to look for caecal cancer and a barium follow-through to evaluate the terminal ileum for Crohn's disease or a lymphoma. Occasionally, a laparotomy may be needed to differentiate these two conditions.

2. The next step would be to explore the common bile duct using a balloon or stone forceps to remove the stone. Once cleared, the common bile duct should be closed over a T-tube. This tube should be left in place for 10–14 days to allow the postoperative swelling to settle and to decompress the biliary tree. After 10–14 days, a T-tube cholangiogram can be performed through the tube to check for any residual stones. If the duct is clear, the tube can be removed. If a stone has been left behind, it can be removed either by ERCP and sphincterotomy or by using a controllable basket introduced into the bile duct along the track of the T-tube.

3. Boerhaave's syndrome is a spontaneous perforation of the oesophagus seen usually in males after a heavy bout of drinking or eating. It follows a period of violent vomiting or wretching and is typified by severe pain in the lower chest, an epigastrium and circulatory collapse. The acute severe presentation may mimic a perforated peptic ulcer or a myocardial infarction. The diagnosis is confirmed by a water-soluble contrast swallow. Once confirmed, urgent surgical repair of the defect is performed through a thoracotomy under antibiotic cover.

Photograph answers

Photograph 1

1. An endoscopic retrograde cholangiopancreatogram.
2. A stone in the common bile duct.
3. Endoscopic sphincterotomy and balloon or basket extraction of the stone.

Photograph 2

1. This is a featureless 'lead pipe colon'.
2. Ulcerative colitis.
3. Complications:
   • toxic dilatation
   • perforation
   • haemorrhage
   • malignant change.

Photograph 3

1. Large bowel obstruction.
2. Sigmoidoscopy (rigid or flexible) plus a barium enema.
3. Perforation leading to faecal peritonitis.

Photograph 4

1. An ultrasound scan of the gallbladder.
2. A gallstone in the gallbladder.
3. Biliary scintiscanning.

Hernias

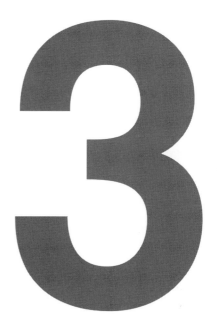

3.1 Hernia formation

An abdominal wall hernia is a protrusion, usually of normal intra-abdominal contents, through its investing fascial and muscular layers. Most present externally as a lump and can contain omentum, small bowel or large bowel.

The four commonest types of hernia are:

- inguinal or femoral (groin hernias)
- incisional hernia
- umbilical hernia
- epigastric hernia.

Most hernias are reducible, i.e. the contents can be returned to the abdominal cavity and the hernial sac emptied by either posture or pressure.

Many hernias are painless and patients will present primarily because they have discovered a lump. Others will complain of a dragging pain associated with the hernia. Surgical repair is indicated in both groups to relieve symptoms and to prevent or treat the development of the following complications:

- irreducibility
- obstruction
- strangulation.

As the hernia develops, it takes with it a protrusion of peritoneum, which forms a sac that invests the hernia contents. The neck of the sac as it passes through the abdominal wall is a narrow point, which will constrict the hernia contents and cause complications. A hernia becomes irreducible when the contents swell secondary to the constriction at the neck of the sac or if they adhere to the sac itself. If the hernia contains a loop of bowel that is irreducible, obstruction can develop (Fig. 31) and strangulation will supervene if the blood supply to the bowel becomes compromised.

3.2 Types of hernia

Groin hernias

Inguinal and femoral hernias are considered together as both present as a lump in the groin. Inguinal hernias are 10 times more common than femoral hernias, and together both account for 80% of all hernias.

A simplified view of the anatomy of the inguinal canal is shown in Figure 32.

Inguinal hernias

There are two types of inguinal hernia:

- indirect
- direct.

Indirect inguinal hernia. These hernias are congenital and develop when the processus vaginalis (the peri-

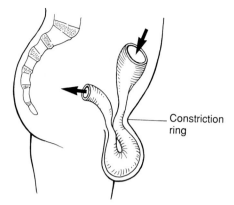

Fig. 31
An obstructed inguinal hernia.

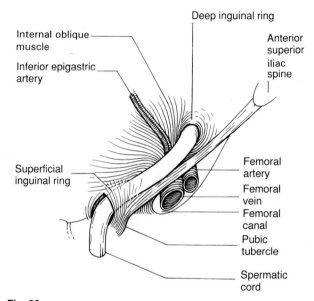

Fig. 32
Anatomy of the inguinal canal (left side) deep to external oblique muscle.

toneal sac through which the testicle descends into the scrotum) remains patent. Although they can occur at any age, they are the most frequent form of hernia found in children and young adults. The processus vaginalis develops into the hernial sac when an increase in intra-abdominal pressure and/or a weakening in the abdominal wall musculature allows abdominal contents through the deep inguinal ring into the inguinal canal and sometimes into the scrotum (inguoscrotal hernia).

Direct inguinal hernia. These are usually smaller than indirect hernias and are less prone to complications. They are formed from a protrusion through the posterior wall of the inguinal canal medial to the inferior epigastric artery (Fig. 32). Occasionally, a combination of both types of hernia can affect the same inguinal canal (pantaloon hernia). Direct inguinal hernias develop in an older age group; they rarely extend into the scrotum. They are associated with a weakness in the abdominal wall musculature and are frequently bilateral.

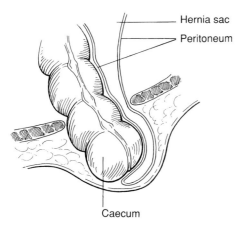

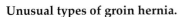

Fig. 33
Sliding type inguinal hernia.

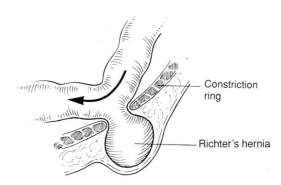

Fig. 34
Richter's hernia.

Unusual types of groin hernia.

Sliding inguinal hernia. In this hernia, part of the wall of the hernial sac is formed by the caecum (right side), pelvic colon (left side) or bladder (both sides) which has slid down extraperitoneally into the inguinal canal (Fig. 33). It is vitally important to recognise this variant at operation in order to prevent injury to the sliding component during ligation of the hernial sac.

Richter's hernia. In this hernia, part of the intestinal wall has become incarcerated in the neck of the hernial sac and may strangulate. The bowel will not be obstructed and the diagnosis may be overlooked (Fig. 34).

Clinical features

Both direct and indirect Inguinal hernias present as a lump in the groin. The various physical signs used to differentiate these two hernias are frequently unreliable. Careful localisation of the neck of the hernia, which *always* lies above and medial to the pubic tubercle (where the hernial sac emerges from the superficial inguinal ring) is more important. This is the key to differentiating an inguinal from a femoral hernia (Fig. 35).

The differential diagnosis of a groin lump includes:

- direct or indirect inguinal hernia
- femoral hernia
- inguinal lymphadenopathy
- undescended testicle.

Treatment

Age is no bar to hernia repair. Most symptomatic hernias can be repaired even in the elderly, using local or regional anaesthetic techniques. Repair should always be considered in order to prevent the risk of complications developing at a later date. Perhaps the only exception is a small obviously direct inguinal hernia, which can be managed with a truss.

Numerous surgical methods of repair have been described. The key steps are:

1. ligation of any indirect hernial sac at the deep inguinal ring

2. strengthening of the posterior wall of the inguinal canal by:

- suturing the conjoint tendon / internal oblique muscle to the inguinal ligament behind the spermatic cord (Bassini type repair)
- repairing any defect in the transversalis fascia in the floor of the inguinal canal in addition to suture of the conjoint tendon / internal oblique muscle to the inguinal ligament (Shouldice type repair)
- implantation of a non-absorbable prolene mesh.

Prognosis

One in 20 hernias will recur. Early recurrence within 2 years is usually a result of an inadequate primary operation. Late recurrence reflects a progression of the underlying neuromuscular weakness that caused the original hernia.

Femoral hernia

A femoral hernia descends through the femoral canal beneath the inguinal ligament to lie medial to the femoral vein (Fig. 35). The neck of the sac is extremely tight and because of this femoral hernias are prone to complications.

Clinical features

Femoral hernias are more common in women than in men. In contrast to inguinal hernias, the neck of the sac is below and lateral to the pubic tubercle in a position corresponding to the femoral canal. These hernias are often irreducible and frequently the primary presentation is with a complication such as obstruction or strangulation.

Treatment

The femoral canal can be approached from above or below the inguinal ligament or even through the posterior wall of the inguinal canal.

Reduction of the hernia, particularly if it is

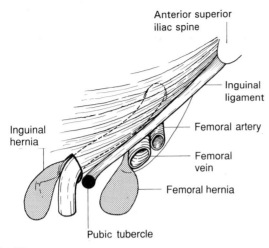

Fig. 35
Femoral hernia – relationship to inguinal hernia.

obstructed, is often difficult because of the tight neck. The surgical aim is to obliterate the femoral canal using non-absorbable sutures. A repair of the hernia will sometimes have to be combined with a resection of gangrenous small bowel or omentum.

Incisional hernia

Incisional (or ventral) hernias develop through a previous operation scar. They are more common in vertical incisions than transverse incisions. In each case there is usually one or more of the following predisposing factors:

- poor surgical technique
- poor perioperative nutritional status
- postoperative wound infection or haematoma
- underlying disease
  — intra-abdominal sepsis
  — malignancy
- postoperative cough
- obesity.

Clinical features
Untreated, these hernias will gradually increase in size. The omentum and intestines are often adherent to the scar tissue associated with these hernias and episodes of obstruction are frequent if these hernias are neglected.

Treatment
Small defects can often be repaired by using non-absorbable sutures to close the defect. Larger hernias may need to be repaired using a non-absorbable synthetic mesh to bridge the defect.

Umbilical and paraumbilical hernia

Umbilical hernia. True umbilical hernias, which develop through the centre of the umbilical cicatrix, are a disorder of childhood. Usually they disappear as the child grows and the rectii muscles develop.

Paraumbilical hernia. In adulthood, a paraumbilical hernia develops through the interlacing fibres of the linea alba that have become weakened with age and obesity. This hernia is much more common in women than men and develops just above the umbilicus. As it enlarges the hernia incorporates the umbilicus in the hernial swelling. The hernial sac is often multiloculated with a tight neck and is prone to complications.

Clinical features
Patients present with a localised swelling through or around the umbilicus that is often irreducible.

Treatment
Surgical repair is usually performed through an elliptical transverse incision with excision of the umbilicus. The most effective repair is obtained if the rectus sheath that forms the border of the defect is overlapped (Mayo's technique).

Epigastric hernia

This hernia often occurs in well-built muscular men. The protrusion develops through the interlacing fibres of the linea alba (in the midline) in the epigastrium.

Clinical features
These hernias are usually small but painful and are tender on examination. Although larger hernias may contain omentum and occasionally loops of intestine, most small hernias only contain extraperitoneal fat.

Treatment
The defect should be repaired with non-absorbable sutures.

Self-assessment: questions

Multiple choice questions

1. The following points relate to hernias in general:
   a. All hernias that strangulate are obstructed
   b. Most hernias are irreducible
   c. hernias are nearly always acquired; they are rarely congenital
   d. Chronic constipation and prostatic outflow symptoms can aggravate a hernia
   e. Every hernia is invested with a layer of parietal peritoneum

2. Direct inguinal hernias:
   a. Are frequently bilateral
   b. Are usually congenital
   c. Generally occur in an older age group than indirect inguinal hernias
   d. Often extend into the scrotum
   e. Have a neck that lies medial to the inferior epigastric vessels

3. A femoral hernia:
   a. Is more common in a woman than an inguinal hernia
   b. Lies lateral to the femoral vein
   c. Can be differentiated from an inguinal hernia by the position of its neck, which lies below and lateral to the pubic tubercle
   d. Rarely strangulates
   e. Rarely recurs

4. Incisional hernias are more common under the following circumstances:
   a. In thin patients
   b. In patients with underlying malignancy
   c. In vertical incisions
   d. After a major wound infection
   e. In severely septic patients

5. A sliding type inguinal hernia:
   a. Can usually be diagnosed preoperatively
   b. Will rarely recur
   c. May contain bladder
   d. If unrecognised can lead to bowel injury
   e. Is usually associated with direct inguinal hernias

Case history

Case history 1

A 54-year-old woman presents with a 2-day history of colicky abdominal pain and vomiting. She has a small painful lump in the left groin. Figure 36 is her plain abdominal X-ray.

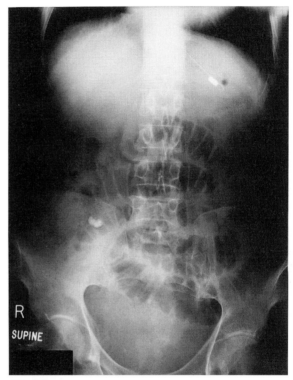

Fig. 36
Plain abdominal X-ray.

1. What is the radiological diagnosis?
2. What is the most likely cause?
3. What is the correct treatment?

Self-assessment: answers

Multiple choice answers

1. a. **False.** Strangulation implies that the blood supply to a loop of bowel or omentum has been compromised. If the hernia contains omentum only or only a part of the circumference of the bowel (i.e. a Richter's type hernia) then strangulation will occur without obstruction.
   b. **False.** Most hernias are reducible. The onset of irreducibility indicates that the hernial contents are trapped by the neck of the sac and cannot return to the abdomen. This will predispose to obstruction and strangulation.
   c. **False.** Indirect hernias are almost always congenital and are caused by failure of the processus vaginalis to obliterate. Although some will present in the neonatal or childhood period, many do not develop until later in life.
   d. **True.** Any condition that intermittently or chronically raises the intra-abdominal pressure can predispose to hernia development.
   e. **True.** As the hernia contents leave the abdominal cavity and enter the fascial defect that constitutes the hernia, they take with them a sac that is formed from the parietal peritoneum.

2. a. **True.** Direct hernias are frequently associated with lax abdominal wall muscles. The weakness is usually symmetrical and results in bilateral muscular defects.
   b. **False.**
   c. **True.** The muscular defects associated with direct hernias are frequently an effect of ageing.
   d. **False.** Direct hernias are usually small and almost never extend into the scrotum. Inguoscrotal hernias usually have a massive sac and are indirect in origin.
   e. **True.** The inferior epigastric vessels are a vital anatomical landmark. By definition, hernias where the neck lies medial to them are direct and hernias where the neck lies lateral to the vessels are indirect in origin.

3. a. **False.** Although femoral hernias are more common in women than men, the overall incidence of inguinal hernias (in both sexes) is far greater. Hence a groin hernia in a woman is still more likely to be inguinal than femoral in origin.
   b. **False.** A femoral hernia passes beneath the inguinal ligament along the femoral canal, which lies medial to the femoral vein.
   c. **True.** The pubic tubercle is an important anatomical landmark. The neck of a femoral hernia lies below and lateral to it whereas the neck of an inguinal hernia lies above and medial to the pubic tubercle.
   d. **False.** The neck of a femoral hernia is small and tight. These hernias are particularly prone to strangulation.
   e. **True.** A recurrence is rare provided the defect is carefully closed.

4. a. **False.** Obesity predisposes to incisional hernia formation by straining the wound during the healing phase.
   b. **True.** Malignancy, particularly when the disease is found to be inoperable, impairs wound healing.
   c. **True.** Vertical incisions are more prone to incisional hernia development than transverse incisions.
   d. **True.** A major wound infection or a post-operative wound haematoma impairs the healing process and predisposes to incisional herniation.
   e. **True.** These patients are usually catabolic and wound healing is impaired.

5. a. **False.** The diagnosis is made at operation when the hernial sac is opened and is found to contain a portion of the viscus or the bladder forming part of the wall and neck of the hernial sac.
   b. **False.** This type of hernia can be technically quite difficult to repair and recurrence is more common compared with an uncomplicated inguinal hernia.
   c. **True.** The bladder, sigmoid colon, caecum and ovary are the most common contents of a sliding type inguinal hernia.
   d. **True.** If this hernia variant is not recognised at operation, the sliding component can be damaged during ligation of the neck of the hernial sac.
   e. **False.** Sliding hernias are a variant of an indirect inguinal hernia.

Case history answers

Case history 1

1. Small bowel obstruction. From the appearance of the X-ray, with multiple loops of distended small bowel, it is probably a distal obstruction.
2. From the history, examination and radiological findings, the small bowel obstruction is likely to be secondary to either a femoral or an inguinal hernia.
3. The obstruction should be relieved by operative repair of the hernia and release of the trapped intestine. A laparotomy may be necessary to resect the segment of intestine involved, which may have been strangulated.

Surgical emergencies

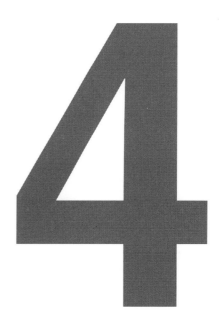

4.1 Trauma

Trauma is the leading cause of death in people under 40 years of age. Many survivors of injury are left with permanent disabilities. The human and economic cost remains enormous despite efforts at accident prevention through education, engineering and enforcement.

Injury patterns and severity

The greater the amount of energy transferred to the injured party, the more extensive and severe the injury. Road traffic accidents and falls from a height are most likely to cause severe and multiple injuries. Knowing the mechanism of the injury makes it easier to predict the pattern of injuries a patient is likely to have. Therefore, a detailed history is as important in trauma patients as elsewhere. The 'dose' of injury a patient has sustained can be quantified by scoring systems: anatomically, using the Injury Severity Score, or physiologically, using the Trauma Score.

Improving the outcome: 'the golden hour'

Some trauma victims die immediately after injury and are probably unsalvageable because of the severity of their injuries (e.g. brainstem tear or a ruptured aorta). Others die later and there is evidence that better early management — especially airway care, control and correction of blood loss, and an early assessment by experienced clinicians — would save many victims and reduce disability among survivors.

The patient's fate is decided by what is done (or not done) during the 'golden hour' of opportunity after injury. Major trauma is best managed by a team of experts drawn from all the relevant fields (especially accident and emergency medicine, anaesthesia and the various surgical specialities) who work together in an appropriate setting such as an accident and emergency department and keep their skills up to date.

Education and training: ATLS

There has been an explosion of interest in how to develop and to maintain the knowledge and skills of those who treat the seriously injured. Advanced trauma life support (ATLS) courses have spread worldwide from the USA because they offer a safe way to assess and resuscitate the seriously injured.

The ATLS principles of early trauma care are:

- do no further harm to the patient
- assess and resuscitate the patient simultaneously and systematically
- develop a rigid order of priority dealing first with the greatest threats to life (the 'primary survey')
- conduct a thorough search for all other injuries ('secondary survey')

- stabilise the patient before transfer to a definitive trauma care facility.

A systematic approach to trauma care

Many patients die because major injuries or their complications are missed or underestimated, often in the 'golden hour'. Having a systematic approach to assessment makes this less likely to happen. The ATLS system offers an easy-to-remember mnemonic:

A — airway (with cervical spine control)
B — breathing
C — circulation (with control of haemorrhage)
D — dysfunction (of the nervous system)
E — exposure and the environment.

The alphabetical order is also that in which complications threaten life. For example, there is no point in operating on a head injured patient to remove an intracranial haematoma while the patient dies from a blocked airway or hypovolaemic shock from uncontrolled haemorrhage. Instead, the management of the patient's head injury should begin by clearing the airway (taking great care to protect the potentially injured cervical spine), ensuring he/she is breathing and then correcting the blood loss causing the hypovolaemic shock.

The following sections systematically outline the core points in trauma management once the 'primary survey' has been completed. Further detailed information is provided in the relevant chapters in this book. In a trauma patient, the injuries, which are often multiple, are best categorised by site:

- head and neck
- thorax
- abdomen
- vascular
- urogenital system
- orthopaedic.

Head and neck injuries

The key points in trauma management are:

1. Provide cervical stabilisation with a collar until cervical X-rays rule out a fracture.
2. Prevent airway obstruction with either an airway or an endotracheal tube.
3. Regularly record neurological status (Glasgow Coma Scale); consider CT scan if status deteriorates; skull X-ray if there has been a loss of consciousness (see p. 165).
4. Remember that vascular, tracheal and oesophageal injuries can occur from blunt or penetrating cervical trauma.

Thoracic injuries

The key points are:

1. Ensure the patient is breathing with unrestricted symmetrical chest movement.

2. Remember the most frequent serious major chest injuries are:

- haemothorax/haemopneumothorax
- flail chest
- tension pneumothorax
- cardiac tamponade.

3. Although the diagnosis will be obvious on a chest X-ray, in a critically injured patient there may not be time and a life will be saved after insertion of a chest drain or pericardiocentesis *after an accurate clinical diagnosis*.

4. Occasionally a life will be saved by urgent thoracotomy in the emergency room to arrest haemorrhage from the heart or lung root.

Abdominal injuries

Parenchymal organs or hollow viscera can be damaged by blunt or penetrating abdominal trauma. A blunt injury may be overlooked in a comatose patient with a head and/or chest injury.

The key points are:

1. Major intra-abdominal blood loss usually follows injury to the liver or spleen (either blunt or penetrating) or a penetrating injury that damages the great vessels or mesentery. If doubt exists, a diagnostic peritoneal lavage will usually identify any intra-abdominal bleeding.

2. Rupture of a hollow viscus can be difficult to detect and may be missed on simple radiological studies. It should be suspected in a patient who becomes septic for no apparent cause or in any patient who develops progressive abdominal signs.

3. The most frequently injured organs are:

- liver: bleeding is the major problem; usually this will stop with tamponade or simple suture. Debridement or formal liver resection is rarely required
- spleen: usually requires splenectomy or occasionally splenorrhaphy to control bleeding
- small bowel and stomach: rupture of any part of the intestine causes peritonitis. Usually a small bowel tear or mesenteric injury can be treated by simple oversew or resection
- colon injury: because of the risks of a postoperative peritonitis caused by faecal leakage or contamination, most surgeons would exteriorise the injured colon to form a colostomy.

Vascular injuries

Worldwide, penetrating injuries caused by gunshot or stabwounds are the most common cause of major arterial injury. Crush injury to the limbs may contuse an artery producing an intimal tear that will impede distal blood flow even though the blood vessel may appear structurally intact. This type of injury frequently accompanies a long bone fracture or dislocation.

Clinical features

Patients may present with an obvious external haemorrhage from a bleeding wound, or the blood loss may be concealed as in a retroperitoneal or thoracic injury, the only clinical evidence being hypovolaemic shock. Alternatively, the patient may present with an ischaemic pulseless limb (pain, pallor, paralysis, paraesthesia, no pulses).

A high index of suspicion is the key to diagnosis, especially in a shocked patient or one with an injury close to a blood vessel or following a fracture/dislocation. Even if distal pulses are present, the proximal vessel can still be injured and if there is any doubt an arteriogram should be performed.

Treatment

Direct compression of a bleeding wound will save a life while emergency resuscitation takes place. Whenever possible, a tourniquet should *not* be used as they can cause further damage to the circulation. Operative treatment involves obtaining control above and below the bleeding vessel, followed by careful exploration of the bleeding point. Sometimes, once the damaged section of vessel has been excised, a primary end-to-end repair can be undertaken. Alternatively, a vein or prosthetic graft can be interposed if the defect is too wide. A careful search should be made for any associated vein or nerve injury.

Urogenital system

Major injury to the renal tract must be suspected in any patient with a loin injury or gross haematuria. An intravenous pyelogram (IVP) is essential.

The kidney should be explored if there are signs of extravasation of urine or continuing haemorrhage. Nephrectomy or partial nephrectomy may be required.

Bladder or urethral injuries may not be so obvious but should be suspected in any patient with a major pelvic injury. Operative repair of the bladder together with suprapubic catheterisation and urinary diversion is the best initial treatment option. Operative reconstruction of a damaged urethra is carried out at a later date.

Orthopaedic injuries

Most orthopaedic injuries can be managed immediately by external splints or external fixation devices which will buy time until other coexisting life-threatening injuries have been dealt with or stabilised. Orthopaedic trauma is dealt with in detail in a different volume of this series.

4.2 The acute abdomen

An acute abdomen can be defined as a non-traumatic, catastrophic event that affects any of the intra-abdominal organs. Acute severe abdominal pain is usually the hallmark. Patients with an acute abdomen require urgent investigation, diagnosis and treatment.

There are numerous causes of an acute abdomen. The most important are listed in Table 9.

Table 9 Causes of an acute abdomen

- Common causes
  —acute appendicitis
  —acute cholecystitis, biliary colic
  —acute pancreatitis
  —acute diverticulitis
  —acute gynaecological problems: salpingitis, ectopic pregnancy, torted ovarian cyst
  —perforated peptic ulcer
  —large or small bowel obstruction
  —ureteric or renal colic
- Less common causes
  —leaking aortic aneurysm
  —mesenteric ischaemia
  —acute colitis or Crohn's disease

Clinical features

Most will present with abdominal pain. Although patients will be distressed, time taken to obtain an accurate history is well spent and will frequently point to the diagnosis.

There are five key points in relation to pain and the acute abdomen, namely:

- location
- onset
- progression
- character
- radiation.

Location

There are usually two components to abdominal pain: visceral and parietal.

Visceral pain. This type of pain is caused by inflammation or distension of a viscus and is often poorly localised:

- pain from organs of the foregut (stomach / liver / gall bladder / duodenum) is usually perceived in the epigastrium
- pain derived from midgut organs (pancreas / small bowel / appendix / ascending colon) is perceived in the centre of the abdomen (periumbilical)
- hindgut pain (transverse / descending and sigmoid colon) is perceived in the hypogastrium / suprapubic areas.

Parietal pain. Eventually the parietal peritoneum becomes inflamed by pus or bile or an adjacent acutely inflamed viscus and pain will localise to that particular part of the abdomen.

Onset

Sudden/explosive pain. This usually heralds an intra-abdominal catastrophe such as a ruptured viscus (e.g. perforated peptic ulcer) or a leaking abdominal aortic aneurysm.

Gradual onset pain. This often implies progressive inflammation of a viscus, as in acute cholecystitis or pancreatitis.

Progression

Acute appendicitis is a classical example of the progression of pain from a visceral to a parietal component and underlines the importance of taking an accurate history. Many patients with acute appendicitis will describe pain originating in the centre of the abdomen (the appendix is a midgut organ) before the pain eventually settles in the right iliac fossa when the parietal peritoneum adjacent to the appendix becomes inflamed. A careful history will lead to the diagnosis, which can be simply confirmed on abdominal examination.

Character

The most important features to determine are:

- is the pain colicky or constant?
- what is the effect of movement?

Colic implies obstruction of a viscus, as in small or large bowel obstruction. Constant pain is in keeping with inflammation of an organ or vascular compromise (e.g. strangulation or ischaemia).

Movement exacerbates pain caused by parietal peritoneal inflammation. A patient with generalised peritonitis caused by a perforated peptic ulcer will lie completely still. In contrast, patients with ureteric or renal colic cannot find a comfortable position and will frequently writhe in agony until they receive adequate analgesia or until the colic subsides.

Radiation

This can often provide an important diagnostic clue. For example, pain from the retroperitoneal organs, such as the pancreas or the aorta, will radiate to the back, whereas pain of biliary origin may radiate to the shoulder tip because of irritation or inflammation of the adjacent diaphragm.

Physical findings

Avoid the temptation to rush to examine the abdomen. The entire patient must be evaluated. Is the patient shocked? Do not forget to examine the chest and cardiovascular system. Resuscitation (see p. 76) may be required while physical evaluation and urgent investigation of the patient continues.

The abdomen

The most important question to answer is: is there an obstruction or peritonitis, or are both present?

In examining the patient, certain key features must be sought.

Inspection. Is the abdomen flat or distended? Does the abdomen move with respiration? A distended abdomen suggests obstruction or the accumulation of ascitic fluid.

Palpation. Is there any tenderness? Is it localised or generalised? Are there any masses? Generalised tenderness with rebound or guarding is in keeping with a generalised peritonitis; occasionally rectus muscle spasm will be induced, causing 'board-like' abdominal rigidity, for example after a perforated ulcer. If the inflammatory process is localised as in appendicitis or acute diverticulitis, careful palpation to elicit the area of maximum tenderness will point towards the most likely underlying cause. A pulsatile abdominal mass is an abdominal aortic aneurysm until proven otherwise.

Percussion. Is the abdomen hyper-resonant or not? A resonant distended abdomen, suggests an obstruction, a dull abdomen, ascites or a mass.

Auscultation. Are there bowel sounds present? Are the bowel sounds obstructive? A silent abdomen is usually a grave sign indicating an intra-abdominal catastrophe, for example generalised peritonitis or severe mesenteric ischaemia. Normal bowel sounds may be reassuring, but in the presence of other significant abdominal findings 'normal' bowel sounds should not lead you into a false sense of security. High-pitched 'tinkling' bowel sounds are indicative of a bowel obstruction.

Rectal and vaginal examination

No abdominal evaluation is complete if a rectal examination is omitted. The pelvic organs, a pelvic mass or abscess, or a pelvic appendicitis are protected by the bony pelvic ring and are inaccessible to abdominal palpation. A rectal examination allows access to the pelvis by *palpation* and will reveal areas of tenderness or a mass that would otherwise be missed. If there is any suspicion that the acute pathology is of gynaecological origin then a vaginal examination is mandatory.

Investigations

Often, simple blood tests and radiological investigations will provide diagnostic evidence and will confirm or refute the clinical findings and diagnosis.

Blood tests. Patients with an acute abdomen should have blood drawn for:

- full blood count
- urea and electrolytes
- serum amylase
- blood grouping (save serum for cross-match).

These tests will detect anaemia, a leucocytosis, electrolyte imbalance or dehydration and will influence the patient's resuscitation. A massively elevated serum amylase will confirm a diagnosis of acute pancreatitis.

Radiological investigations.

Erect chest X-ray. The most important feature to look for is subdiaphragmatic gas. Its presence indicates a perforated viscus. Occasionally, a chest X-ray will demonstrate an unexpected cause of a patient's abdominal pain, such as a right-sided basal pneumonia, which clinically had been mistaken for an attack of acute cholecystitis.

Plain abdominal radiology. A single supine abdominal film will identify a small or a large bowel obstruction. Critical features such as caecal dilatation with impending perforation or a toxic colonic dilatation will also be identified. Occasionally abnormal calcification in the gallbladder (gallstones), pancreas (pancreatitis) renal tract (ureteric or renal colic) or outlining a dilated aorta (aneurysm) will point to the underlying diagnosis.

ECG. Many patients with an acute abdomen will require surgical intervention. An ECG may be required in view of a forthcoming anaesthetic. Sometimes an underlying cardiac cause for an acute epigastric pain (e.g. an atypical myocardial infarction) will be discovered.

A treatment plan

Much will depend on the diagnosis. Sometimes, despite careful clinical evaluation and investigation, no firm conclusion is reached. Those patients who do not respond to resuscitation and conservative measures will require a diagnostic laparoscopy or laparotomy to establish and treat an elusive diagnosis.

The key management points are:

- resuscitate
- antibiotics
- analgesia
- monitor the response.

Resuscitation. Several immediate steps are necessary: establish an intravenous fluid infusion and replace volume deficits with crystalloid, colloid or blood as appropriates; administer supplemental oxygen therapy.

Antibiotics. Many patients will have intra-abdominal sepsis. Until culture and sensitivity reports are to hand (often only as a result of specimens obtained during urgent surgery), antibiotics will have to be chosen based on the likelihood of the infecting organisms. Usually broad-spectrum cover is required to include Gram-negative and Gram-positive aerobes plus anaerobic organism cover. Take blood cultures first.

Analgesia. Adequate *parenteral* analgesia is essential and should not be withheld once a preliminary assessment has been completed. A carefully titrated analgesic dose will not mask significant abdominal findings but instead will often facilitate abdominal examination by relaxing the patient.

Monitor the response. Fluid resuscitation, antibiotic therapy and adequate analgesia form the cornerstone of conservative management. The patient's vital signs and urine output are a sensitive indicator of the response to treatment.

Getting better?

Some causes of an acute abdomen will respond well to conservative measures, e.g. acute cholecystitis or acute pancreatitis. For others, an initial response to conservative treatment simply indicates that resuscitation has been adequate and that the patient is now optimised and ready for surgical treatment (e.g. a perforated duodenal ulcer). Any untoward delay and the benefits of resuscitation will be lost as sepsis supervenes and compromises the outcome of surgery.

No improvement or a worsening clinical condition?

A falling blood pressure, rising pulse rate and dwindling urine output all indicate a failure to respond to conservative measures. In these patients, the initial diagnosis may have been incorrect or a complication may have supervened (e.g. rupture of a diverticular abscess causing generalised peritonitis). Patients in this category usually require aggressive resuscitation prior to surgical intervention.

Surgery inevitable?

In a third group of patients, the need for surgical intervention is obvious from the outset once a diagnosis has been reached (e.g. perforated peptic ulcer, leaking aortic aneurysm). In this group of patients, conservative management is limited to providing the necessary resuscitation to optimise the patient's condition prior to operation.

4.3 Major gastrointestinal haemorrhage

Haemorrhagic shock is the most common form of shock encountered by surgeons. The clinical picture depends on the extent of blood loss (see Table 10). Patients with a massive, exsanguinating haemorrhage will need a rapid overall evaluation with resuscitation taking priority over a full history and physical examination.

Resuscitation

The initial resuscitation is the same, regardless of the site of blood loss. The key steps are:

1. Ensure adequate ventilation and oxygenation.
2. Establish venous access using multiple peripheral sites if necessary.
3. Pass a nasogastric tube.
4. Obtain blood for cross-match, baseline haemoglobin and coagulation profile.

5. Resuscitate with colloid plasma expanders (e.g. Haemaccel) or crystalloid solutions until matched whole blood is available. In an exsanguinating patient, it may be necessary to use group O negative blood.
6. Monitor response by vital signs; catheterise patient to observe urine output.
7. Consider urgent surgical intervention in any patient who does not respond to 2–3 litres fluid resuscitation.
8. Invasive monitoring using central venous access and pressure monitoring is best left until resuscitation is established and the circulating volume restored.

Overall, bleeding stops spontaneously in 80% of patients and these steps will effectively resuscitate most patients and allow time for diagnostic evaluation.

Causes

The main causes of massive upper gastrointestinal haemorrhage are:

- Common
  — peptic duodenal or gastric ulceration
  — oesophageal varices
  — acute gastritis
  — Mallory–Weiss tear

- Uncommon
  — gastric or oesophageal cancer.

The main causes of massive lower gastrointestinal haemorrhage are:

- Common
  — diverticular disease
  — angiodysplasia
  —acute colitis of any cause

- Uncommon
  — colon carcinoma
  — haemorrhoids.

On the rare occasions the small intestine is the site of major gastrointestinal blood loss, angiodysplastic lesions or a Meckel's diverticulum are usually responsible.

Clinical features

Haematemesis implies a brisk upper gastrointestinal bleed either from oesophagus, stomach or duodenum. Melena, the passage of black tarry stools, indicates blood loss from any point of the gastrointestinal tract as

Table 10 Clinical features of haemorrhagic shock

Blood loss	Physical findings
Mild shock vasoconstriction (< 20% loss of blood volume)	Periphery pale, cold
Moderate shock (loss of 20–40% blood volume)	As above plus oliguria, postural hypotension
Severe shock (loss of > 40% blood volume)	As above plus restlessness, supine hypotension

far as the caecum. Haemorrhage from the colon, rectum and anus is characterised by fresh rectal bleeding or passage of dark altered blood per rectum.

Several points in the case history are particularly important:

- drug history
  - — anti-inflammatory agents
  - — anticoagulants
  - — aspirin
- alcohol intake.

Diagnostic difficulties arise because:

- not all upper gastrointestinal bleeds are associated with haematemesis; some present with melena alone
- rapid upper gastrointestinal bleeding may present as rectal haemorrhage rather than melena because of rapid transit through the intestines. These patients are usually profoundly shocked.

The essential diagnostic steps are:

- urgent gastroscopy for all suspected upper gastrointestinal bleeds plus those patients with shock and rectal haemorrhage

- colonoscopy for all patients with suspected lower gastrointestinal bleeds
- selective mesenteric angiography in patients who continue to bleed despite negative endoscopic evaluation.

Treatment

This will depend upon the underlying cause and is covered in detail in Chapter 2. The most frequent urgent procedures are:

- sclerotherapy for bleeding oesophageal varices
- sclerotherapy or surgery for bleeding peptic ulcers
- colonic resection for angiodysplasia or diverticular disease
- subtotal or total colectomy for acute colitis.

Outcome

Approximately 80% of acute bleeds of whatever cause will stop and these patients will survive provided resuscitation is adequate. For the remainder, the outcome will depend on the cause of the bleed. Those at greatest risk are the elderly or those patients who bleed for a second time (rebleeding) after the initial haemorrhage has stopped.

Self-assessment: questions

Multiple choice questions

1. The following points relate to the early management of trauma:
   a. The first priority in a critically injured patient is to establish intravenous access
   b. Cervical fractures are usually obvious
   c. Supine hypotension usually indicates a greater than 40% loss of blood volume
   d. Mediastinal injury is likely in patients with bilateral rib fractures
   e. Diagnostic peritoneal lavage will reliably detect visceral rupture in the comatose patient

2. Major peripheral arterial injuries:
   a. Inevitably cause loss of peripheral pulses distal to the injury
   b. Are reliably diagnosed by arteriography
   c. Are rarely accompanied by vein or nerve injury
   d. Frequently accompany fracture/dislocations of the long bones
   e. Should have a tourniquet applied to them to obtain initial control of the blood loss

3. The following points relate to abdominal pain:
   a. The visceral component of duodenal pain is perceived in the periumbilical area
   b. Patients with renal colic can often alleviate their symptoms by lying very still
   c. Shoulder tip pain is a characteristic of a perforated peptic ulcer
   d. Mesenteric thrombosis is rarely associated with colicky abdominal pain
   e. Parietal pain is often preceded by visceral pain

4. A supine plain abdominal radiograph often provides useful diagnostic information in the following conditions:
   a. Abdominal aortic aneurysm
   b. Perforated peptic ulcer
   c. Acute appendicitis
   d. Acute cholecystitis
   e. Large bowel obstruction

5. In patients with upper gastrointestinal bleeding:
   a. The bleeding point is frequently beyond the ligament of Treitz
   b. Angiodysplastic lesions are a common cause
   c. The patients always present with haematemesis
   d. Diagnostic endoscopy is best deferred for at least 24 hours
   e. Selective mesenteric angiography is the key diagnostic step

6. Patients with a major rectal haemorrhage:
   a. Should have a gastroscopy
   b. Almost always require surgery
   c. Frequently harbour a colorectal cancer
   d. Have angiodysplastic lesions most frequently found in the caecum
   e. Should have an emergency barium enema as the key investigation

Case histories

Case history 1

A 24-year-old man is brought into a casualty department after falling off his motorcycle. He was not wearing a crash helmet. The ambulance officer tells you he was conscious for a time after the injury but then became unrousable. He has an obvious fracture of his left femur and marked bruising over his pelvis. His blood pressure is 100/60 mmHg with a pulse rate of 96/minute.

1. What are the key points in this patient's initial evaluation and management that would be undertaken before embarking on any investigations?
2. What would be the most useful diagnostic tests for this patient and how would they be prioritised?

Case history 2

A 75-year-old man is admitted after a collapse at home. He tells you that he had felt light-headed when he went to the toilet and fainted after he passed a black, offensive-smelling tarry stool. He looks grey and sweaty and his pulse rate was 126/minute; he has a systolic blood pressure whilst lying down of 90 mmHg.

1. What key features in the history and physical examination would you look for?
2. What is the most likely differential diagnosis?
3. What would be your initial management plan for this patient?
4. What diagnostic steps would you take?

Case history 3

An 82-year-old woman who has previously had a coronary artery by-pass graft and has a long history of intermittent claudication affecting both legs is admitted with severe abdominal pain. The discomfort she describes is poorly localised, constant not colicky, but was of sudden onset. It is agonising and the patient tells you it is the worst pain she has ever had. On examination she is thin and looks dehydrated and she has a diffusely tender abdomen. You note she does *not* have an aortic aneurysm and that her bowel sounds are scanty. She is mildly hypotensive.

1. What do you think is the likely differential diagnosis?
2. What urgent diagnostic tests would be useful in this difficult case?

Two hours after admission, the patient's condition deteriorates further. Her pain increases and she develops rebound tenderness and guarding. The bowel sounds are now absent.

3. What possible management options are there?

Case history 4

A 62-year-old woman is admitted urgently with a short history of cramp-like lower abdominal pains. The discomfort is centred in the hypogastrium. There is no history of vomiting, nor has she had any previous surgery. On examination she has a tympanitic, grossly distended abdomen and appears mildly tender in the right iliac fossa. She has high-pitched tinkling bowel sounds.

1. What other points in her case history and physical examination would you seek in order to establish the most likely diagnosis?
2. What diagnostic steps would you take?
3. What, if any, is the potential significance of this patient's right iliac fossa tenderness?

Self-assessment: answers

Multiple choice answers

1. a. **False**. The first priority is to secure the patient's airway. A patient will die of asphyxia before he exsanguinates.
   b. **False**. Cervical spine X-rays are essential to detect a fracture or dislocation. All major trauma victims should be considered to have a cervical fracture until proven otherwise by radiology. For this reason all these patients should have their cervical spine stabilised immediately with a cervical collar.
   c. **True**. Supine hypotension indicates a major loss in the circulating blood volume, usually in excess of 40%.
   d. **True**. Bilateral rib fractures indicate a severe injury to the chest. This group of patients are at a high risk of mediastinal injury.
   e. **False**. Peritoneal lavage is most effective at determining intraperitoneal bleeding: the lavage returns pink or blood-stained.

2. a. **False**. There may still be partial blood flow despite the injury or there may be a transmitted pulsation along the vessel wall.
   b. **True**. This is the key diagnostic step where major arterial injury is suspected. There is no substitute.
   c. **False**. Veins and nerves frequently accompany arteries in a neurovascular bundle. Injury to these structures should always be sought in any major arterial injury.
   d. **True**. This is one of the most common mechanisms that lead to vascular trauma in association with a blunt soft tissue injury. For example, the popliteal artery can be stretched and damaged during a posterior dislocation of the knee.
   e. **False**. A tourniquet is the last resort. It may further damage the blood supply to the distal tissues and will enhance any venous bleeding by obstructing the venous return. Direct pressure over the bleeding point is the best method of providing control.

3. a. **False**. The duodenum is a foregut structure. The visceral component of foregut pain (caused by distension, inflammation, etc.) is perceived in the epigastrium. Midgut pain is perceived in the periumbilical area.
   b. **False**. Renal or ureteric colic is characterised by pain in which *no* position is comfortable. Patients frequently 'writhe in agony'.
   c. **True**. This is caused by diaphragmatic irritation from released gastric contents, which track up to lie beneath the diaphragm.

d. **True**. The pain of mesenteric ischaemia is characteristically severe, constant and diffuse.
e. **True**. Parietal pain develops as a consequence of inflammation of the parietal peritoneum by an inflamed viscus, intestinal contents or pus. It may be preceded by a visceral type pain, e.g. in acute appendicitis (periumbilical pain (visceral); right iliac fossa pain (parietal)).

4. a. **True**. The wall of the aneurysm may be calcified and this will be detected on a plain abdominal X-ray.
   b. **False**. A plain abdominal X-ray may be normal. The most useful non-invasive test in a suspected perforated ulcer is an erect chest X-ray; this will detect subdiaphragmatic gas in 8 out of 10 patients.
   c. **False**. This is essentially a clinical diagnosis. A plain abdominal film will not add to the diagnosis.
   d. **True**. Radio-opaque gallstones will be detected in 10% of cases.
   e. **True**. This is a key diagnostic step in these patients and will confirm or refute the diagnosis.

5. a. **False**. The ligament of Treitz is sited at the duodenal–jejunal flexure. Gastrointestinal bleeding beyond this point presents as melena or rectal haemorrhage (depending on the rate of blood loss).
   b. **False**. Angiodysplastic lesions are extremely uncommon in the stomach and duodenum. Peptic ulcers, gastric and duodenal erosions and oesophageal varices are the main causes of upper gastrointestinal haemorrhage.
   c. **False**. Some patients will present with melena alone. The combination of haematemesis and melena usually implies a more major bleed.
   d. **False**. The detection rate of the underlying cause of an upper gastrointestinal bleed declines markedly after 24 hours. All these patients should undergo a gastroscopy within the first 24 hours.
   e. **False**. Gastroscopy is the key step. Selective mesenteric angiography is reserved for those patients who continue to bleed but from no obvious source.

6. a. **True**. This is an important part of their work-up. Occasionally a major acute bleed from an upper gastrointestinal source will present as a rectal haemorrhage. The large volumes of blood released are an irritant to the gastrointestinal tract and stimulate a rapid transit through the small and large bowel.
   b. **False**. Overall 80% of patients with rectal haemorrhage will settle on conservative treatment.

c. **False.** A major bleed is rarely caused by colorectal cancer. Occult bleeding or small amounts of blood loss with stools would be more likely. Angiodysplasia or diverticular disease are the most common causes of a major rectal haemorrhage.

d. **True.** They can be detected during colonoscopy or by mesenteric angiography.

e. **False.** A barium enema will provide the least information in a patient with an acute bleed. It will not detect any angiodysplastic lesions and may even mislead: diverticular disease is a common finding on any barium enema study and is not necessarily the cause of bleeding.

Case history answers

Case history 1

1. The Advanced Trauma Life Support (ATLS) systematic approach can be used to assess this patient and perform a 'primary survey' in order to deal first with the greatest threats to the patient's life.

    A. Airway. The airway should be clear with no blood, saliva, vomit or broken teeth likely to cause an obstruction. Before moving the head and clearing the airway, ensure that the cervical spine is stabilised with an external collar in case the patient has fractured his cervical spine. It may be necessary to provide the patient with an artificial airway.

    B. Breathing. Check there is respiratory movement and symmetrical chest expansion with air entry into both lungs. If not the will would require intubation and ventilation.

    C. Circulation. Check the patient has a cardiac output (carotid pulsation) and start regular monitoring of pulse and blood pressure. If there is no cardiac output, cardiopulmonary resuscitation will need to be started. Set up an intravenous infusion. Carefully examine the abdomen, catheterise the patient and carry out a diagnostic peritoneal lavage. These steps will detect any major intra-abdominal bleeding.

    D. Dysfunction. A quick neurological examination should be made, concentrating on consciousness level, pupillary response, peripheral reflexes and limb movements. These will form a baseline for the patient's Glasgow Coma Scale observations.

    E. Exposure. The patient should be totally undressed and a complete physical examination carried out to check for any other injuries.

2. The patient has signs of major trauma with a head injury, pelvic injury and limb fracture. He is mildly hypotensive and from the distribution of his bruising may have a fractured pelvis in addition to his broken left femur. Also, there has been a deterioration in his consciousness level since the time of injury suggesting he might have a progressive intracerebral injury.

Blood should be drawn for cross-matching and baseline haematological and biochemical indices.

He needs an urgent X-ray of his cervical spine (to exclude a cervical fracture / dislocation), chest (to exclude a mediastinal injury / haemothorax / rib fractures), plain abdominal film and pelvis (to exclude a pelvic fracture) and left femur. Depending on the result of the diagnostic peritoneal lavage and the stability of the patient's condition the next priority would be a cerebral CT scan.

Case history 2

1. The history is in keeping with a gastrointestinal bleed with the patient passing a melena stool. The patient should be asked if he has a history of dyspeptic symptoms (epigastric pain, nausea, indigestion) or if he is taking anti-inflammatory drugs, aspirin or anticoagulants, all of which can predispose to a gastrointestinal haemorrhage. His alcohol intake should be established.

    This patient has supine hypotension and has clearly had a major gastrointestinal bleed. A quick chest and abdominal examination should be performed once it has been established that the patient is haemodynamically stable. This examination would look for signs of epigastric tenderness, and a rectal examination would confirm the presence of melena.

2. The history suggests a major upper gastrointestinal haemorrhage. The most likely cause would be one of the following:
    - duodenal or gastric ulcer
    - duodenal or gastric erosions
    - oesophageal varices.

    As there is no history of vomiting it is unlikely this bleed has been caused by a Mallory–Weiss tear.

3. Initially, intravenous access should be established using one or two wide-bore cannulae and blood taken for urgent cross-match and baseline haematological and biochemical studies and for a coagulation screen. The patient is hypotensive with a tachycardia. While waiting for cross-matched blood to arrive, an artificial plasma expander such as Haemaccel can be used to resuscitate the patient.

    The patient should be catheterised and his vital signs monitored at least every 15 minutes to monitor the response to treatment. A nasogastric tube should be passed to decompress the stomach or empty it of blood. A satisfactory outcome would be indicated by restoration of his blood pressure and a fall in pulse rate in the presence of a good urine output (greater than 30 ml / hour).

    If the patient does not respond to 1–2 litres of fluid / blood resuscitation, then a central venous line will be required to monitor the patient's further resuscitation; consideration should be given to the need for urgent therapeutic intervention.

4. An urgent upper gastrointestinal endoscopy is the key investigation. This should be performed within the first 24 hours of admission or earlier if the patient continues to bleed and is unstable. The oesophagus, stomach and duodenum should be carefully evaluated. Active bleeding from ulcers or varices can be treated by injection sclerotherapy during the endoscopy. If this fails, surgical intervention will be required, the procedure depending on the cause and site of the bleeding.

Case history 3

1. This patient is an arteriopath, having previously undergone a coronary artery by-pass graft and presently has symptoms of intermittent claudication. She may have atheromatous disease affecting her mesenteric vessels. The history and physical signs suggest there has been an intra-abdominal catastrophe.

   The most likely diagnoses are:
   - generalised peritonitis caused by a perforated viscus
   - acute pancreatitis
   - acute mesenteric vascular occlusion
   - intestinal strangulation.

2. The following blood tests would be important:
   Serum amylase. A massive elevation would be in keeping with a diagnosis of pancreatitis.
   White cell count. Although this is a non-specific marker of an inflammatory process, a leucocytosis would be in keeping with serious intra-abdominal sepsis.
   Baseline haematology and biochemistry. These are would be important aids to planning resuscitation.
   Radiology. An erect chest X-ray and plain abdominal film would be important to rule out a perforation or an unexpected obstruction.

3. The patient now has signs of generalised peritonitis. There is little to be gained from further non-invasive exploration. The patient should be resuscitated and prepared for an exploratory laparotomy.

Case history 4

1. The history and abdominal findings are highly suspicious of a large bowel obstruction. It would be important to know of any recent alteration in bowel habit, passage of blood or mucus per rectum. Also, it would be vital to know when the patient's bowels last moved or if there has been a stoppage in the passage of flatus. A rectal examination should be performed. This might detect a mass, faecal impaction or a distended empty rectum.

2. A plain abdominal radiograph should be diagnostic. The absence of haustral folds would help distinguish a large bowel obstruction from a small bowel obstruction. The characteristic features of a large bowel volvulus would also be detected.

   A sigmoidoscopy should also be performed in order to identify an obstructing recto-sigmoid cancer.

   Before any surgery is undertaken it is important that the level and cause of the obstruction within the colon are identified in order that the most appropriate operation can be planned. Whenever possible, these patients should have a preoperative barium enema.

3. Tenderness in the right iliac fossa in a patient with large bowel obstruction can indicate that the caecum is distended. The thin-walled caecum is at risk of perforation if the obstruction is unrelieved and this can lead to a lethal faecal peritonitis. Caecal dilatation is usually seen in patients with a closed-loop large bowel obstruction (caused by a competent ileocaecal valve preventing reflux or overflow of obstructed colonic contents back into the small intestine) and is an indication for urgent surgical intervention. The diagnosis can be confirmed on a plain abdominal X-ray, which will clearly show any caecal distension.

Peripheral vascular surgery

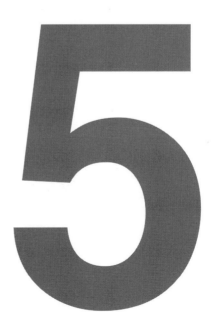

5.1 Arterial disease

Atherosclerosis

Atherosclerotic occlusive disease is common; it affects at least 40% of males over 50 years of age. Currently, 50% of all deaths are caused by circulatory diseases: principally myocardial infarction and stroke. Up to 10% of all adults have evidence of *peripheral* atherosclerotic occlusive disease (PAOD).

Atherosclerosis is a diffuse disease process that affects most blood vessels. In many patients with peripheral atherosclerotic disease, it is often the coexisting cardiac component that causes death.

Epidemiology
The main epidemiological factors are:

- diabetes
- smoking
- hypercholesterolaemia
- hypertension
- family history
- geographic considerations.

Patients with multiple risk factors from this list are at a greater risk of developing atherosclerosis than those with a single risk factor.

Pathophysiology
Atherosclerosis is an inflammatory response to the deposition of lipids within an arterial wall. It is commonly found in areas of maximum blood flow turbulence, principally at vessel bifurcations. The following is the most likely sequence of disease progression:

1. fatty streaks or patches
2. intimal lipid deposits
3. superficial fibrosis, overlying the lipid deposit
4. atheromatous plaque formation producing:
   — stenosis/occlusion causing distal ischaemia
   — disruption/ulceration causing embolisation.

Symptom patterns
This varies depending upon the region of the body most affected by the disease:

- coronary artery disease leads to a cardiac symptomatology
- lower limb disease causes claudication and limb ischaemia.

The reason why one area of the body should be affected more than another is unknown. There are also interesting local geographic variations, even within the UK. One region may have a very high coronary arterial problem (e.g. West of Scotland) whereas other areas have a relatively higher incidence of lower limb disease (e.g. Tayside, Scotland).

The rate of development of atherosclerosis is also extremely important. Slowly developing disease allows compensating mechanisms to develop (e.g. a collateral arterial supply). This can reduce symptoms to an extent that they are barely noticed. In contrast, acute occlusion of an otherwise relatively healthy artery causes severe symptoms.

5.2 Lower limb arterial disease

Classification
The Fontaine classification is most widely used:

Fontaine I: asymptomatic lower limb arterial disease
Fontaine IIa: claudication > 200 metres
Fontaine IIb: claudication < 200 metres
Fontaine III: rest pain
Fontaine IV: ulceration and/or gangrene.

Clinical features
A detailed history and examination paying particular attention to the cardiovascular system is essential. The key points are:

- history of stroke, transient ischaemic attack
- angina, myocardial infarction
- shortness of breath
- smoking history
- claudication distance, ability to climb stairs, etc

It is important to ascertain how much a patient's symptoms interfere with his/her lifestyle and to gauge the quality of life.

Claudication. The most common clinical presentation of PAOD is pain during exercise, a symptom known as claudication. Typically, claudication occurs most often in the calf, but may also involve the thigh or buttocks. Frequently, two or even three muscle regions become symptomatic. The pain is cramp-like, only comes on with exercise and is relieved by rest. It is exacerbated by walking quickly, climbing hills, cold weather and some medications (e.g. beta blockers). Claudication is an extremely common symptom.

Physical examination
It is important to evaluate the entire cardiovascular system, not only the peripheral circulation. Listen to the heart; look for signs of right or left heart failure. Measure the blood pressure. Examine for an aneurysm and check for vascular bruits particularly in the abdomen and neck.

Clinical examination of the peripheral vascular system includes careful assessment of femoral and distal pulses together with a search for hair loss, temperature differences, ulceration or any other features of chronic ischaemia.

The detection of iliac and/or femoral bruits is also

important. Reduced femoral pulses or bruits indicate aorto-iliac disease.

Although palpation of pulses can be unreliable, it is a widely recognised method of assessment. Pulses can be documented as either present or absent, but it is more useful to grade pulses according to the following system:

- +++ aneurysmal pulse
- ++ normal pulse
- + diminished pulse
- 0 absent pulse.

Unfortunately, most patients with significant claudication have absent distal pulses, and it is often impossible to discriminate between a limb that is not in any particular danger and a 'threatened' limb with critical ischaemia solely on the basis of absent pulses.

Diagnosis

Routine blood tests. All patients with peripheral vascular disease should have a full blood count, urea and electrolyte, serum glucose and serum cholesterol assay.

ECG and chest X-ray. These investigations should be performed in patients who are to undergo arteriography with a view to intervention, as many will have occult cardiac disease. Also, as these patients are usually heavy smokers there is an increased risk of finding coexisting respiratory disease, especially carcinoma of the bronchus.

Doppler-derived arterial pressure measurements. These should always be made to confirm the presence of arterial disease. Usually, they will be performed with the pressure cuff on the thigh, calf and ankle (Fig. 37). In some patients (e.g. diabetics) arterial calcification of the vessel media renders the vessels incompressible and causes false 'high' readings. In these patients, toe pressure measurements will be of value. The sensitivity of pressure measurements may be enhanced by exercising the patient for 1 minute on a treadmill and assessing the recovery time following exercise.

Arteriography. This is mandatory if any form of therapeutic intervention is being considered. Preliminary colour duplex scans can be used to identify regions of stenosis that might be treated during the initial arteriography. Arteriography (Fig. 38) is usually performed by a retrograde Seldinger technique. This involves passing a catheter percutaneously from the common femoral artery up into the aorta. Using this technique, day-case and outpatient angiography is easy to perform and the risk of complications is minimal. The arteriographic image may be enhanced by intra-arterial or intravenous digital subtraction techniques.

Treatment

There are two options:

- conservative management
- intervention by angioplasty or surgery.

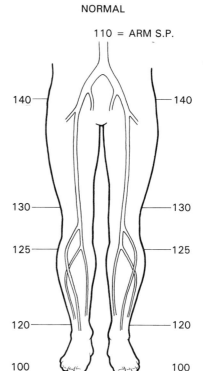

Fig. 37
Doppler-derived arterial pressure measurements in mmHg.

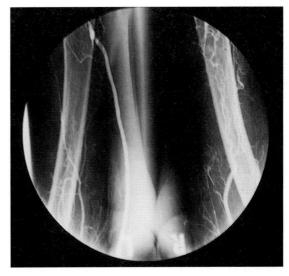

Fig. 38
Arteriogram showing right common femoral occlusion.

Conservative management. The key points are:

- all patients must be encouraged to stop *smoking*
- optimise medical control of hypertension
- institute cholesterol-reduction programmes: a simple modification of dietary intake seems to benefit many patients
- encourage exercise in all patients: a gradual exercise programme will substantially increase a patient's claudication distance over a period of time.

Percutaneous transluminal angioplasty. Percutaneous transluminal angioplasty (PTA) has revolutionised the management of patients with aorto-iliac disease and/or some types of superficial femoral artery disease. Localised stenosis or complete occlusion of the common iliac artery or the external iliac artery can be recanalised with excellent immediate results and 5-year patency rates of more than 70%. Where disease is limited to the superficial femoral artery, PTA may still be used, although long-term patency rates are not as good as bypass surgery (see below).

Technique. PTA is usually carried out under local anaesthesia in the X-ray suite. An angioplasty catheter is passed percutaneously from the groin into the narrowed area and a sausage-shaped balloon is placed across the stenosis or occlusion and inflated. In some cases, a metallic stent may be used to maintain luminal integrity after the dilatation. Patients usually go home the day after angioplasty and are kept on low-dose aspirin therapy as an antiplatelet agent.

Infra-inguinal bypass surgery. This is usually reserved for patients who have very severe ischaemia or who have a severely restricted lifestyle. Most infra-inguinal bypasses (Fig. 39) are performed under regional anaesthesia. Patency rates at 1 year are between 70% and 80%. There is always a small but finite risk of limb loss if a bypass graft fails, so surgery should not be undertaken lightly. Modification of a patient's expectations is often an easier option than surgical intervention.

Aorto-femoral/iliac bypass. Where severe aorto-iliac occlusion is present that is not amenable to PTA, aorto-femoral (or iliac) bypass (Fig. 40) is an option. Although 5-year graft patency rates of > 90% may be obtained, the operative mortality and morbidity with this major surgery are considerable.

Prognosis

The natural history of claudication is difficult to determine. Approximately 25% will deteriorate with time and up to 10% of patients ultimately develop critical limb ischaemia. Of the remainder, some improve, although many suffer repeated cycles of symptom regression/improvement owing to the stepwise progression of the disease.

Up to one-third of all claudicants will die within 5 years of diagnosis, principally from coincidental cardiac disease.

Critical limb ischaemia (CLi)

Critical limb ischaemia (CLi) can be defined as a limb in which the ankle systolic pressure is less than 50 mmHg or the toe pressure is less than 30 mmHg when measured using Doppler techniques. Without intervention these limbs will be lost.

Clinical features

These patients present with:
- rest pain
- gangrene
- ulceration
- a combination of these symptoms.

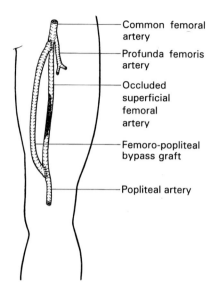

Fig. 39
Infra-inguinal bypass.

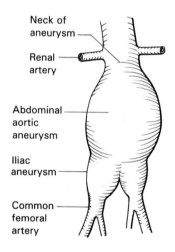

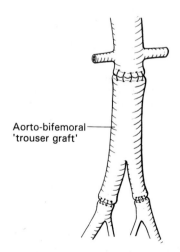

Fig. 40
Aorto-femoral bypass: 'trouser graft'.

Rest pain. This means pain that affects the toes and/or forefoot and is worse when the patient lies horizontally. In this position, the net perfusion pressure to the foot is significantly decreased. Rest pain is worse at night and, in severe cases, patients will sleep upright to avoid discomfort. Rest pain is relieved by standing up and taking a few steps around the bed. Eventually, secondary orthostatic oedema sets in and perfusion is further compromised.

Gangrene. Gangrene means tissue necrosis caused by an inadequate blood supply. Usually this is *dry* and affects the most distal extremities (the toes) first. *Wet* gangrene develops if infection supervenes. Wet gangrene spreads rapidly and leads to a severely compromised limb, systemic sepsis and death if there is no intervention. Such a sequence of events is more likely to occur in a diabetic patient.

Ulceration. The following factors predispose to ulceration:

- neuropathy (e.g. diabetes)
- poor nutrition
- severe ischaemia
- prolonged bed-rest
- infection.

Ulceration is most commonly seen over pressure areas such as the heel, tips of the toes and the first metatarsal head. Although the intact foot may withstand markedly reduced skin perfusion, an ulcerated lesion requires a greatly enhanced blood flow to heal; therefore, many ulcers fail to heal where critical ischaemia exists.

Assessment of critical ischaemia
This can be difficult because distal pulses will invariably be absent and it can be hard to tell which limbs are critically ischaemic and warrant urgent investigation and treatment in contrast to those limbs that have chronic *sub*critical ischaemia, which require less urgent management.

Femoral pulses. Palpation of the femoral pulses is essential and will indicate whether there is aorto-iliac disease, which in turn often determines subsequent management. Treatment of aorto-iliac disease alone may sufficiently improve the inflow of blood to the limb so that it is no longer critically ischaemic.

Investigations. Doppler pressure measurements and urgent angiography are carried out. In the latter, if a digital subtraction technique is used, the distal pedal/ankle vessels may be visualised. Non-visualisation of these vessels on angiography does not always mean they are absent, but the outcome after surgery is likely to be much worse.

Treatment
This depends upon the fitness of the patient, surgical expertise and the availability of an autologous vein from the patient that can be used as a bypass graft.

The treatment options for patients with established critical limb ischaemia are:

- conservative (i.e. analgesia and general supportive measures) (10%)
- primary amputation (10%)
- thrombolysis/angioplasty (10%)
- surgical revascularisation (65–70%).

All patients require vigorous treatment of any coexisting medical disorders. In many cases, improving the cardiac output alone will produce a sufficient increase in peripheral perfusion to abolish rest pain. However, when ulceration or gangrene is present, it is nearly always necessary to improve the blood supply with either angioplasty or surgery.

Acute limb ischaemia

Acute limb ischaemia may be either acute or 'acute-on-chronic'. The latter is more common. The most frequent causes are:

- embolism: (look for evidence of atrial fibrillation, recent cardiac infarct, proximal arterial disease, aortic aneurysm, no collateral circulation)
- acute-on-chronic thrombosis (underlying PAOD), may have a good collateral circulation
- thrombosis of a peripheral aneurysm (e.g. a popliteal aneurysm)
- thrombosis of a previous bypass graft (e.g. femoro-popliteal bypass)
- trauma (direct or indirect)
- intra-arterial injection (e.g. drug abusers).

Clinical features
Classically, an acutely ischaemic limb presents abruptly with severe distal ischaemia characterised by the 'five Ps', although not all will necessarily be present:

pain:	constant and with muscle tenderness
pulseless	
pallor:	white limb which eventually mottles suggesting irreversible ischaemia
paraesthesia:	indicates inadequate circulation for survival
paralysis:	a late sign that suggests underlying muscle necrosis; some limbs with foot drop alone can be salvaged if revascularisation is promptly carried out.

The acutely ischaemic limb will also be cold when compared with the other side.

Treatment
Most of these patients are extremely ill. However, active intervention is usually justified. The first-line *management* is:

- adequate parenteral analgesia
- full anticoagulation with heparin
- optimise cardiovascular status.

If the ischaemia is present for longer than 24 hours, consideration should be given to primary amputation.

If revascularisation appears possible, this should be achieved by:

- thrombolysis
- embolectomy/bypass
- a combination of these methods.

Thrombolysis. This technique is ideal as it allows:

- initial visualisation of the disease by angiography
- lysis of the clot
- angioplasty, if necessary.

Lysis is best achieved using recombinant tissue plasminogen activator or streptokinase infused via an intra-arterial catheter directly into the clot and the affected artery. If the artery remains blocked after 12 hours of treatment, surgical intervention may be required. Close cooperation between surgeon and radiologist is essential.

Surgery. Surgery for limb salvage is a major undertaking. Often an operation that sets out to be a simple 'embolectomy' will fail and only a distal bypass procedure (e.g. a bypass from the femoral artery to the posterior tibial artery) will save the limb. The surgeon must be able and willing to undertake this technically demanding procedure from the outset should embolectomy be unsuccessful. True emboli are less common; many suspected emboli turn out to be an acute or chronic arterial thrombosis.

Anaesthesia. Local anaesthesia is rarely suitable for these procedures, which should be undertaken under regional anaesthesia. If revascularisation is successful, the affected limb may swell acutely (the postoperative compartment syndrome). For this reason, decompression fasciotomies may be required at the time of the original operation to prevent this complication, which can endanger a satisfactorily revascularised limb.

Reperfusion syndrome. The greatest danger to these patients after successful revascularisation is the 'reperfusion syndrome'. This is caused by the release of toxic metabolites and oxygen free radicals into the systemic circulation from the ischaemic limb. This can cause a profound cardiovascular collapse with renal and sometimes respiratory failure.

Prognosis

The duration of limb ischaemia is crucial to the final outcome. If it is less than 6 to 8 hours, a good result can be expected. Any longer and the limb may suffer irreversible damage. Up to 25% of patients with an acutely ischaemic leg will die without leaving hospital. Of the remainder, up to 20% will require a major amputation.

Amputation

Incidence

Peripheral arterial occlusive disease and/or diabetes is the cause of >90% of major limb amputations in Western Europe. In the UK, between 5000 and 7000 major limb amputations are performed annually. Up to 40% of amputees die within 2 years of amputation and a further 30% may develop critical ischaemia in the remaining limb that requires either a second amputation or limb salvage surgery.

Indications

Although unsuccessful revascularisation procedures carry a high perioperative morbidity, primary amputation should only be offered when revascularisation is considered inappropriate; for example:

- in bed-ridden patients
- in a functionally useless limb
- in patients with life-threatening sepsis
- where revascularisation is technically impossible.

Amputation may also have to be considered if revascularisation fails leaving a patient with:

- gangrene/necrosis of part of a limb
- severe ulceration
- rest pain
- a combination of these features.

Investigations

Most patients considered for amputation should have already had an arteriogram and have been seen by a vascular surgeon with consideration given to salvaging the limb.

Major amputations. Above knee amputation (AKA) or 'transfemoral amputation' is associated with a much poorer outcome. After a below knee (BKA) or 'transtibial amputation', up to 80% of patients become independently mobile because the knee joint is preserved and also because a lighter prosthesis is used.

Minor amputations. Toe and transmetatarsal resections are rarely possible in the presence of critical ischaemia without first revascularising the limb. In some diabetic patients, with little or no large vessel involvement (e.g. diabetic neuropathy or osteomyelitis), minor amputation may alone be successful.

Treatment

Patients who require amputation are usually elderly, have end-stage peripheral vascular disease and frequently have life-threatening coexistent medical conditions. The key points in their *management* are:

- a careful preoperative cardiovascular renal and pulmonary evaluation
- amputation under regional anaesthesia
- antibiotic prophylaxis
- aggressive treatment of any established infection.

Early fitting of a temporary prosthesis and early mobilisation in an acute rehabilitation unit (with the aid of occupational therapists and physiotherapists) will maximise the chance of a successful independent return to the community.

Prognosis

Emergency amputation carries a mortality of up to 50% because of severe sepsis and the effects of tissue necrosis.

5.3 Cerebrovascular disease

Epidemiology

Stroke (a cerebrovascular accident or CVA) is the third most common cause of death in Western society and causes an enormous financial and sociological burden to the community. Currently, strokes are becoming less common because of dietary improvements and better control of systemic hypertension.

Up to 25% of patients will die following their first stroke. Of the remainder:

- one-third recover fully
- one-third have a non-disabling deficit
- one-third require permanent support.

Of these survivors, one-third will have a second CVA within 5 years and almost one-half will die from myocardial ischaemia during the same period.

Aetiology

There are three major causes for CVAs:

- small vessel intracerebral disease (arteriosclerosis) usually secondary to hypertension (50%)
- extracranial cerebrovascular cause (30%): of this group, the vast majority have carotid bifurcation disease
- haemorrhage (20%), either subarachnoid or intracerebral.

The major risk factors for CVA are:

- hypertension
- smoking
- hyperlipidaemia
- diabetes.

A combination of these risk factors places an individual at a much greater risk of having a stroke than any single factor.

Pathophysiology

Carotid disease causes CVAs mainly by acting as a source for distal emboli (Fig. 41), which damage the cerebral circulation. The brain can tolerate slowly progressive carotid disease remarkably well and sometimes both the internal carotid and the vertebral arteries can be completely occluded with minimal symptoms! In contrast, acute occlusion or embolisation to an important area (e.g. speech) can be devastating. Major carotid stenoses are associated with compound haemorrhagic plaques and intimal disruption and, hence, an increased risk of embolisation.

Clinical features

Cerebrovascular disease can present in several different ways:

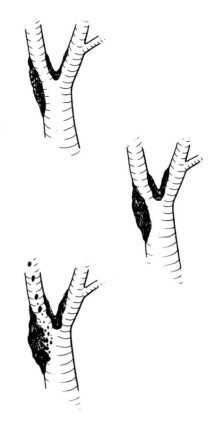

Fig. 41
Carotid plaque causing stenosis and giving rise to distal emboli.

Asymptomatic carotid artery stenosis. Usually detected by eliciting a carotid bruit in an otherwise asymptomatic patient. Frequently these bruits are caused by external carotid artery disease.

Amaurosis fugax. A transient monocular loss of vision, often described as 'a veil' coming down across the eye. Acute permanent loss of vision in one eye is caused by occlusion of the central retinal artery or a retinal vein thrombosis. Eye signs are a frequent finding in cerebrovascular disease because the ophthalmic artery is the first branch of the internal carotid artery.

Transient ischaemic attacks (TIAs). These are defined as localising and usually lateralising symptoms where the motor and/or sensory deficit lasts less than 24 hours. Although there are other causes of TIAs, embolisation from the carotid bifurcation is of the greatest importance because it can be effectively treated.

Stroke. This is the first symptom for many patients with cerebrovascular disease, although close questioning will often elicit preceding symptoms.

Dizziness, vertigo and fainting. These are very poor indicators of cerebrovascular disease and only a few patients with these non-localising symptoms will have significant carotid artery disease.

Diagnosis

A careful case history and physical examination is the key step in evaluating patients who have had symptoms or signs of a cerebral insult. Only patients who appear to have carotid disease should be subject to further carotid investigation.

All patients with suspected carotid disease should have their blood pressure and cardiac status evaluated fully and treated.

Duplex scanning is the key diagnostic test. The technique combines B-mode ultrasound with pulsed Doppler wave-form analysis and has almost replaced the need for carotid angiography even when surgery is contemplated. Duplex scanning enables an accurate evaluation of the degree of stenosis and plaque morphology. The method is cheap, non-invasive and easily repeatable.

Treatment

The form of treatment depends on the results of these investigations. The aim of surgery is prophylaxis, i.e. to prevent a stroke. Unless contraindicated, all patients should receive aspirin.

1. Patients with a symptomatic stenotic lesion of over 70% should undergo carotid endarterectomy if their life expectancy is more than 1 year.
2. Asymptomatic patients with over 70% stenosis may be offered carotid endarterectomy in certain cases.
3. Surgery should not be undertaken for stenoses of less than 30%.

The correct treatment for symptomatic stenoses between 30% and 70% (either conservative measures or carotid endarterectomy) remains uncertain.

Prognosis

The major causes of death in these patients are either a catastrophic cardiac event or a perioperative stroke. Patients at highest risk are those with previous CVAs or severe contralateral carotid disease. However, it is this group of patients who are most likely to benefit from surgery.

5.4 Aneurysms

An aneurysm is a localised or a diffuse dilatation of an artery. There are two types of aneurysm:

- true aneurysm, where the wall is made up of diseased arterial tissue
- false (or pseudo) aneurysm, where the wall is made up partly of artery and partly with compressed surrounding tissue.

Aneurysmal disease is associated with peripheral vascular disease, hypertension and advancing age. It is not clear why some patients develop occlusive vascular disease while others develop aneurysmal disease.

Abdominal aneurysms

Abdominal aortic aneurysms (AAAs) are frequent and invariably fatal if untreated after rupture. Aneurysms account for 1–2% of male deaths in Western Europe and are five times more common in men than in women. Up to 10% of all patients with peripheral vascular disease will have a detectable AAA. Some will also have a peripheral aneurysm.

The natural history is unpredictable: some gradually increase in size over a number of years; some expand in a stepwise fashion; while others remain static.

Clinical features

Most AAA's present either as an asymptomatic finding on routine examination (a pulsatile abdominal mass) or as an acute rupture causing collapse and hypotension. Other symptoms include distal embolisation by clot originating from the aortic sac and non-specific abdominal and/or loin pain and backache.

The majority of patients with AAAs > 5 cm will have a palpable abdominal mass in the epigastrium that is pulsatile; in some obese patients, even very large AAAs may be impossible to detect.

Over 95% of AAAs arise from below the renal arteries. Aneurysms that extend above the renal arteries are more difficult to repair and there is an increased morbidity.

Diagnosis

Ultrasound is the simplest definitive test. It allows accurate sizing of the aneurysm although the proximal extent is usually poorly visualised. A CT scan may provide important preoperative information about the neck of the aneurysm in relation to the renal arteries. Also, in stable patients with backache a CT scan may confirm if a leak has taken place.

Treatment

Symptomatic aneurysms of any size require urgent or emergency surgery. Rupture is much more common if the transverse diameter of the AAA is greater than 5.5 cm. Surgery should be offered for all *asymptomatic* patients with an AAA of more than 5.5 cm who are fit enough to withstand major surgery.

The role of elective surgery in small aneurysms (between 4 cm and 5.5 cm) is currently being evaluated.

The operation involves replacing the aneurysmal segment of the aorta with a straight tube prosthetic graft or a bifurcated ('trouser') graft if the iliac vessels are involved in the aneurysm.

Complications. The main complications after surgery are:

Early
- haemorrhage
- myocardial infarction
- renal failure
- distal embolisation

Late
- colonic ischaemia
- graft infection.

Prognosis

The mortality rate from elective surgery varies from 2% to 6%, depending upon the selection criteria: older patients with larger aneurysms are at higher risk of perioperative death, especially if they have coexistent cardiac disease. The mortality rate increases dramatically after rupture to 30–50%.

After successful AAA surgery, most patients return to a normal lifestyle and a near normal life expectancy.

Peripheral aneurysms

These are often multiple. The more common sites for peripheral aneurysms are:

- popliteal: often bilateral
- femoral: often a pseudo-aneurysm
- iliac: isolated iliac aneurysms are uncommon, they are often associated with an aortic aneurysm
- carotid: rare
- splenic: associated with pregnancy; best treated by therapeutic embolisation
- renal: relatively benign.

If any single aneurysm is identified, a careful search should be undertaken to ensure another potentially more serious aneurysm does not coexist.

Popliteal aneurysms. These are the most frequent type of peripheral aneurysm and most should be repaired if greater than 2 cm in size. Untreated they may thrombose or embolise causing acute limb ischaemia. Occasionally they will rupture. Simple ligation and bypass is all that is required.

Femoral aneurysms. True femoral aneurysms are uncommon and most are secondary to previous vascular surgery. Repair can be difficult as an underlying graft infection may be the cause.

5.5 Other peripheral arterial diseases

Visceral artery vascular disease

Renal artery atherosclerosis

This is usually asymptomatic. Occasionally it causes hypertension or renal failure. These patients are usually high-risk surgical candidates and are frequently unsuitable for surgery. The diagnosis is often made as part of a work-up for other vascular disease.

The treatment options are:

- angioplasty
- bypass grafting
- endarterectomy.

Although the renal failure often responds to treatment, the hypertension frequently persists.

Mesenteric arterial vascular disease

Although quite common, this diagnosis is often made too late, either at laparotomy or at postmortem examination. Acute mesenteric ischaemia may result from:

- embolus
- thrombosis
- acute-on-chronic arterial thrombosis.

Clinical features

In an acute case, the abdominal findings are often minimal although the presence of significant arterial disease elsewhere (e.g. the legs) is a clue. Weight loss may be marked in acute-on-chronic cases and is often erroneously attributed to malignancy. *Chronic* mesenteric ischaemia (abdominal angina) is much less common. It is characterised by:

- weight loss
- postprandial pain
- evidence of generalised peripheral vascular disease
- obvious abdominal bruits on auscultation.

Many of these patients will have had long-standing undiagnosed abdominal pain and have been investigated extensively without a diagnosis.

Diagnosis

The definitive diagnosis is made by:

- mesenteric angiography
- laparoscopy
- laparotomy.

In acute mesenteric ischaemia, a high degree of clinical suspicion is required in order to clinch the diagnosis in time to save the patient. Any delay in reaching the diagnosis may mean that bowel necrosis will supervene and the patient will become inoperable. In acute cases with an embolus, the opportunity for intervention is only a few hours.

In chronic disease, there is sufficient time for mesenteric angiography to be performed. In these cases usually at least two of the three main visceral arteries (coeliac, superior and inferior mesenteric arteries) are occluded.

Treatment

Management must be aimed at revascularisation with or without resection of any non-viable small bowel. In most cases this is achieved by constructing an aorto-coeliac or aorto-superior mesenteric artery bypass using either vein or a synthetic graft. Very occasionally, an embolectomy will be possible. Often, a 'second look' laparotomy after 24 hours will be necessary to ensure the bowel remains viable. A small bowel resection alone is rarely enough to ensure a patient's survival.

Uncommon causes of mesenteric ischaemia

Non-occlusive mesenteric infarction. This can develop in patients who have cardiac low output syndrome (e.g. hypovolaemia, cardiogenic shock, sepsis). There is usually extensive patchy necrosis of the entire gut and no evidence of mesenteric insufficiency on an arteriogram. Treatment is directed toward correcting the underlying problem.

Mesenteric venous thrombosis. This condition presents in a similar way and in the same group of patients. Full heparinisation is the cornerstone of treatment. Outcome depends upon the extent of the venous thrombosis and the amount of secondary arterial infarction.

Thoracic outlet syndrome

This is a group of symptoms linked together because of a common aetiology: compression at the thoracic outlet.

Most present with neurological signs and symptoms of the upper arm while one in 10 have symptoms secondary to compression of the subclavian artery or vein. A cervical rib is the most common cause of these symptoms although in some patients without a cervical rib, adhesions resulting from fibrous scalene muscle bands may be responsible.

Clinical features

Symptoms reflect the principle nerve root(s) involved from C8 to T1. Complaints include:

- pain in the shoulder or arm
- tingling down a dermatome
- weakness in a muscle group
- loss of fine movement in a hand.

Occasionally, where the artery is compressed, upper arm claudication may occur or, very rarely, a stenosed segment may give rise to distal emboli.

Diagnosis

History and examination are crucial steps to the diagnosis as there is no definitive test to confirm that where a cervical rib exists *it is responsible* for the symptoms. Exclusion of local nerve compression problems such as carpal tunnel syndrome or ulnar nerve compression is important. The presence of cervical spondylosis would suggest that this may be the most likely cause for symptoms.

Treatment

Conservative treatment. Conservative measures should be tried first. A supervised exercise programme is used to improve posture and shoulder girdle movements. Where a neurological deficit is already present, treatment is urgent and is aimed at avoiding further deterioration.

Surgical treatment. Where pain is excessive or everyday activity limited, surgical correction may be required. The cervical rib is excised often together with a first rib resection by either a transaxillary or a supraclavicular approach. The results of surgical decompression can dramatically benefit this group of patients.

Arteriovenous malformations

These are a spectrum of disorders in which there are abnormal connections between the venous and arterial systems. The classification is complex and depends upon their histopathology and the nature of their development. Almost all are congenital, although many lie dormant for long periods. Some are soft with predominantly venous elements. Others comprising mainly arterial elements are almost aneurysmal. Invariably they are all far more extensive than apparent clinically and their management and treatment is highly specialised.

Clinical features

The lesions are usually:

- warm
- pulsatile
- compressible
- painless.

Some are slow growing and never become a significant problem to the patient: these can be safely left alone. Others will have spurts of growth (typically at adolescence and during pregnancy) but may otherwise be dormant. Others have an aggressive course with gross enlargement and involvement of a major part of the body.

Complications. These include:

- development of high output cardiac failure
- limb hypertrophy and distortion
- skin necrosis
- major bleeding.

Diagnosis

These malformations are usually confirmed by arteriography and magnetic resonance imaging.

Treatment

The treatment has changed dramatically over the last 10 years as our understanding of these lesions has improved. Excision should rarely be performed unless for a limb-threatening or life-threatening complication. Likewise, ligation of a 'feeder' artery is not only of little value but also destroys a route of access for therapeutic embolisation, which has become the mainstay of treatment. Embolisation is carried out usually in stages and can be repeated if regrowth occurs.

Raynaud's disease and Raynaud's phenomenon

Raynaud's 'disease' was originally described as signs and symptoms caused by an over sensitivity to the sympathetic nervous drive. The exact pathophysiology of the disorder is still uncertain.

The term 'Raynaud's disease' has been superseded by the classification of this syndrome into primary and secondary Raynaud's phenomenon.

Primary Raynaud's phenomenon

This is an episodic, vasospastic disorder of the extremities causing hypersensitivity of the hands and feet to cold and stressful stimuli. Attacks are irregular and unpredictable and are characterised by digital blanching followed by cyanosis and reactive hyperaemia as the vasospasm abates. This rewarming is accompanied by quite severe pain in the affected digits. The whole attack generally lasts less than 30 minutes. The symptoms are usually bilateral and patterns of digital involvement are symmetrical. Primary Raynaud's phenomenon is extremely common and affects up to 5% of young women. It is a self-limiting benign condition and probably never leads to digital necrosis or ulceration. A few of these patients will, in time, be shown to have secondary Raynaud's phenomenon.

Treatment

Management for primary Raynaud's phenomenon is supportive such as heated gloves and socks. Nifedipine (a calcium channel blocker that relaxes vascular smooth muscle) is used to provide maintenance therapy, with increased doses for acute exacerbations.

Secondary Raynaud's phenomenon

This is more serious and implies an underlying pathology, usually a collagen vascular disease (vasculitis). Common causes are:

- scleroderma
- rheumatoid arthritis
- systemic lupus
- vibration white finger (prolonged use of vibrating tools, e.g. road drills)
- atherosclerosis
- malignancy.

Treatment

The management of secondary Raynaud's phenomenon is directed at treating the underlying pathology, when known. Severe exacerbations require hospitalisation, especially during the winter months, in order to treat digital ulceration and/or necrosis. Intravenous prostacycline relieves the symptoms in some of these patients, who sustain a benefit of up to several months with just one infusion course.

Acrocyanosis

This is one form of the spectrum of vasospastic disorders where there is a more constant cyanotic element to the extremity. This is quite common in young patients. Treatment is as for Raynaud's.

Erythromelalgia

This is another sympathetic nerve disorder, where the prevailing symptom is a burning (painful) extremity that is hyperaemic.

Vibration white finger syndrome

This is caused by protracted exposure and sensitivity to many types of vibration tool, as used in industry.

Establishing this diagnosis is important because morphological changes in the arterioles and nerves will eventually supervene, with long-standing symptoms. It is recognised as an occupational disease and attracts many claims for compensation.

5.6 Venous disease

Varicose veins

Primary varicose veins and deep venous insufficiency are the main venous diseases that present to the surgeon. Varicose veins are common and affect up to half the population at some time during their life. Curiously, varicose veins are almost non-existent in many non-western countries.

Varicose veins can be classified as primary (idiopathic) or secondary.

Secondary varicose veins are a consequence of deep venous insufficiency. In order to understand the management of venous disease, it is important to have a working knowledge of the anatomy, physiology and pathophysiology of the venous system.

Anatomy and pathophysiology

There are two venous systems in the leg:

- superficial veins that drain the skin and subcutaneous tissue; the long and short saphenous veins are the major vessels
- deep veins that drain the muscles of the leg.

Both systems are connected by numerous perforating veins, which normally have competent valves that allow blood to flow from the superficial to the deep systems only. Normally, the superficial system drains into the deep system at the sapheno-femoral junction (long saphenous vein) and at the sapheno-popliteal junction (short saphenous vein).

Sustained high venous pressure in the superficial veins is prevented by:

- the muscle pump effect (when walking), which squeezes blood from the distal venous system proximally
- deep vein valves and perforator vein valves which prevent retrograde flow into the superficial venous system.

Together, these mechanisms facilitate flow from the superficial venous system into the deep venous system. Failure of either the perforator valves or the deep venous valves allows blood to flow back into the superficial system and will cause a high superficial venous pressure.

Deep venous insufficiency develops when the deep valves are incompetent. This creates a constant high deep venous pressure, known as ambulatory venous hypertension.

Clinical features

Cosmetic problems, aching, discomfort or a sensation of heaviness of the legs on standing are the main complaints. Severe pain is not usually a symptom unless there is evidence of superficial phlebitis. Four out of five of all patients are women.

Careful assessment of all patients with 'primary' varicose veins is extremely important. Any history suggestive of a previous deep venous thrombosis (DVT) should be elicited. Evidence of possible underlying deep venous insufficiency should be sought, e.g. leg swelling (especially if it is unilateral), haemosiderin staining of the skin and a history of previous or current leg ulceration. If there is any doubt, a more detailed investigation with photoplethysmography and/or venography will be required.

Physical examination should identify saphenofemoral reflux either using a finger to palpate a thrill or using a hand-held Doppler probe to detect reflux in the groin and popliteal regions.

Investigations

Trendelenburg test. Finger tip or tourniquet control of the sapheno-femoral junction can be used to demonstrate sapheno-femoral incompetence.

Photoplethysmography. This can be used to assess venous refilling time after mild exercise. This non-invasive technique correlates well with direct venous pressure measurements. Application of superficial tourniquets and repetition of this test may allow isolation of the region of the leg in which perforator incompetence is present.

Treatment

There are four treatment options for primary varicose veins:

- reassurance
- injection sclerotherapy
- compression stockings
- surgery.

Reassurance. Conservative management with or without support stockings is often possible once patients with minor varicosities realise there is no absolute need for treatment.

Sclerotherapy. The original concept was to inject sclerosant at sites of perforator incompetence. However, accurate identification of these sites is often difficult. The benefit of treatment mainly relates to the obliteration of superficial varicosities. Sclerotherapy is performed on an outpatient basis and may require multiple courses of injections. The technique is useful for minor below knee varicosities and residual varicosities after surgery but not for major varicosities. There is a risk of damage to the deep veins by the highly irritant sclerosant which may cause permanent deep venous insufficiency.

Compression stockings. These are specially manufactured stockings that provide graduated compression from the foot to the thigh and should be worn during periods of prolonged standing; because they lose their elasticity, they should be renewed at least every 6 months.

Surgical treatment

Surgery for primary varicose veins involves three steps:

1. sapheno-femoral ligation
2. above knee saphenous stripping
3. multiple avulsion of varicosities.

With meticulous surgery, the results are excellent (less than 5% recurrence rates). If the primary treatment is inadequate, recurrence rates may be over 20%. Surgery is best performed under regional anaesthesia and the patient allowed home the following day. Selected cases may be carried out as day-case surgery. After surgery, patients are advised to wear support stockings for 3 to 6 weeks to minimise bruising and maximise comfort.

Complications. These are uncommon. Leg ulceration is rarely the sequel to primary varicose veins. Superficial thrombophlebitis is more common with severe varicosities and may be mistaken for a deep venous thrombosis. It is treated with anti-inflammatory drugs and support bandages. Only if thrombophlebitis extends to the sapheno-femoral junction is there any danger of pulmonary embolisation. Urgent saphenofemoral ligation may be required.

Deep venous insufficiency

Deep venous insufficiency exists when the deep valves have been previously damaged, usually by a deep vein thrombosis (DVT). It is particularly common after limb fractures, major surgery, pregnancy and prolonged bed rest. In many cases, the previous DVT will have been asymptomatic and the clinical features of deep venous insufficiency can take 10–20 years to manifest.

Patients may present with various symptoms:

- common
  - leg swelling
  - secondary varicose veins
  - eczema
  - thickened sclerotic skin (lipodermatosclerosis)
- less common
  - ulceration
  - venous claudication (very rare).

Diagnosis

The key investigations are: venous plethysmography, duplex scanning of veins and venography.

Treatment

The management of deep venous insufficiency depends upon the symptoms. In fit patients, surgery to coexisting superficial varicose veins combined with long-term compression stockings is the optimum treatment.

Venous ulceration

Ulceration is most likely in patients who have constant ambulatory venous hypertension. Where ulceration is present, Doppler arterial pressures should be checked to ensure there is no coexisting arterial component. The mainstay of treatment to *pure* venous ulceration is the application of sustained compression therapy to improve deep venous flow and reduce superficial venous stasis. The most consistent and reliable compression pressures will be obtained with support stockings placed over appropriate dressings.

Venous ulceration accounts for 80–90% of all leg ulcers and accounts for a considerable amount of time lost from work. The exact pathophysiology of ulceration secondary to venous disease is uncertain but it is probably caused by a combination of factors leading to hypoxia in the skin itself. The medial aspect of the calf is most frequently affected.

Other causes of lower limb ulcers are:

- arterial
- neuropathic
- malignant.

Arterial ulcers are usually sited on the toes or lateral aspect of the calf above the malleolus. It is important to differentiate them as compression treatment will make them worse. Neuropathic ulcers occur in weight or pressure bearing areas (e.g. sole of the foot); they are aggravated by impaired sensation (e.g. in diabetes). In any ulcer which refuses to heal the possibility of malignant change should be considered and a biopsy will be necessary.

Treatment

Healing can be extremely slow, but is improved by:

- foot elevation
- compression
- local treatment of infection.

  Occasionally, skin grafting (especially pinch skin grafting) may speed up healing. Antibiotics are only used if there is evidence of systemic sepsis or severe cellulitis in the limb.

Once an ulcer is healed, the patient will need to wear support stockings for life to prevent recurrence.

Self-assessment: questions

Multiple choice questions

1. Atherosclerosis:
   a. Is caused by being overweight
   b. Is more common in non-western countries
   c. Is most commonly found in the radial arteries
   d. May be found in the arteries of children
   e. Is more common in men

2. In the management of intermittent claudication:
   a. Quality of life is more important than absolute walking distance
   b. The absence of femoral pulses suggests inoperability
   c. Arteriography should always be performed
   d. Most patients should be offered surgery
   e. Exercise should always be encouraged

3. In critical ischaemia:
   a. Rest pain may be relieved by taking a few steps around the bed
   b. Rest pain may be found in the calf muscles
   c. The diagnosis is confirmed by the absence of pulses
   d. Most patients will require revascularisation
   e. Primary amputation of gangrenous toes is usually successful

4. The following points relate to drugs commonly used in vascular disease:
   a. Beta blockers can improve muscle blood flow
   b. Aspirin reduces cardiac mortality
   c. Tissue plasminogen activator is a major cause of acute thrombosis
   d. Anticoagulation with warfarin should aim for an INR (international normalised ratio) of > 10
   e. Sensitivity to heparin can cause thrombosis

5. In patients with cerebrovascular disease:
   a. Most strokes are caused by intracerebral haemorrhage
   b. Carotid surgery should always be carried out for stenosis > 50%
   c. About one in four stroke patients will die from their initial CVA
   d. Dizziness is a common symptom of carotid disease
   e. Duplex ultrasound is the investigation of choice for carotid disease

6. Deep venous thrombosis:
   a. Is best diagnosed clinically
   b. Is always preventable by subcutaneous heparin
   c. Is common after pelvic surgery
   d. May lead to venous ulceration in later life
   e. Should usually be treated with a vena cava filter

7. Varicose veins:
   a. Are a rare cause of pulmonary embolus
   b. Usually are asymptomatic
   c. Are best dealt with by surgery
   d. Are generally secondary to deep venous insufficiency
   e. Affect 2% of the population

8. The following features are characteristic of venous ulcers:
   a. They are never painful
   b. They are usually found on the medial aspect of the lower leg
   c. They are best treated with high compression (class III) support hose
   d. They usually require hospitalisation
   e. They are 10 times more common than arterial ulcers

9. The following statements relate to aortic aneurysms:
   a. They never rupture if less than 3 cm in diameter
   b. They are more common in men
   c. Repair should be undertaken if they are > 5.5 cm in diameter
   d. Most are found incidentally in patients
   e. They are associated with a > 10% elective operative mortality

10. Raynaud's phenomenon is:
    a. Extremely common in young women
    b. Best treated with cervical sympathectomy
    c. Usually secondary to an underlying disorder
    d. Also known as acrocyanosis
    e. Is associated with a benign course in most patients

11. Which of the following statements concerning peripheral vascular disease are true?
    a. Treatment of hypertension reduces the risk of stroke
    b. Diabetics are less likely to require amputation for arterial disease
    c. Atherosclerosis is more common in diabetics than in non-diabetics
    d. Amputation for critical limb ischaemia is best performed above the knee
    e. Balloon angioplasty of the iliac arteries is generally unsuccessful

Case histories

Case history 1

A 60-year-old man is brought into casualty with a 6-hour history of severe pain in his right foot with numbness and paralysis. He is a lifelong smoker and attended the casualty department 3 days previously with central chest pain.

1. What is the likely diagnosis?
2. How would you proceed to investigate the problem?
3. How should he be managed?
4. What is his prognosis?

Case history 2

An 80-year-old man is brought into A & E with a history of sudden collapse associated with severe back pain 2 hours previously. On admission, his blood pressure is 90/60 mmHg; his pulse rate is 110/min and he is cold and sweaty. Examination reveals a tender abdomen and left flank with the suspicion of a mass.

1. Describe your initial management.
2. What is the likely differential diagnosis?
3. What tests should be performed?
4. What is his prognosis?

Short notes

Write short notes on:
1. popliteal aneurysms
2. mesenteric ischaemia
3. deep venous insufficiency
4. atherosclerotic risk factors.

Photograph question

Photograph 1 shows the angiogram of a 62-year-old woman who was admitted with severe claudication in both legs.
1. Describe the appearance.
2. What is the diagnosis?
3. What further investigations should be performed?
4. How should she be managed?

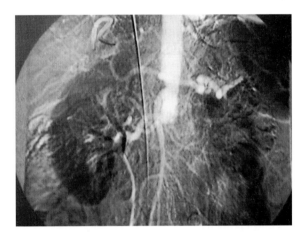

Photograph 1

Self-assessment: answers

Multiple choice answers

1. a. **False**. Excess fat is not a cause of atherosclerosis although it may be a secondary phenomenon.
   b. **False**. It is a disease of Western environments and perhaps genetic make-up.
   c. **False**. It is most commonly seen at bifurcations and in the lower limbs.
   d. **True**. Atheroma has been detected in the arteries of children before their teens.
   e. **True**. Atherosclerosis is more frequently seen in men.

2. a. **True**. The patient's existing quality of life is the most important determinant for intervention in claudication.
   b. **False**. Femoral pulses may often be absent (indicating aorto-femoral disease); these patients are usually operable.
   c. **False**. Arteriography should only be performed if intervention is being considered.
   d. **False**. Most patients are treated conservatively.
   e. **True**. By encouraging exercise with a graduated exercise programme many patients will develop an improvement in their claudication distance and the need for surgery will be obviated.

3. a. **True**. In critical ischaemia, rest pain is paradoxically relieved by standing out of bed and taking a few steps.
   b. **False**. True rest pain occurs in the toes and the foot.
   c. **False**. Absent pulses are a common finding in arterial disease and do not necessarily signify critical ischaemia.
   d. **True**. Revascularisation is usually the only option if the critically ischaemic limb is to be saved.
   e. **False**. Primary toe amputations rarely heal in the absence of pure diabetes; preliminary revascularisation of the limb is usually required.

4. a. **False**. Beta blockade reduces muscle blood flow.
   b. **True**. Aspirin has been clearly shown to reduce both the frequency of myocardial infarction and the mortality following infarction.
   c. **False**. Tissue plasminogen activator is a naturally occurring thrombolytic agent and may be given by the intra-arterial or intravenous route to achieve thrombolysis.
   d. **False**. An INR of > 10 is extremely dangerous: doses should aim at a therapeutic range of between 2 and 3.5 depending upon the indication.
   e. **True**. Hypersensitivity to heparin can induce thrombocytopenia; this is an uncommon but extremely important cause of intravascular

thrombosis as the treatment is cessation of heparin. Watch out for a platelet count of < 100 000 during prolonged heparin therapy.

5. a. **True**. Most strokes are caused by intracerebral haemorrhage or infarction; only some are caused by extracranial carotid disease producing thrombosis or embolism.
   b. **False**. Carotid endarterectomy should be carried out for symptomatic stenoses > 70% in those who are fit. Most patients with a 50–70% stenosis can be treated conservatively.
   c. **True**. About 25% of stroke patients will die from their initial CVA.
   d. **False**. Non-localising/non-lateralising symptoms such as dizziness are rarely caused by carotid artery disease.
   e. **True**. Duplex ultrasound is the gold standard investigation in carotid disease; it has replaced angiography as the procedure of choice.

6. a. **False**. Clinical evaluation is inaccurate; a DVT is only present in 25–50% of clinically suspicious limbs. A duplex scan is the best diagnostic tool.
   b. **False**. Although subcutaneous heparin administration reduces the incidence of a DVT and may reduce the incidence of a fatal pulmonary embolism, these conditions are not completely prevented.
   c. **True**. A DVT is particularly common after pelvic or major orthopaedic surgery.
   d. **True**. A DVT may lead to chronic deep vein insufficiency which may progress to venous ulceration.
   e. **False**. Inferior vena cava filters should only be used if there is a contraindication to anticoagulation or in patients who have suffered pulmonary emboli despite apparently adequate anticoagulation.

7. a. **True**. Varicose veins are an extremely uncommon cause of pulmonary emboli. Very occasionally they are a source if there is thrombophlebitis involving the sapheno-femoral junction.
   b. **True**. Most varicose veins are asymptomatic. Cosmetic problems or an ill-defined ache are the most common reasons for referral for surgery.
   c. **True**. In patients with varicose veins whose symptoms warrant treatment, surgical treatment is the best line of management.
   d. **False**. Most varicose veins are primary or 'idiopathic' and not secondary to underlying deep venous insufficiency.
   e. **False**. At least 10% of the population at any given time have varicose veins.

8. a. **False**. Venous ulcers are rarely painful. Discomfort usually develops when infection supervenes.
   b. **True**. They are usually found on the medial aspect of the ankle and lower calf. Arterial ulcers, in contrast, are often sited on the lateral aspect of the calf or on the foot.
   c. **True**. Extrinsic compression using specially designed support stockings is the best management.
   d. **False**. Patients with venous ulcers rarely require hospitalisation and can be treated on an ambulatory basis.
   e. **True**. Venous disease is the most common cause of lower limb ulceration in Western civilisation. It is about 10 times more common than arterial ulceration.

9. a. **False**. Any aortic aneurysm carries a risk of rupture, although aneurysms of less than 3 cm are very unlikely to rupture.
   b. **True**. They are five times more common in men than in women.
   c. **True**. All aneurysms should be repaired if they are greater than 5.5 cm in diameter provided the patient is fit enough to undertake the operation. The incidence of rupture dramatically increases in aneurysms above this size.
   d. **True**. Most aneurysms are found on accidental examination. Some present with lower abdominal or back pain and others with acute collapse or death after rupture.
   e. **False**. Although the overall mortality for ruptured aneurysms is approximately 50%, the operative mortality for elective aneurysms should be 5% or less.

10. a. **True**. Raynaud's phenomenon is a very common finding in young women.
    b. **False**. Cervical sympathectomy is no longer recommended even in severe cases. Although a temporary improvement was sometimes obtained after this operation, recurrence was frequent within a year.
    c. **False**. Raynaud's phenomenon is usually primary or 'idiopathic'. Only a small number are secondary to an underlying disorder, usually a collagen vascular disease.
    d. **False**. Acrocyanosis is a distinct entity characterised by a persistant cyanosis of the extremities.
    e. **True**. Primary Raynaud's phenomenon has a benign course.

11. a. **True**. Careful treatment of hypertension substantially reduces the risk of stroke in later years. This has been one of the main reasons for the reduction in incidence of cerebrovascular accidents.

   b. **False**. Diabetes is one of the major causes of lower limb amputation.
   c. **True**. Atherosclerosis is much more common in diabetics. Many diabetics who require amputation have a combination of diabetic microangiopathy and atherosclerosis.
   d. **False**. When amputation is necessary for critical limb ischaemia, it should be carried out below the knee (transtibial) if at all possible. Successful rehabilitation is much more likely after a below-knee amputation compared with an above-knee amputation.
   e. **False**. Transluminal angioplasty of the iliac arteries is very successful. Eight out of 10 vessels so treated will remain patent 5 years after the procedure.

Case history answers

Case history 1

1. An acute thrombotic or embolic event to the right leg is likely. The presence of two or more of the following clinical features would support this:

   - pain
   - pallor
   - paralysis
   - paraesthesia
   - absent pulses.

   The recent attendance with chest pain raises the possibility of a cardiac source of emboli such as atrial fibrillation/flutter or myocardial infarct. A past history of claudication may suggest underlying PAOD.
2. Doppler pressure studies will confirm arterial occlusion. A careful cardiac assessment is essential. Particularly important is an ECG to exclude a recent myocardial infarction (which might produce a mural thrombus) and the evaluation of any rhythm disturbance.
3. Absence of sensation and/or movement in the limb heralds limb loss unless surgery is urgently undertaken. There are several options: emergency angiography followed by thrombolysis or thrombo-embolectomy and/or bypass.
4. If the patient has had a recent myocardial infarct, the risks during operative intervention will be considerable.

Case history 2

1. The first step in this patient's management is to determine whether the collapse results from cardiac or intra-abdominal causes. Venous access should be immediately established using a wide-bore cannula. A careful history and physical examination should be performed to exclude, as far as possible, a cardiac

cause for his collapse, followed by a thorough abdominal examination.

During his initial assessment and resuscitation, his vital signs should be monitored at frequent intervals and a urinary catheter should be passed to allow measurement of his urinary output.

2. The key differential diagnoses are:
   - leaking aortic aneurysm
   - myocardial infarction
   - mesenteric infarction
   - visceral perforation with peritonitis.

   Careful examination of the abdomen should elicit the cardinal signs of peritonitis if a perforated viscus is present. The detection of a tender diffuse pulsatile mass in the abdomen would be virtually diagnostic of a leaking abdominal aortic aneurysm. These patients require urgent surgery.

3. The following tests should be undertaken:
   a. blood should be drawn for urea and electrolytes, full blood count and group and cross-match of 6 units
   b. an ECG should be performed to look for evidence of a myocardial infarction
   c. if time permits, a chest X-ray and plain abdominal X-ray should be performed
   d. in a few cases where the patient is stable, an urgent CT scan may be helpful in the diagnosis.

4. The survival rate for ruptured aortic aneurysm after surgery is approximately 50%. Most deaths are caused by severe postoperative complications such as bleeding, renal or respiratory failure, stroke or myocardial infarction.

Short notes answers

1. Popliteal aneurysms are the most common peripheral arterial aneurysms. They are usually asymptomatic and are frequently bilateral. Acute symptoms are usually caused by thrombosis of the aneurysm, which may cause acute ischaemia of the limb either directly or by producing emboli. Popliteal aneurysms rarely rupture. Once detected, a careful search should be undertaken for other aneurysms, e.g. iliac or aortic aneurysms, which are frequently associated with popliteal aneurysms and are potentially lethal.

   B-mode ultrasound is a simple non-invasive diagnostic test for popliteal aneurysms. A local popliteal bypass is the treatment of choice.

2. Mesenteric ischaemia is a common intra-abdominal catastrophe in elderly patients, particularly if they have coexisting peripheral vascular disease. It can be extremely difficult to make a clinical diagnosis as there are no specific diagnostic tests. A high index of suspicion is required in patients who have unexplained abdominal pain and peripheral arterial disease.

   Mesenteric ischaemia may be classified as:

   - acute ischaemia
   - acute-on-chronic ischaemia
   - chronic ischaemia.

   Acute ischaemia is a catastrophic event that often results in complete infarction of most or all of the small or large intestine. Survival is very unlikely as most patients will not have their operation in time to salvage the intestines.

   The outcome in patients with acute-on-chronic ischaemia is marginally better as they have an extensive collateral intestinal blood supply that will sustain the bowel.

   Patients with chronic mesenteric ischaemia present with abdominal angina, weight loss and fear of eating. In these cases, the diagnosis is best made using mesenteric angiography.

   In all three groups of patients, the optimum treatment involves revascularisation of the coeliac and/or superior mesenteric arteries coupled with resection of non-viable bowel.

3. Deep vein insufficiency is a functional disorder of the deep veins of the lower limb where there is incompetence of some or all of the valves in the veins. Deep venous insufficiency develops as a result of previous deep venous thrombosis. In some patients who have had a 'silent' deep vein thrombosis, there may be no significant previous history.

   Clinical symptoms include leg swelling, secondary varicose veins and skin changes, including venous ulceration in more severe cases. The diagnosis is best established on a combination of clinical and laboratory criteria. Venous photoplethysmography and in some cases ascending and descending lower limb venography will demonstrate valvular incompetence.

   Patients with deep venous insufficiency have ambulatory venous hypertension, i.e. permanent high pressure in the superficial venous system because of failure of the muscle pump system. In the long term, damage to the skin microcirculation occurs. Lifelong support compression stockings, which are worn during the day, are the best management option. This treatment will alleviate, though not cure, the superficial venous problem. There is little role for surgery.

4. All patients who present with vascular disease should be assessed and counselled about their risk factors. The most important risk factor is a family history, which of course cannot be modified. However, there are several risk factors that can be modified in most patients. These include smoking, high serum cholesterol, poor diabetic control (where relevant), high blood pressure, sedentary lifestyle, previous cardiovascular events and obesity.

   Although the greatest benefit derived from altering these risk factors is obtained in younger patients, there is evidence that reducing smoking, treating hypertension, plus administration of aspirin in selected cases, will significantly improve both cardiac and cerebrovascular morbidity and mortality in all age groups.

Photograph answer

1. This is an intravenous digital subtraction angiogram of the aorta and iliac arteries. There is a complete occlusion of the aorta at the level of the inferior mesenteric artery which can be seen as a large tortuous vessel communicating with the superior mesenteric system proximally. The common iliac arteries are not really seen and are probably occluded. The external iliac arteries are just visible where they have been reconstituted by collateral flow.

2. The patient has a bilateral iliac occlusion. This is likely to be a chronic occlusive rather than an acute occlusive episode because of the widespread collateral blood supply, which would have gradually developed over a long period of time.

3. Further investigations include a Doppler pressure assessment and a full cardiac and pulmonary assessment.

4. Depending upon the severity of this patient's symptoms and the effect this has on her quality of life, there are several options:
   a. it may be possible to manage this patient conservatively
   b. alternatively, an aorto-iliac or aorto-femoral bypass will be required
   c. because of the extent of the disease, angioplasty or intravascular stenting is unlikely to help.

Urology

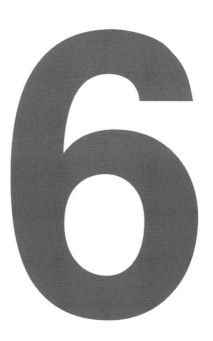

6.1 Structure, function and symptoms

Disease of the urinary tract accounts for a substantial proportion of emergency and elective surgical admissions. The most important disorders of the urinary system, which will be discussed here, are infection, urinary stones, obstruction and malignant tumours.

The central role of the urinary system is the maintenance of fluid and electrolyte balance by the kidneys. The ureters, bladder and urethra together are responsible for continent storage and disposal of urine.

Kidneys

The two kidneys lie against the posterior abdominal wall musculature in a retroperitoneal position, flanking the abdominal aorta and vena cava. Important anatomical relations include the adrenals, the duodenum, the retroperitoneal colon, the spleen and the liver. The kidneys receive a very substantial blood supply—about 20% of the cardiac output. The functional renal unit is the nephron, each consisting of glomerular vessels and Bowman's capsule, and the vasa recta and the renal tubule. There are about one million nephrons per kidney. Filtration of blood at the glomerulus, followed by selective reabsorption and secretion of certain electrolytes and solutes by the renal tubule results in the production of urine.

The renal parenchyma is in two parts; the cortex consists of the glomeruli, the convoluted parts of the tubules and the short tubular loops (of Henle); the medulla consists of the long loops of Henle and the collecting tubules, grouped together to form the renal pyramids (Fig. 42). The collecting system of the kidneys is formed by the calyces, (each calyx cupping one or more renal papillae) and the renal pelvis.

Important congenital anomalies:

- renal agenesis or hypoplasia
- simple or crossed ectopia
- infantile polycystic disease
- adult polycystic disease
- horseshoe kidney.

Ureters

The ureters are completely retroperitoneal in their course. Important bony landmarks of the normal course of the ureter are the tips of the transverse processes of the lumbar vertebrae, the sacroiliac joints and the ischial spines. The ureters transport urine to the bladder by peristalsis, and reflux of urine from the bladder is normally prevented by a valvular mechanism at the vesicoureteric junction.

Important congenital abnormalities:

- pelviureteric junction obstruction
- complete or incomplete ureteric duplication

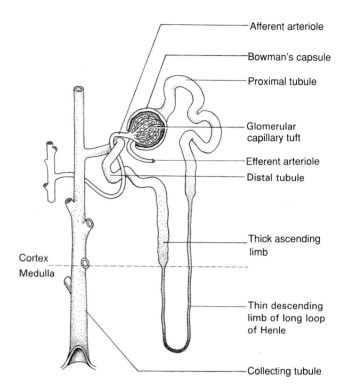

Fig. 42
A nephron.

- vesicoureteric reflux
- megaureter.

Bladder

The empty bladder lies within the true pelvis but rises into the abdomen with filling. The bladder provides a highly compliant reservoir for urine, the pressure within rising only very slightly during normal filling and not normally exceeding urethral pressure except during voluntary voiding. Like the ureter and the pelvicalyceal system of the kidney, the bladder is lined with a transitional cell epithelium.

Congenital anomalies. An important congenital abnormality of the bladder is extrophy, where the anterior abdominal wall, anterior bony pelvis and bladder fail to close properly.

Prostate

The prostate is a male organ that has no normal counterpart in the female. It is a pale firm structure, part muscular and part glandular, lying posterior to the lower part of the symphysis pubis at the neck of the bladder, where it surrounds the proximal part of the urethra (the prostatic urethra). The fibromuscular part of the gland is complex and is concerned with seminal emission, ejaculation and urinary continence. The prostate also has an exocrine secretory function, which is incompletely understood.

Urethra

The proximal urethra and bladder neck form part of the continence mechanism.

Congenital anomalies (of the male urethra):

- posterior urethral valve causes bladder outflow obstruction in the male
- hypospadias, where the ventral part of the anterior urethra fails to close properly.

Testis

Although strictly not part of the urinary tract, disorders of the male gonad and its associated structures, epididymis and vas deferens, are considered part of urology.

Important congenital anomalies. Most important congenital disorders are those of infant hydrocele and maldescent. Two main types of maldescent are recognised:

- incomplete descent: the testis is arrested at some point in the normal path of descent
- ectopic testis: the testis has left the normal path of descent.

Urinary symptoms

A clear understanding of certain symptoms with which urological disorders may present is essential in diagnosis.

Voiding symptoms

Patients may admit to difficulty passing urine:

- poor flow: stream is prolonged and weak
- hesitancy: there is a delay before stream begins
- feeling of incomplete bladder emptying.

Patients may complain of:

- increased frequency in passing urine during the day
- need to get up to pass urine at night (nocturia).

Pain

Dysuria. Lower urinary tract pain during or just after voiding, suggests inflammation in the bladder or urethra.

Loin pain. Renal or ureteric pain may radiate to the scrotum, whereas testicular pain may radiate to the loin.

Incontinence of urine

Involuntary loss of urine per urethra occurs when the pressure in the bladder exceeds urethral resistance. These conditions occur during normal voiding, of course, but should not occur at other times in health.

Stress incontinence. This is caused by a deficiency of the mechanisms that maintain urethral resistance; the incontinence is abrupt and typically occurs after a cough or sneeze.

Urge incontinence. This is the result of inappropriate contraction of the detrusor and is preceded by an urgent sensation of imminent wetting.

Overflow incontinence. Typically, this is a continuous dribbling incontinence, worse at night and caused by chronic retention.

Haematuria: blood in the urine

Haematuria may be:

- painless or accompanied by abdominal or flank pain, or by pain while voiding
- microscopic (undetectable to the naked eye)
- frank: blood can be seen with the naked eye and clots may be seen too (bladder pathology is more likely to be found).

If haematuria is frank, then it may be initial (blood is seen only in the first part of the stream) or terminal (blood is seen in the last part of the stream) or total (throughout the whole stream). Initial and terminal haematuria suggest that the bleeding has occurred distal to the kidneys, possibly from the urethra or bladder neck.

Urethral bleeding, where blood passes from the urethral meatus when urine has not been voided, can usually be distinguished from true haematuria.

6.2 Infections and stones

Urinary infection

Bacterial infection in the urinary tract is common. It may be localised (cystitis, epididymitis) or may pass along the urinary tract as a diffuse urine infection. The effects depend on the extent and site, and range from asymptomatic to life-threatening.

Acute bacterial cystitis

Occasional infection of the bladder urine occurs in otherwise healthy women, but in men and children some other urinary abnormality is likely.

Symptoms

Symptoms are those of vesical inflammation: dysuria and frequency, sometimes with fever or haematuria. The urine may be cloudy or have a strong odour.

Treatment

Treatment should be started only after obtaining a midstream urine specimen for culture. Fluids are encouraged, and a simple antibiotic is prescribed pending culture results. Bowel flora (e.g. *Escherichia coli* (most common), *Streptococcus faecalis*, *Klebsiella* or *Proteus* spp.) are usually involved.

Recurrent urinary infection

Recurrent urinary infection requires investigation to look for a causative urinary abnormality, although in women a structural abnormality is not often found. Important aetiological factors include those that induce local stasis of urine:

- incomplete bladder emptying caused by obstruction
- urinary calculus
- urothelial tumour
- radiation injury.

Acute pyelonephritis

Acute renal infection may result from the ascent of a lower urinary tract infection or, less frequently, from haematogenous spread from elsewhere in the body. Destruction of renal tissue occurs and is especially severe if there is renal obstruction.

Symptoms

Symptoms are of loin pain and tenderness, high fever and tachycardia, which may obscure those of the associated bacterial cystitis. There may be a sympathetic pulmonary effusion or abdominal guarding.

Differential diagnosis

Several differential diagnoses should be considered:

- pulmonary infection
- acute cholecystitis
- appendicitis
- diverticulitis
- aortic aneurysm
- pancreatitis.

Treatment

Aggressive treatment is required (to prevent or treat septicaemia and to minimise renal damage) including intravenous fluids and parenteral antibiotics once blood and urine are obtained for culture. Intravenous urogram (IVU) or renal ultrasound with plain abdominal radiograph to include kidneys, ureters and bladder (KUB) is required to exclude obstruction or calculus. An obstructed infected kidney should be drained promptly, usually percutaneously.

Outcome of an acute infection

The common outcome of an acute infection is resolution with no damage; scarring can occur, especially when there was obstruction.

Less often the outcome can be suppuration, abscess or pyonephrosis, or granuloma formation.

Chronic pyelonephritis

Chronic pyelonephritis is the cyclic sequence of post-infective scarring in the renal parenchyma and recurrent infection leading to further scarring. Accumulating

damage leads to serious loss of renal function and accounts for a fifth of all cases of end-stage renal failure. Predisposing causes should be treated, and infection eradicated by appropriate antibiotics, including long-term low-dose antibiotics. In children, vesicoureteric reflux is a treatable cause that should be excluded by performing a micturating cystourethrogram, and can be treated by surgical means to re-establish the ureterovesical valve mechanism.

Urinary tract stones

The incidence of urinary tract stones is increasing. It is more common in men and more common with a refined diet.

Pathogenesis

Urinary calculi form by the crystallisation of urinary solutes. Certain systemic conditions and local anatomical changes in the urinary tract predispose to stone formation. The main factors are increased concentration of solute, local urine stasis and an abnormal surface to form a nucleus on which crystallisation can begin.

Idiopathic occurrence. For many calcium oxalate and calcium phosphate stones, no cause can be found, or hypercalciuria may be found with no identifiable cause.

Infective causes. *Proteus mirabilis* splits urea in urine to ammonia; this increases urinary pH and favours the crystallisation of magnesium ammonium phosphate ('triple phosphate stone'). Such stones can enlarge massively to fill the pelvis and calyces ('staghorn' calculus) and may be bilateral.

Other infections encourage stone formation by providing infective debris as a nucleus for crystallisation.

Metabolic causes. Certain conditions result in urinary solutes exceeding saturation. Though none of these conditions is common and some are rare, they are important because treatment reduces recurrence:

- uncommon
  — hypercalcaemia caused by hyperparathyroidism
  — gout: uric acid stone (may be radiolucent)
- rare
  — hyperoxaluria
  — xanthinuria
  — cystinuria.

Management of the acute episode

The pain of ureteric colic can be very severe and should be treated promptly. Next the size and position of the stone are determined, the obstruction treated and, lastly, removal of the stone is planned if spontaneous passage is unlikely.

Analgesia. Prostaglandin synthetase inhibitors such as diclofenac or indomethacin are more effective than opiates but both may be required, sometimes with an antiemetic.

Assessment:

- plain KUB film shows most (90%) calculi
- ultrasound may show dilatation
- IVU gives most information in the acute phase.

If imaging shows no obstruction, or obstruction with a small stone (less than 5 mm), conservative management is reasonable initially, since most small stones will pass spontaneously. Indications for intervention are:

- fever: suggesting infection and obstruction
- persisting pain
- persisting obstruction without progress of stone.

Decompression of the obstruction. Decompression relieves symptoms and minimises further renal damage. It is achieved by:

- direct percutaneous drainage of the obstructed system
- bypassing the obstruction with a ureteric stent
- displacement or removal of the obstructing stone.

Stenting. Plastic self-retaining tubes (stents) can be passed endoscopically into the ureter to prevent reobstruction with a pelvic stone or to encourage passage of a ureteric stone. These can be left in place for several weeks while treatment of the stone is planned but will themselves eventually become encrusted with stone.

Removal of stones

Small stones may pass spontaneously but larger stones often require intervention.

Open surgery. Classical open surgery for renal and ureteric stones is still occasionally required but has become infrequent with the development of less invasive methods.

Percutaneous nephrolithotomy (PCNL). Direct puncture of the renal collecting system and dilatation of the puncture tract allows endoscopic disintegration and removal of renal stones.

Extracorporeal shockwave lithotripsy (ESWL). ESWL uses focused shock waves to disintegrate renal stones without requiring anaesthesia, but fragmented stone is left to be passed. Treatment of large stones requires combined techniques with PCNL and stenting.

Ureteric calculi. A calculus stuck in the ureter can be snared and removed under direct vision with a ureteroscope, or fragmented using an ultrasound probe or a pulsed dye laser via a fibre passed along the ureteroscope. Alternatively, an upper ureteric stone can be 'pushed back' into the kidney for ESWL.

Bladder calculi. Although renal stones may pass into and remain in the bladder, enlarging there to cause bladder symptoms, some stones arise in the bladder and are often multiple. There is usually bladder outflow obstruction and stasis, perhaps complicated by diverticulae or even squamous carcinoma arising in the chronically irritated urothelium. The stone can be crushed and removed through the urethra, but the associated pathology must also be treated.

Investigation after the acute episode

Once a renal stone is dealt with, investigation is directed at identifying treatable causes of recurrence:

- urine microscopy, culture and pH
- stone analysis
- urea and creatinine
- serum calcium, urate, phosphorus
- 24-hour urine collection for calcium and phosphate.

All patients should be advised to maintain high fluid intake to dilute urine.

6.3 **Renal obstruction and tumours**

Renal obstruction

Obstruction to the passage of urine from the kidneys may occur at any level and, if unrelieved, results in impairment of renal function. The clinical picture depends on the level of obstruction.

Upper urinary tract obstruction

Upper tract obstruction occurring at points between the renal medulla and the bladder lumen is usually unilateral, except with extrinsic causes. The renal pelvis and ureter above the level of the obstruction become distended (hydronephrosis and hydroureter). Acute obstruction usually causes loin pain but chronic obstruction can be 'silent' and if bilateral may present with signs of renal failure.

The causes of obstruction are many:

Intraluminal causes:

- calculus: by far the most common
- clot
- renal papillary necrosis.

Intramural causes:

- urothelial tumour of ureter or bladder
- congenital pelviureteric junction obstruction
- ureteric stricture
- ureterocele.

Extrinsic causes:

- ureteric injury, most often iatrogenic
- direct invasion from carcinoma of cervix, uterus, prostate or bladder
- retroperitoneal fibrosis, which may be malignant, inflammatory or idiopathic
- pregnancy.

Treatment

Treatment depends on the cause, but the dilated collecting system proximal to the obstruction can be drained with a percutaneous cannula (nephrostomy) under ultrasound or radiographic control, to provide temporary relief of the obstruction. This protects renal function while the level and cause of the obstruction is determined and definitive treatment planned. It also permits antegrade urography, which may be very useful in diagnosis. If the cause is known to be untreatable pelvic malignancy, the decision to relieve obstruction needs to be taken with care, to avoid compromising best palliation.

Lower urinary tract obstruction

Obstruction occurring distal to the bladder (infravesical obstruction) causes voiding difficulty initially. Such bladder outflow obstruction is very common and of great importance in urology.

The acquired causes in the adult may be structural:

- urethral stricture
- benign prostatic hyperplasia
- carcinoma of the prostate
- other pelvic tumour
- bladder neck hypertrophy.

Alternatively, the causes may be functional:

- bladder neck and sphincter dysynergia.

Clinical features and treatment
The clinical features of bladder outflow obstruction will be discussed below in the section on benign prostatic hyperplasia (the most common cause in men). Treatment of this and the other causes are discussed in the relevant sections.

Tumours

Nephroblastoma

Wilm's tumour accounts for 10% of child malignancies. The prognosis is now much improved as a result of new treatment protocols.

Clinical features
Patients may present with signs and symptoms of the primary tumour, those of secondary spread, or systemic manifestations.
Features seen frequently are:

- palpable abdominal mass
- systemic symptoms.

Features seen less often are:

- haematuria
- pain
- associated anomalies in 15% of patients.

Tumours may be very large; 5% are bilateral and 20% are metastatic at presentation. Differentiation is variable, and the tumour may contain muscle, cartilage and epithelial elements if well differentiated.

Differential diagnosis
The diagnosis may be:

- polycystic kidney
- hydronephrosis
- neuroblastoma.

Treatment
Treatment should be carried out according to a precise protocol and will include nephrectomy, or partial nephrectomy and combination chemotherapy. It may also include radiotherapy.

Prognosis
Prognosis is now 80% survival at 5 years.

Renal adenocarcinoma

This is the most common adult renal malignancy. It is also known as hypernephroma, Grawitz tumour and clear cell carcinoma.

Clinical features
The clinical presentation of renal adenocarcinoma is very variable; it normally presents with the 'classic triad':

- flank pain
- abdominal mass
- haematuria.

However, it may also present with:

- anorexia and weight loss
- anaemia
- hypertension
- fever
- other paraneoplastic syndromes
- symptoms from metastases.

The tumour spreads by direct invasion through the renal capsule, venous invasion to the renal vein and vena cava, and haematogenous spread to bone and lungs.

Diagnosis
IVU shows calyceal distortion and a soft tissue mass. Ultrasound differentiates the tumour from a cyst.
CT scan and cavography can be useful in preoperative planning to determine the extent of venous invasion.

Treatment
Treatment is surgical, by radical nephrectomy, and is considered worthwhile even with major venous invasion, or in patients with limited metastatic disease who have symptoms from the primary tumour. Rare spontaneous regression of metastases occurs. There is little effective treatment for metastases, but immunotherapy and progestogens are used.

Prognosis

Although average survival at 5 years is 40%, individual prognosis is very unpredictable, with occasional long survival with extensive disease.

Urothelial tumours

Malignant tumours of the lining transitional cell epithelium (urothelium) can occur in the urinary tract at any point from renal calyces to the tip of the urethra. The tumour type is most often transitional cell carcinoma, and the bladder is the site most frequently involved (90%). In some parts of the world where schistosomiasis is endemic, squamous cell carcinoma of the bladder is common, but this tumour type is infrequently seen elsewhere. The most important presenting feature is haematuria, which should always be investigated urgently.

Causes

Exposure to many chemical carcinogens have been implicated. An occupational history should be taken in all patients with urothelial tumours.

The most important agents are:

- azo dyes
- tobacco smoke
- chemicals used in rubber manufacture.

Pathology and staging

Transitional cell carcinoma is more common in males and incidence increases with age. Most tumours are superficial and papillary but may be papillary or solid, single or multiple, superficial or deeply invasive. Superficial tumours are mostly well differentiated, but muscle-invasive tumours tend to be of higher grade. Spread is by direct invasion, and by lymphatics and bloodstream.

Transitional carcinoma in situ is an important variant that can progress rapidly to invasive disease.

Staging of the local bladder tumour is based on the invasive level (Fig. 43):

T1: invasion is superficial to bladder muscle
T2: invasion of superficial muscle
T3: invasion of deep muscle or perivesical fat
T4: fixed mass or invading adjacent organ
CIS: carcinoma in situ, which appears as a flat red patch of high-grade non-invasive tumour, is a special case that if extensive progresses rapidly.

Clinical features

Although patients may occasionally present with symptoms resulting from invasive or metastatic disease, by far the most frequent presenting symptom is painless haematuria. This can be frank, reported by the patient, microscopic, detected by the doctor or it can also present with recurrent urine infection, or irritative bladder symptoms (dysuria and frequency).

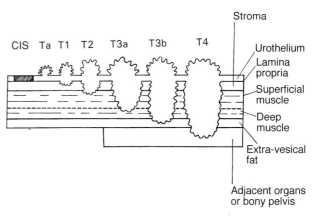

Fig. 43
Staging of bladder cancer.
CIS = carcinoma in situ.

Investigation of haematuria

Investigation of frank haematuria should be urgent and requires a minimum of upper tract imaging (intravenous urogram or ultrasound scan) and cysto-urethroscopy. Urothelial tumours may be seen as filling defects on contrast radiography.

Exfoliative urine cytology can be useful, especially for upper tract tumours and carcinoma in situ of the bladder, but false negatives are common.

Bladder tumours are diagnosed, staged and treated by cystoscopy and endoscopic resection.

Treatment

Appropriate treatment depends on clinical stage and histological grade of tumour.

In the bladder, superficial (Ta or T1) tumours can be managed by endoscopic resection. Follow-up by prolonged endoscopic surveillance is required. Intravesical chemotherapy is used for multiple recurrent superficial lesions. Invasive (T2–T3) bladder tumours require either radiotherapy or radical cystourethrectomy, or both.

In the upper tracts nephro-ureterectomy has been traditionally used for unilateral disease, since tumours are often multifocal on one side. More conservative surgery is now considered for unifocal disease and for bilateral disease.

Prognosis

Prognosis is dependent on stage and grade, with the most superficial tumours having 90% survival at 5 years; this halves to 45% for muscle invasive disease.

6.4 Prostate and urethra

Prostate: benign hyperplasia

Benign prostate hyperplasia (BPH) is detectable in nearly all men over the age of 40 years, and in later years many will develop some degree of bladder outflow obstruction as a result. Currently only one in 10 men come to require surgical treatment, but with the advent of potentially effective drug therapies, both symptomatic presentation and treatment rates are rising.

Clinical features

Benign prostatic hyperplasia is the most common cause of bladder outflow obstruction in men. The clinical presentation of bladder outflow obstruction is very variable.

Early symptoms. These are frequency, nocturia, hesitancy and poor stream, or of secondary urinary infection. Such symptoms may be tolerated for many years, and patients may not complain at all until retention of urine occurs.

Retention of urine. This may be acute retention, with an apparently sudden and distressing inability to pass urine. The bladder is tender and tensely distended, and the patient is well aware of a desperate urge to pass urine. Alternatively, the bladder may undergo gradual progressive dilatation and this results in painless chronic retention and eventually overflow incontinence. The stretched and weakened detrusor gives way in places to form diverticulae, which come to contain stagnant infected urine and often urinary stones. This insidious presentation is more serious since bladder function may not recover completely.

Neglected obstruction. More importantly though, untreated obstruction can lead eventually to bilateral upper tract obstruction and consequent renal impairment (obstructive uropathy). Patients may then present for the first time with signs of established chronic renal failure with polyuria, anorexia, vomiting, hypertension and impaired consciousness.

Diagnosis

Investigation depends on the stage at which the patient presents.

Patients presenting with early outflow symptoms require careful assessment to exclude other causes of similar symptoms (described below), especially bladder cancer and prostate cancer:

- urinalysis and rectal examination are essential
- uroflowmetry gives an objective measure of poor flow
- ultrasound can measure incomplete bladder emptying sensitively
- a plain film is useful to exclude stones.

If there is incomplete bladder emptying, serum creatinine should be checked and an upper tract ultrasound examination performed, since conservative management may be contraindicated.

Treatment

Patients presenting with acute retention require relief with urethral (or percutaneous suprapubic) catheterisation. Most will subsequently require surgical treatment, but if there is no good preceding history of outflow symptoms then a trial removal of catheter may be followed by a return to voiding, allowing elective assessment of the bladder outflow.

Surgery. Transurethral prostatic resection (TURP) remains the current standard treatment.

Early complications can occur:

- haemorrhage
- septicaemia
- 'TUR syndrome'.

Delayed complications can also occur:

- secondary haemorrhage
- urethral stricture
- incontinence.

Retropubic (open) prostatectomy is reserved for very large glands.

Alternative 'minimally invasive' treatments:

- transurethral microwave thermotherapy (TUMT)
- transurethral laser coagulation
- prostatic stents
- balloon dilatation.

Medical treatment. Alpha-adrenergic blockers inhibit contraction of the prostate capsule and bladder neck, which can improve mild symptoms.

5α-Reductase inhibitors can cause gradual shrinkage of the prostate, but their place in treatment is not established.

Prostate: carcinoma

The incidence of adenocarcinoma of the prostate is increasing worldwide, but there is great geographical and racial variation. In the UK, it is now the third most frequent malignant tumour to present in males, and subclinical disease is present in the majority of elderly men. No convincing aetiology factors have been established.

Clinical features

About one half of patients have locally advanced or metastatic disease at presentation. The most frequent metastatic site is the axial skeleton, especially pelvis and lumbar spine.

The most common symptoms are:

- bladder outflow obstruction
- retention of urine.

Symptoms seen less often are:

- bone pain
- ureteric obstruction
- anaemia.

Diagnosis

Histology. The histological diagnosis is established by transurethral resection of the prostate when there are outflow symptoms, but by needle biopsy otherwise.

Markers. The serum tumour markers prostatic acid phosphatase or prostate-specific antigen (PSA) may be elevated, or sclerotic metastases may be seen in bone on plain radiograph.

Grade and stage. Tumour grade (differentiation) and stage have a bearing on prognosis and both are important in deciding the best treatment. Staging of a local tumour (Fig. 44) is most often by digital rectal examination:

T0: no evidence of primary tumour
T1: tumour not detectable by palpation; microscopic foci found incidentally at prostatic resection
T2: clinically detectable, not breaching capsule
T3: beyond capsule, invading bladder neck or seminal vesical, not fixed
T4: fixed or invades other local structures.

Metastatic staging is usually established by radioisotope bone scan, since metastasis to bone is the most common clinically important site.

Treatment
Opinion on the best treatment for prostate cancer is divided, but the treatment chosen will depend on the symptoms, the age and general health of the patient and on the tumour stage.

Clinically localised tumour in a younger patient. Treatment includes radical radiotherapy to the prostate and/or radical prostatectomy. The aim is to cure and both treatments are controversial. An alternative approach is 'watchful waiting'.

Symptomatic advanced disease at any age. Four out of five prostatic cancers are 'androgen dependent' and advanced disease will regress well for a time if the source of circulating testosterone is removed by orchiec-

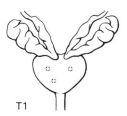
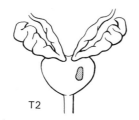
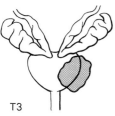
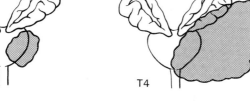

Fig. 44
Staging of prostate cancer.

tomy or the secretion or action of testosterone is blocked by drugs. The main current alternatives are:

- orchiectomy (subcapsular or total)
- LHRH (luteinising hormone releasing hormone) analogues (stop testosterone release)
- antiandrogens (block testosterone action).

Oestrogens have been widely used but are now obsolete because of their cardiovascular side effects.

Asymptomatic locally advanced or metastatic disease. Hormonal treatment may be given immediately or 'deferred' until the symptoms emerge. The timing is controversial as many elderly men with advanced disease die of other causes, without ever becoming symptomatic.

Hormone-relapsed disease. Secondary hormone treatment is ineffective and treatment is aimed at palliation of symptoms.

Recurrent prostatic obstruction can be treated by repeat transurethral resection.

Focal bone pain is palliated by external beam radiotherapy.

Diffuse pain is palliated by hemibody radiotherapy or bone-seeking isotope therapy.

Opiate analgesia may be required.

Prognosis
Prognosis is very variable but can be predicted by stage.

With metastatic disease at presentation, one half of patients die within 2 years. When there is no metastatic disease at presentation, one half will die within 4 years.

Urethra: stricture

Stricture results from contraction and fibrosis occurring during healing of urethral injury or inflammation.

Traumatic causes:

- major pelvic fracture: urethral rupture
- perineal trauma: a 'fall astride'
- iatrogenic: instrumentation or catheterisation.

Infective and inflammatory causes:

- gonococcal urethritis (now less common than in the past)
- non-specific urethritis.

Complications of urethral stricture. Complications are generally those of long-term bladder outflow obstruction:

- common complications
  — urine infection
  — epididymitis
- rare complication
  — squamous carcinoma.

Diagnosis
Urethral stricture should be suspected in a young man with poor urine flow. The urine flow rate has a charac-

teristic 'plateau' appearance. The diagnosis is confirmed by urethroscopy and further assessed by contrast urethrography.

Treatment
Urethral dilatation has been in use for centuries but provides temporary relief only and has to be repeated at intervals.

Endoscopic incision (optical urethrotomy) can be curative and can be supplemented by intermittent self-catheterisation by the patient.

Formal urethroplasty (open urethral repair) is required for recurrent or dense strictures.

6.5 Testis and penis

Testicular malignancy

Incidence and aetiology
Testicular cancer is one of the most common cancers in young men, with a peak incidence in the third decade. There is some racial variation, with a higher risk in Caucasians. Risk is also higher in testicular maldescent, but the aetiology is unknown.

Clinical features
Presentation is usually as a painless lump and less often as:

- tender inflamed swelling
- history of trauma
- symptoms from metastasis.

Diagnosis
Any lump in the testis is considered a testicular tumour until proved otherwise and should be explored through a groin incision and, unless another diagnosis is evident, the testis removed. Preoperative ultrasound is sometimes helpful in confirming that the abnormality actually lies within the testis itself.

Tumour markers. Blood for tumour markers is taken immediately before and serially after surgery. The markers tested for are:

- AFP (α-fetoprotein)
- β-hCG (human chorionic gonadotrophin).

Pathology
The pathology is very variable. Germ cell tumours of various types predominate. The previous distinction between seminoma and teratoma has now been superseded by classifications that consider the variable amounts of differentiation present. Testicular lymphoma is relatively rare and is seen in an older age group, peaking in the sixth decade.

Carcinoma in situ. Carcinoma in situ is sometimes seen in testicular biopsies for infertility and, if present, there is a 50% risk of invasive cancer developing within 5 years.

Spread. Spread is by local invasion to adjacent structures and by lymphatic invasion to para-aortic lymph nodes.

Nodal staging. Nodal staging is important to treatment and is determined by CT scanning, sometimes augmented by lymphangiography. The Royal Marsden Hospital staging system is widely used:

Stage I: disease is confined to the testis
Stage II: infradiaphragmatic nodes involved
Stage III: supradiaphragmatic nodes involved
Stage IV: extralymphatic disease.

Treatment
Treatment depends on the pathology and the stage but follows detailed national protocols:

- low-stage disease with negative test results for markers:
  — orchiectomy and surveillance or
  — radiotherapy
  — prophylactic chemotherapy

- nodal disease, persistent tumour markers or relapse on surveillance:
  — combination chemotherapy

- persistent nodes:
  — salvage node dissection
  — repeat chemotherapy.

Prognosis
Prognosis is extremely good for early-treated disease. The prognosis is much worse if nodal disease persists after combination chemotherapy.

Benign scrotal disorders

Testicular torsion
The testis can occasionally twist on its vascular pedicle and become ischaemic. Torsion should be considered in any acute tender scrotal swelling, especially before puberty, and early exploration is needed to save the testis. Both testes should be sutured to prevent further episodes.

Differential diagnosis:
- acute epididymitis
- torsion of testicular appendage.

Hydrocele
Accumulation of fluid in the tunica vaginalis may be idiopathic, but it may also be secondary to inflammation or tumour.

Treatment. Treatment of secondary hydrocele is that of the underlying cause. For the idiopathic hydrocele, simple aspiration may be used but there is a risk of bleeding and infection and the fluid tends to reaccumulate.

Surgical excision or eversion and plication of the hydrocele sac offers the best chance of lasting cure.

Penile carcinoma

Penile carcinoma is uncommon and only affects uncircumcised men. The tumour is a squamous cell carcinoma that most often affects the inner aspect of the foreskin and the glans. Spread is by local direct infiltration and by the lymphatics to the inguinal and then iliac nodes. Inguinal nodes are palpable in 50% at presentation, but this is often the result of secondary infection and only one third are actually involved by the tumour.

Staging
The London Hospital classification is most useful:

Stage I: confined to foreskin and glans
Stage II: early invasion of shaft
Stage III: proximal shaft involved
Stage IV: inguinal nodes involved.

Treatment
Treatment depends on the stage.

Stages I and II. Treatment is by radiotherapy or partial amputation.

Stage III. Treatment is by radical amputation, including the scrotum and testes.

Stage IV. Treatment is by radiotherapy or by radical block node dissection.

Prognosis
The 5-year survival is up to 90% with Stages I to III, falling to 50% for Stage IV and to 20% if iliac nodes are involved.

Self-assessment: questions

Multiple choice questions

1. A man aged 60 years who denies other symptoms reports a single episode of frank painless total haematuria:
   a. If culture shows urine infection, bladder tumour is very unlikely
   b. Cystoscopy is indicated even if urine cytology shows no abnormality
   c. The most likely serious cause is renal adenocarcinoma
   d. There is a 20% chance that cystoscopy and IVU will reveal a bladder tumour
   e. Cystoscopy is indicated if the IVU is reported to show a normal bladder outline

2. The following statements relate to prostatic cancer:
   a. Prostate cancer is present in most men over 80 years of age
   b. A serum PSA greater than 100 μg/litre suggests skeletal metastases
   c. A serum PSA of 15 μg/litre is diagnostic of prostate cancer
   d. Early disease can often be cured by bilateral orchiectomy
   e. Abnormal uptake on bone scan can be disregarded if radiographs of the same area are quite normal

3. A man aged 74 years presents with a history of passing no urine for 12 hours. He denies previous urinary symptoms but on direct questioning admits that he has needed to get out of bed two or three times each night to pass urine for several years. He is now very restless and uncomfortable, with a constant urge to pass urine:
   a. Catheterisation should be deferred until renal function has been assessed by urgent blood biochemistry
   b. The bladder should be decompressed slowly to avoid causing heavy haematuria
   c. The retention may have been precipitated by antidepressant medication
   d. The most likely cause is benign prostatic enlargement
   e. Blood should be taken for PSA assay within 24 hours

4. The following statements are true of transitional cell carcinoma:
   a. Most patients have advanced disease at first presentation, requiring radical treatment
   b. It is more common in cigarette smokers
   c. The bladder is affected more frequently than are the ureters
   d. Even if there is no evidence of recurrence after 10 years, follow-up is still justified
   e. Carcinoma in situ involving the whole bladder usually runs a long benign course

5. A boy of 13 years presents with a 4-hour history of pain, swelling and redness of one side of the scrotum:
   a. He is likely to have epididymitis
   b. He should have early surgical exploration to exclude testicular torsion
   c. A diagnosis of testicular lymphoma should be considered
   d. If the affected testis is infarcted, the unaffected side should be left alone
   e. A twisted appendix testis may be responsible

6. Ureteric obstruction:
   a. Is most often caused by calculus
   b. Cannot be caused by calculus if the plain KUB radiograph is normal
   c. May be asymptomatic
   d. Usually causes an increase in blood urea
   e. Should always be relieved when complicating advanced pelvic malignancy

7. An overweight 45-year-old mother of four has used pads to control leakage of urine for 5 years. She has a 'smoker's cough'. She is now finding it difficult to afford the pads and asks for treatment:
   a. Most women with incontinence of urine do not seek medical help
   b. Her incontinence is almost certainly the result of weakness of the pelvic floor
   c. She may be helped by drug treatment
   d. If she passes urine in small volumes, frequently and urgently, bladder instability may be present
   e. If she has genuine stress incontinence she should have surgery without delay

8. A 23-year-old woman has had repeated episodes of frequency and dysuria, occurring every few weeks for 18 months. She left her parents' home shortly before the attacks began and now lives with her boyfriend:
   a. She probably has an underlying urinary tract abnormality
   b. Urine should be collected for culture before commencing treatment at each attack
   c. The social history is irrelevant
   d. A vulval disinfectant will not help reduce the number of attacks
   e. She should be advised to decrease her fluid intake and empty her bladder before intercourse

Case histories

Case history 1

A man aged 62 years presents with a single episode of painless total haematuria. He has no other voiding symptoms but admits that he had a mild ache in the left loin a few weeks before.

1. How should he be investigated, and why?

Before investigations begin he presents to casualty with a 5-hour history of severe pain in the left flank, which started abruptly and now radiates to the left groin. He has vomited, is sweating and pale and finds it difficult to lie still to be examined. Urine testing shows microscopic haematuria.

2. What is now the most likely diagnosis, and how can it be confirmed? What important differential diagnosis must be excluded?

Imaging shows a 9 mm radio-opaque calculus at the pelviureteric junction, with complete obstruction of the left kidney.

3. Outline the steps in clinical management.

Case history 2

A man of 44 years presents with a 3-year history of increasing frequency of micturition. For the past year he has needed to wake about five times each night to pass urine. He admits that the stream of urine has become weaker and prolonged. About 6 years ago he was involved in a fight and was kicked in the perineum. Examination shows a mild phimosis. Rectal examination reveals a normal prostate. Urinary flow rate is a maximum of 4 ml per second, and it takes 90 seconds for him to pass 200 ml.

1. What is the most likely diagnosis?
2. What other investigations should he have?
3. How might he be treated initially?
4. Should he have a circumcision and if so why?

Case history 3

A man of 76 years presents with increasing difficulty passing urine over the past 3 months. He has had a 'bad back' for years, but over the last month, the pain is much worse and he has had difficulty sleeping, despite taking regular paracetamol and codeine. Examination reveals some tenderness to percussion over the lower lumbar spine, and the prostate is irregular, fixed and stony hard. A PSA done by the GP is 580 µg/litre and a plain radiograph of the lumbar spine shows osteosclerotic deposits.

1. What is the likely diagnosis and how can it be confirmed?
2. If the diagnosis is confirmed, what is the disease stage?
3. What is the prognosis?
4. What initial treatment options are there, and what is the likelihood of remission?

Two weeks later his back pain has resolved and this improvement is maintained although he complains of some 'hot flushes'. The PSA falls to 10 µg/litre within 3 months of starting treatment, but by the end of the year has increased to 150 µg/litre. Fifteen months after initial treatment the back pain has returned, with new pain in the left hip that cannot be controlled by simple analgesics.

5. What treatment options remain?

Viva questions

1. The presentation of renal adenocarcinoma is very variable, but what are the three classic features?
2. Give three causes of bladder outflow obstruction.
3. What conditions predispose to recurrent urine infection?
4. What stage is given to a bladder cancer which is invading superficial muscle?
5. What are the possible complications of prostatectomy?
6. Give three causes of acquired urethral stricture.
7. What tumour markers are useful in the management of testicular tumours?
8. What type of malignant tumour commonly affects the bladder?

Self-assessment: answers

Multiple choice answers

1. a. **False.** 40% of patients with bladder tumours have proven urinary infection.
   b. **True.** False negatives are common with cytology of urine.
   c. **False.** The most likely serious cause is transitional cell carcinoma of the bladder.
   d. **True.**
   e. **True.** Many bladder tumours are not seen on IVU.

2. a. **True.** But most men have an asymptomatic microscopic focus.
   b. **True.** 80% will have a positive bone scan.
   c. **False.** A PSA at this level is probably caused by benign hyperplasia only.
   d. **False.** Orchiectomy and other types of hormonal manipulation can produce useful remission of advanced disease but are never curative. Such treatments are not indicated for early asymptomatic disease.
   e. **False.** Although bony secondaries are usually sclerotic, this combination is also diagnostic of metastases.

3. a. **False.** This presentation is of acute retention and early relief by catheterisation takes priority over investigation.
   b. **False.** Although bleeding can occur from the bladder after decompression by catheterisation, this is more common after chronic retention and, furthermore, is not prevented by slow decompression.
   c. **True.** Any drug with anticholinergic action can precipitate retention.
   d. **True.**
   e. **False.** The PSA level may be spuriously elevated soon after retention or catheterisation.

4. a. **False.** Superficial disease is most common and is amenable to local endoscopic treatment.
   b. **True.** Smoking is thought to produce a urinary carcinogen in susceptible individuals.
   c. **True.** 95% occur in the bladder, and the pelvicalyceal system is affected more frequently than the ureter or urethra.
   d. **True.** Most authorities support lifelong endoscopic follow-up, since recurrence is not unusual even after 10 years.
   e. **False.** Carcinoma in situ tends to progress to muscle invasive disease, especially if extensive.

5. a. **False.** Infective causes are unlikely.
   b. **True.** This is a classic presentation and should be dealt with as an emergency to avoid loss of the testis.

   c. **False.** Testicular neoplasms are rare at this age, and lymphoma is seen in a much older age group.
   d. **False.** If the affected testis is infarcted, the 'unaffected' side may also be vulnerable to torsion and should be sutured to prevent torsion.
   e. **True.** This is often only diagnosed at operation, but removing the infarcted appendix testis (a Müllerian duct remnant) speeds recovery.

6. a. **True.** 90% of cases are caused by stone.
   b. **False.** Not all urinary stones are radio-opaque.
   c. **True.** Especially when of gradual onset.
   d. **False.** If the other kidney is normal and unobstructed, as is usually the case, blood biochemistry is unchanged.
   e. **False.** Each individual patient should be considered carefully, but it is often considered wrong to relieve a painless terminal complication and then expose the patient to a painful death from other causes.

7. a. **True.** Unfortunately.
   b. **False.** About one half of women with urinary incontinence have detrusor instability. Cystometry is essential to diagnose the mechanism of incontinence.
   c. **True.** If she has an unstable bladder she may benefit from anticholinergic drug treatment.
   d. **True.**
   e. **False.** Weight reduction, stopping smoking and physiotherapy will cure many such women and should always be tried before surgery.

8. a. **False.** Investigation of women in this age group rarely shows any abnormality.
   b. **True.** It is important to obtain a sample to establish the responsible organism and its antibiotic sensitivity before starting treatment, although a 'best guess' antibiotic should be commenced while awaiting the result.
   c. **False.** Sexual activity is often implicated in the initiation of urinary infection in women.
   d. **True.** Alteration of the natural vulval flora will often make the situation worse.
   e. **False.** She should increase her fluid intake. The bladder is better emptied after intercourse to 'flush out' any vulval organisms that may have been introduced.

Case history answers

Case history 1

1. Despite the history of loin pain, the most likely important diagnosis to exclude is still urothelial

neoplasm of the bladder. Investigation should include urine culture, cystoscopy and upper tract imaging with intravenous urogram, and if these are normal renal tract ultrasound to exclude hypernephroma.

2. The most likely diagnosis is ureteric colic, caused by calculus. Although a plain abdominal film and ultrasound may be useful, an intravenous urogram gives most useful information in the acute phase. In a man of this age the most important differential diagnosis is of a leaking abdominal aortic aneurysm.

3. Pain should be relieved using non-steroidal anti-inflammatory agents, such as diclofenac, and antiemetics. A stone of this size is unlikely to pass spontaneously. The obstructed kidney should be decompressed as an emergency, either by percutaneous nephrostomy or by passing a ureteric catheter to the level of the stone and flushing the stone back into the kidney. A ureteric stent should be left in place. The stone can then be electively fragmented by extracorporeal shockwave lithotripsy (ESWL) or removed by percutaneous nephrolithotomy if ESWL is not available.

   Once the acute episode is over, the patient should be investigated to exclude a treatable cause for stone.

Case history 2

1. Symptomatic benign prostatic hyperplasia is only occasionally seen at this age, with functional bladder neck obstruction being rather more frequent. This history and findings are, however, most suggestive of obstruction caused by traumatic urethral stricture.

2. A midstream urine specimen should be collected for culture, since obstruction is often complicated by infection. The probable diagnosis is best confirmed by flexible (fibreoptic) cystoscopy, although the actual length and position of any urethral stricture may be better defined by contrast urethrography. Urinary tract ultrasound may be indicated if there is evidence of incomplete bladder emptying, and plain abdominal radiograph will exclude bladder calculus.

3. Urethral strictures can be managed initially by dilatation with urethral sounds, but endoscopic incision of the stricture (optical urethrotomy) has better long-term results.

4. No; circumcision should be avoided if possible, since long or recurrent strictures may come to require urethroplasty and the preputial skin may be required to form a urethral patch.

Case history 3

1. The likely diagnosis of advanced metastatic prostate cancer should be confirmed without delay. Since this

patient has troublesome bladder outflow symptoms, these may be improved temporarily by transurethral prostatic resection, which would also provide a tissue diagnosis. Alternatively, the histology could be confirmed by a needle biopsy of the prostate, which can be performed under local anaesthetic if required.

2. If the histology is confirmed, the stage is T4 M1.

3. For men with metastatic disease at presentation, the 2-year survival is 50%, (half die within 2 years).

4. This patient has symptoms from metastases and so, after full discussion with the patient, hormonal treatment ('androgen deprivation') should be initiated by either orchiectomy, or by the medical alternatives of LHRH analogues or antiandrogens. A very useful response is seen in 80% of patients, and the remission lasts on average for about 18 months.

5. Palliative radiotherapy can provide very effective temporary relief of symptoms from bone pain. This can be administered by external beam to the affected sites or, if the painful lesions are widespread, by either external beam hemi-body irradiation or intravenous administration of a radioactive bone-seeking strontium isotope. Analgesics should be increased, using non-steroidal anti-inflammatory agents and opiates if needed, until the radiotherapy has been allowed to work. Secondary hormonal treatments are of no significant benefit.

Viva answers

1. Flank pain, abdominal mass and haematuria.

2. Common causes are benign prostatic hyperplasia, carcinoma of the prostate and urethral stricture. Less often it can be caused by bladder neck hypertrophy, sphincter dyssynergia. In young boys, it can (rarely) be caused by abnormalities of the posterior urethral valve.

3. Any condition that causes incomplete bladder emptying or local urine stasis, such as those listed in Viva Question 2, and also urothelial tumour and urinary calculus.

4. T2.

5. Early complications include haemorrhage, septicaemia and 'TUR syndrome'. Delayed complications are secondary haemorrhage, urethral stricture and incontinence.

6. Traumatic, from major pelvic fracture and urethral rupture, perineal trauma from a 'fall astride' and iatrogenic from instrumentation or catheterisation. Also gonococcal and non-specific urethritis.

7. Alpha-fetoprotein (AFP) and beta human chorionic gonadotrophin (β-HCG).

8. Transitional cell carcinoma is the most common (squamous cell carcinoma is more common in some parts of the world where schistosomiasis is endemic).

Breast and endocrine surgery

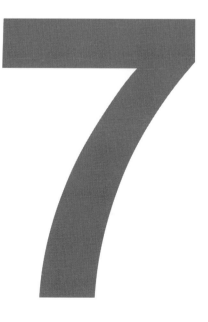

7.1 Benign breast disease

There are five important benign breast conditions that frequently present as surgical problems:

- fibrocystic breast disease
- fibroadenoma
- breast sepsis
- gynaecomastia
- nipple discharge.

Fibrocystic disease

Fibrocystic disease, fibroadenomatosis and cystic mastalgia are interchangeable terms used to describe the triad of pain, nodularity and cyst formation in the female breast. Symptoms are often cyclical and worse in the premenstrual period. The peak incidence occurs between 35–45 years of age. The condition is rare after the menopause and may be hormonally linked.

Clinical features
Clinical features include pain, breast lumps and recurrent breast cysts. Occasionally, a nipple discharge occurs.

Classically, the symptoms vary from one menstrual cycle to another.

Diagnosis
The initial management consists of:

- a careful physical examination
- fine needle aspiration cytology (FNAC) of any discrete lump
- mammography in any woman over 35 years of age.

Treatment
Reassurance and psychological support are often all that is needed once cancer or an underlying breast infection has been ruled out.

Breast cysts can be aspirated and the fluid sent for cytological analysis. Cysts that recur or solid lumps with worrying cytological features should be excised. In some patients, pain is the predominant symptom. Often this responds to simple measures, which include:

- reassurance
- physical measures (such as a brassière which provides firm support)
- gamma-linoleic acid (evening primrose oil).

A few patients will have severe pain. Completion of a pain chart over a period of 3–6 months will give an indication of the pattern of the symptoms. Severe cyclical mastalgia will sometimes respond to a sex hormone inhibitor, such as danazol which suppresses pituitary gonadotrophin secretion.

Prognosis
Relapses and remissions characterise this condition.

Long-term follow-up is often necessary to provide the necessary psychological support. Usually symptoms resolve spontaneously as the menopause approaches.

Fibroadenoma

This is the most common cause of a breast lump in women under 30 years of age. It is rare after the menopause. About 20% will resolve spontaneously with time, although the condition can recur at other sites or in the contralateral breast. Malignant change is extremely uncommon. Occasionally, a giant fibroadenoma develops which grows rapidly.

Clinical features
This is a clinical diagnosis. A fibroadenoma is characterised by a firm, painless, smooth often highly mobile lump in the breast.

Diagnosis
Mammography is unhelpful. The breasts of young women are extremely radiodense and this prevents accurate radiological resolution of any breast lumps.

Fine needle aspiration cytology. This is of limited help as there are no diagnostic features of a fibroadenoma on FNAC.

Treatment
Usually a fibroadenoma is excised, although some surgeons prefer conservative treatment for cosmetic reasons, to avoid scarring the breast in a young woman.

Infection in the breast

Infection can develop in the peripheral glandular mass of the breast or in relation to the nipple (subareolar infection).

Peripheral sepsis
This infection involves one or more segments of the breast and can occur in the lactating and in the non-lactating breast. Most of these infections are staphylococcal or anaerobic in origin.

Clinical features. The typical features of acute inflammation are present. The breast is painful and tender with areas of erythema and induration. Without treatment, the cellulitis will progress to a breast abscess and it then presents as a fluctuant mass.

Treatment. During the cellulitic stage, before suppuration supervenes, infection can often be resolved with an appropriate course of antibiotics (flucloxacillin plus metronidazole). A breast abscess requires:

- incision and drainage
- culture of any pus
- biopsy of the abscess wall (this will rule out the occasional cancer which presents as an abscess).

Subareolar infection
A subareolar infection can develop from:

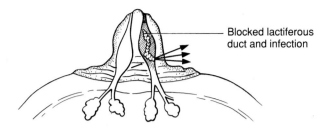

Blocked lactiferous
duct and infection

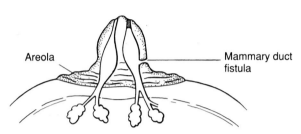

Areola

Mammary duct
fistula

Fig. 45
Mammary duct fistula.

- cuts or abrasions on the nipple caused by breast feeding
- an infected sebaceous gland (Montgomery's tubercle)
- a blocked lactiferous duct (this can spontaneously discharge through the areola and lead to a mammary duct fistula (Fig. 45).

In older women, dilatation of the nipple duct system associated with a surrounding chronic inflammatory cell infiltrate leads to a condition called mammary duct ectasia or plasma cell mastitis. Chronic inflammation and scarring will lead to indrawing and inversion of the nipple. If secondary infection supervenes, a mammary duct fistula can also develop.

Treatment. An acute subareolar abscess requires incision and drainage. Chronically diseased ducts in mammary duct ectasia or a mammary duct fistula require subareolar excision.

Gynaecomastia

Gynaecomastia is caused by hypertrophy of the male breast tissue. It can be unilateral or bilateral and is sometimes painful. In order of decreasing frequency, the three main causes are:

1. physiological, at puberty
2. drug-induced, e.g. by cimetidine, spironolactone, digoxin
3. disease-induced, e.g. by cirrhosis, hyperthyroidism, Kleinfelter's syndrome, pituitary tumour.

Treatment
Physiological gynaecomastia usually resolves sponta-

neously. Surgical excision should be reserved for cosmetic reasons when gynaecomastia persists.

Nipple discharge

In the non-lactating breast, the four most common causes of nipple discharge in order of decreasing frequency are:

- fibrocystic breast disease
- mammary duct ectasia
- intraduct papilloma
- breast cancer.

Clinical features
It is important to determine whether the discharge is:

- unilateral or bilateral
- from a single duct or from multiple ducts
- bloodstained.

The discharge associated with fibrocystic breast disease is usually green/brown in colour, has the associated features of fibrocystic breast disease outlined above and may issue from multiple ducts or from both breasts. Mammary duct ectasia also causes a similar discharge. A serous or serosanguinous discharge from a single duct is more likely to be caused by an intraduct papilloma or a carcinoma. A frankly bloodstained discharge from one or more ducts with an underlying breast mass is usually caused by breast cancer.

Diagnosis
Mammography. This is essential in all women over 35 years of age with a nipple discharge, in order to rule out an underlying cancer.
Fine needle aspiration cytology. It is vital that any associated breast lump be fully evaluated.
Cytological analysis of any discharge. This will occasionally reveal cancer cells.

Treatment
Treatment depends on the cause of the nipple discharge and can involve:

1. Exploration and excision of a single lactiferous duct (microdochectomy) to remove an intraduct papilloma.
2. Subareolar resection of one or more ducts for mammary duct ectasia.
3. The appropriate management of any underlying breast disease, e.g. fibrocystic disease or carcinoma.

7.2 Breast cancer

Carcinoma of the breast is the most common cancer occurring in women. In the UK it causes more than 10 000 deaths each year. It is the leading cause of death in women aged between 40–50 years. Currently between 1 in 10 and 1 in 15 women can expect to develop the disease during their lifetime.

Aetiology

Several factors are known to be important. Breast cancer is more common in:

- women whose mothers and sisters have had breast cancer
- nulliparous women or those who have a late first pregnancy, or a late menopause
- women who have had endometrial cancer
- women who smoke.

Despite these 'high-risk' groups, the disease is unexpected in most women. This has led to the introduction of self-examination programmes for women aimed to promote early detection of cancer, together with nationwide mammography screening programmes to detect impalpable cancers.

Pathology and staging

Most breast cancers grow slowly and may take several years before they enlarge enough to become palpable. By local growth, they will eventually invade the underlying pectoral muscles and chest wall and the overlying breast skin. Lymphatic dissemination occurs early to the axillary and internal mammary nodes and later to the supraclavicular nodes. Distant spread by bloodstream occurs to the liver, lungs and bones.

Because survival and treatment options are closely related to the extent of disease at presentation, accurate staging of the disease is essential. The two most commonly used systems are outlined in Table 11.

Table 11 Methods of classifying breast cancer

System 1

Stage	Description	5-Year survival (%)
1	Growth confined to breast; no axillary lymph node involvement	80
2	Growth confined to breast; mobile, ipsilateral, involved axillary lymph glands	60
3	Growth spread beyond edges of breast; growth fixed to pectoral muscles; fixed, ipsilateral, involved axillary lymph glands	
4	Advanced cancer; evidence of distant metastases	

System 2

T,N,M Classification (tumour, nodes, metastases)

This complex classification takes into account the size of the tumour, the extent of any lymph node involvement and the presence or absence of distant metastases.

Clinical features

Most painless breast lumps are discovered by the patient either by accident or during routine self-examination.

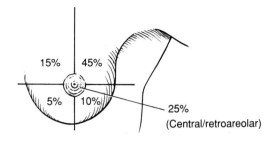

Fig. 46
Distribution of breast cancer.

The most frequent distribution within the breast is shown in Figure 46. Nationwide breast-screening programmes have led to the earlier detection of some cancers and some women now present with radiologically detected evidence of cancer without a lump.

Less frequently, nipple discharge or retraction, nipple crusting or itching, or breast pain will be the presenting symptom. A few patients still present with an advanced fungating cancer often fixed to the chest wall.

Careful inspection and palpation of the breast and axilla provide the key to the clinical diagnosis.

Inspection. The most important features on inspection are:

- breast asymmetry
- skin tethering
- nipple indrawing
- skin oedema or peau d'orange.

Palpation. The most important features on palpation are:

- a non-tender, hard lump
- a poorly defined edge between lump and surrounding breast tissue
- a bloody nipple discharge
- fixity to underlying pectoral muscles
- the presence or absence of axillary or supraclavicular lymphadenopathy.

Further examination. The opposite breast must also be carefully examined; in 1% of women a second breast cancer may be present. Finally, a search should be made for more distant metastases particularly lung, liver and spine.

Diagnosis and disease staging

Clinical suspicion must be confirmed by fine needle aspiration cytology and by mammography.

An irregular radiodense breast mass with a spiculated border, which sometimes contains areas of fine 'pepper pot' calcification (microcalcification) is the hallmark of a breast cancer. The surrounding breast architecture may also be distorted. FNAC may reveal malignant cells.

If the results of these investigations are equivocal, biopsy excision of the lump is mandatory to confirm or refute the diagnosis. Once cancer is proven, evidence of distant metastases should be sought by:

- chest X-ray
- ultrasound or isotope liver scan
- isotope bone scan.

   Differential diagnosis:
- benign breast disease (see p. 120)
- traumatic fat necrosis.

Traumatic fat necrosis may closely mimic a breast cancer in appearance. Despite the name, there may be no history of injury. Although the condition spontaneously resolves, excision biopsy is usually necessary to exclude a cancer.

Unusual clinical forms of breast cancer

Ductal carcinoma in situ

Ductal carcinoma in situ is a tumour which develops within the glandular ducts and has not yet invaded the surrounding parenchyma. It is usually detected following biopsy of areas of microcalcification identified on mammography. As a result of screening programmes this type of breast cancer is being diagnosed more frequently. Untreated it may progress to invasive breast cancer in some but perhaps not all cases. Because the tumour is often multifocal total mastectomy is the best treatment. Usually only one breast is affected.

Inflammatory breast cancer

This is a highly aggressive form of breast cancer. Women present with a tender, inflamed, erythematous painful breast, which can be mistaken for a breast abscess. These appearances are caused by lymphatic invasion by the cancer. The disease is often widely disseminated and beyond surgical resection by the time of presentation. Survival is poor even after aggressive treatment with a combination of radiotherapy and chemotherapy.

Paget's disease of the breast

Paget's disease occurs in 1 in 50 breast cancers. These patients present with symptoms of nipple disease. They complain of itching, weeping or bleeding of the nipple, which appears excoriated or covered with a scaly rash on examination. Although an underlying breast mass is rarely present in the early stages of the disease, these patients invariably have an associated ductal carcinoma in situ and if untreated will go on to develop breast cancer.

   The diagnosis is confirmed by nipple biopsy and mammography, with treatment as for carcinoma of the breast.

Breast cancer in pregnancy and lactation

This is uncommon but the outcome is poor. The disease is often detected late because it may be masked by the physiological changes occurring in the breast. The same principles of treatment apply as for breast cancer in non-pregnant or non-lactating women.

Lobular breast cancer

This uncommon variant of breast cancer is frequently bilateral. Some surgical authorities recommend bilateral mastectomy once the diagnosis is made in either breast.

Cancer of the male breast

Of all breast cancers, 1 in 100 occur in men. Because the breast is small, spread occurs early to the lymph glands and to the chest wall. As a result, the disease is often advanced by the time of presentation and the outcome after surgery in men is not as good as in women.

Treatment of breast cancer

There is still much controversy regarding the best way to treat breast cancer. Earlier radical breast surgery has been replaced by more conservative techniques that provide a better cosmetic result without increased risk of recurrence. Since more than one half of patients with breast cancer who have no evidence of distant disease at the time of diagnosis will ultimately die of distant metastases *without* evidence of local recurrence, a variety of adjuvant therapies are used in an attempt to kill *occult* metastases that are present at the time of surgery.

Treatment of early breast cancer: Stages 1 and 2 disease

Until recently, total mastectomy plus axillary clearance was the treatment of choice for women with this extent of disease. However, studies within the last few years have shown that a segmental mastectomy (preserving the breast after a wide local excision of the tumour) plus an axillary lymph gland clearance when combined with radiotherapy to the remaining breast tissue is just as effective. There is no greater risk of a local recurrence and long-term survival is similar. As the bulk of the breast is preserved, there is a considerable cosmetic benefit.

   Large tumours in a small breast are an exception and these are better treated by total mastectomy and axillary clearance.

Adjuvant therapy
This is a complex issue and its final role in breast cancer is not yet defined. Both chemotherapy and hormonal therapy are used (see Table 12). The following factors are taken into account before deciding on adjuvant therapy in any woman:

- axillary lymph node status
- is the patient pre- or postmenopausal?
- oestrogen receptor status of the tumour.

Table 12. Chemotherapy* and hormonal therapy in breast cancer

Oestrogen receptor status	Lymph gland involvement	Adjuvant treatment
Premenopausal women		
Negative	Negative	None
Positive	Negative	Tamoxifen or *chemotherapy or both
Negative	Positive	*Chemotherapy
Positive	Positive	*Chemotherapy
Postmenopausal women		
Negative	Negative	Tamoxifen
Positive	Negative	Tamoxifen
Negative	Positive	*Chemotherapy
Positive	Negative	Tamoxifen

*Usually combination chemotherapy regimens are used, such as:
CMF—cyclophosphamide, methotrexate, 5-fluorouracil
CHOP—cyclophosphamide, hydrodoxorubicin, oncovin (vincristine), prednisolone

The goal of this systemic therapy is to prevent death from recurrence resulting from distant metastases.

Treatment of advanced breast cancer: Stages 3 and 4 disease

Patients with locally advanced cancer, metastatic or recurrent disease fall into this category. As treatment is palliative, it must be individualised to provide the maximum benefit with the minimum morbidity for each patient.

Treating the primary cancer
Radiotherapy or hormonal manipulation are used in preference to chemotherapy, which has greater side effects. Sometimes it will be necessary to perform a toilet' mastectomy in order to control locally advanced but resectable disease and to prevent fungation.

Treating the metastases
Bone and soft tissue metastases usually respond well to hormonal manipulation. Visceral metastases (e.g. liver) respond better to chemotherapy. Radiotherapy is particularly useful in treating isolated painful bone metastases (e.g. in the femur).
  The choice of hormonal agent for either primary or metastatic disease depends on the menstrual status of the patient.
  For **premenstrual patients** the order of choice is:

1. antioestrogen therapy: tamoxifen
2. ovarian ablation: either surgical or by radiotherapy
3. medical adrenalectomy: aminoglutethamide, which inhibits adrenal corticosteroid synthesis.

  For **postmenopausal patients** the order of choice is:

1. antioestrogen therapy: tamoxifen
2. chemotherapy.

Breast cancer follow-up
Close follow-up of all breast cancer patients is essential to provide the necessary psychological support, to detect recurrence and to screen for cancer in the remaining breast.

Prognosis
The 5-year survival figures vary from 80% to 10% depending on the stage of the disease at presentation (see Table 11). However, despite aggressive and appropriate treatment, many women will ultimately die of their disease.

7.3 Thyroid disease

Patients with thyroid disease present most commonly with one or a combination of the following:

- signs of hyperthyroidism (thyrotoxicosis)
- signs of hypothyroidism (myxoedema)
- a lump in the neck which is of thyroid origin (a goitre).

Thyrotoxicosis

Thyrotoxicosis is caused by excess circulating thyroid hormones (usually thyroxine (T_4), occasionally tri-iodothyronine (T_3) coupled with a loss of control of the feedback mechanisms regulating hormone secretion.
  Most cases of thyrotoxicosis are autoimmune in origin and produce a diffuse smooth swelling of the thyroid gland (Graves' disease). Less often, thyrotoxicosis develops in a multinodular goitre.

Clinical features
There is usually a distinctive combination of symptoms and signs:

- irritability, fatigue, palpitations
- weight loss, increased appetite
- menstrual irregularities

- tremor, tachycardia
- goitre with a bruit
- eye signs: lid lag, exophthalmos.

Diagnosis

The clinical diagnosis is confirmed by radioimmuno-assay of the circulating thyroid hormone levels, which reveals:

- elevated serum T_4 or T_3 levels
- normal or reduced thyroid-stimulating hormone (TSH) levels.

Treatment

There are three treatment options:

- antithyroid drugs
- radioiodine
- subtotal thyroidectomy.

Antithyroid drugs. Carbimazole and propyl-thiouracil are the drugs of choice. Both act by interfering with thyroid hormone synthesis. Their use is best restricted to young patients with mild disease and small goitres. Treatment is continued for 1–2 years in the hope of inducing long-term remission. Recurrent thyrotoxicosis occurs in three out of four patients. Permanent agranulocytosis is an occasional but serious side effect of these drugs.

Radioiodine (^{131}I) therapy. Radioiodine is taken up by the thyroid follicles and destroys the acinar cells, thus reducing T_3 and T_4 production. Its use is avoided in children and pregnant women because of the potential irradiation hazard. It is a highly effective treatment but in the long term leads to hypothyroidism and most patients ultimately need thyroid hormone-replacement therapy.

Subtotal thyroidectomy. Thyroidectomy controls thyrotoxicosis by reducing the functional mass of thyroid gland tissue. It is especially helpful in patients who do not comply or respond to antithyroid drug therapy or in patients who have a goitre. It has the advantage that long-term hypothyroidism does not occur. As the posterior part of the gland is left undisturbed, the risks to the recurrent laryngeal nerves and parathyroid glands are minimal. The conditions for surgery are optimised preoperatively by administering Lugol's iodine orally to reduce the vascularity of the gland, and by beta-adrenergic blockade using propranolol to block the cardiovascular and central nervous system symptoms of thyrotoxicosis.

Post-thyroidectomy complications. There are three important complications following thyroid (or parathyroid) surgery:

- recurrent laryngeal nerve injury, causing vocal cord paralysis and hoarseness
- postoperative haemorrhage, causing respiratory distress by tracheal compression
- hypocalcaemic tetany caused by damage or inadvertent excision of the parathyroid glands.

Thyroid goitres

A goitre is an enlargement of the thyroid gland. Goitres may be toxic or non-toxic (simple) depending whether or not there is any associated thyrotoxicosis. There are three main types:

- diffuse
- multinodular
- solitary thyroid nodules.

Diffuse goitre

These are usually physiological, the gland increasing in size during times of increased demand, e.g. during puberty or pregnancy.

Multinodular goitre

If the stimulus causing the goitre is prolonged, some areas of the gland will involute and others will enlarge, leading to a multinodular goitre. In areas where there is a dietary lack of iodine, this may lead to an endemic goitre; this can affect 20% or more of the population of that area.

Solitary thyroid nodules

There are five main causes of a single thyroid nodule:

- a prominent nodule within a multinodular goitre
- a thyroid cyst
- a benign thyroid neoplasm
- thyroid cancer
- thyroid adenoma.

Clinical features

A neck swelling is the primary complaint of most patients with a goitre. Other important symptoms are dysphagia and stridor (caused by local pressure effects on the oesophagus or trachea) or symptoms of thyrotoxicosis. Hoarseness or pain are rare and may indicate malignant infiltration from a thyroid cancer.

Goitres are midline in origin and move on swallowing but not on tongue protrusion. The type of goitre can be determined by palpation, either nodular or smooth. A special check should be made for evidence of:

- tracheal deviation
- cervical lymphadenopathy
- signs of thyroid over- or underactivity
- a thyroid bruit.

Diagnosis

There are four key steps in the evaluation of a thyroid goitre or nodule:
- test thyroid function
- X-ray the thoracic inlet to detect tracheal compression/deviation
- isotopic thyroid scan

— hot areas denote areas of secretory overactivity and are rarely malignant
— cold areas denote areas of underactivity caused by either cysts or malignancy
● fine needle aspiration cytology (FNAC) is used to evaluate cold areas.

Treatment

A diffuse physiological goitre rarely requires surgical intervention. These patients are euthyroid and the goitre frequently regresses once the physiological stress (such as puberty or pregnancy) has passed. The most common operation performed for a multinodular goitre is a subtotal thyroidectomy, the main indications for surgery being:

● pressure symptoms in the neck
● cosmetic reasons
● thyrotoxicosis.

The treatment of a single nodule is more complex. Some thyroid cancers present as a single nodule and aspiration cytology is mandatory. Nodules that are not simple cysts require surgical removal—either a thyroid lobectomy (e.g. for a functioning adenoma) or a more radical surgical removal, depending upon the type of thyroid cancer (see below).

Carcinoma of the thyroid gland

Thyroid cancer is uncommon compared to breast, colon and lung cancer. It accounts for 1% of all cancers in adults. There are four types of thyroid cancer. Although they all have similar clinical features initially, they differ in biological behaviour and response to therapy.

Papillary carcinoma. This is the most common cancer and has the best prognosis. Disease spread is to the lymph nodes and by direct invasion into the neck. Distant metastases are infrequent.

Follicular carcinoma. This tumour develops later in life than papillary cancer. Spread is mainly via the bloodstream with distant metastases to the bones, liver and brain.

Medullary carcinoma. This uncommon cancer develops from the calcitonin-secreting parafollicular cells in the thyroid gland. It is sometimes associated with tumours in the parathyroid and adrenal glands (*multiple endocrine adenomatosis*, MEN Type 2 syndrome).

Undifferentiated carcinoma. This is the most aggressive thyroid malignancy. It is locally invasive to vital structures in the neck and has a poor prognosis.

Clinical features

Almost all thyroid cancers present as a solitary mass or nodule in the thyroid gland of a euthyroid patient. They rarely develop in a multinodular goitre. There is often a history of irradiation to the head and neck during childhood.

Examination will reveal a hard mass, which may be fixed, with or without cervical lymphadenopathy. Patients are usually euthyroid.

Diagnosis

The investigations carried out are:

● thyroid function tests
● X-ray of the thoracic inlet
● isotopic thyroid scan
● fine needle aspiration cytology.

Treatment

Near-total or total thyroidectomy are the main treatment options. A near-total thyroidectomy leaves a thin rim of thyroid capsule overlying the recurrent laryngeal nerves and parathyroid glands and minimises the risk of postoperative vocal cord paralysis and hypoparathyroidism. It is used most frequently for papillary cancer.

In follicular or medullary cancers, where complete removal of the gland is more important because of the poorer prognosis in this group of tumours, total thyroidectomy is the treatment of choice.

Undifferentiated cancers are usually inoperable and are treated by radiotherapy or chemotherapy.

Recurrent thyroid cancer either in the neck or in distant sites will often respond to treatment with radio-iodine therapy (see p. 125).

In order to suppress the cellular activity of any remaining thyroid tissue, patients with thyroid cancer are given sufficient amounts of thyroxine to maximally suppress their endogenous thyroid-stimulating hormone production.

Prognosis

Survival ranges from 80% at 10 years for papillary cancer to 15% at 10 years for an undifferentiated cancer.

7.4 Parathyroid gland disease

Usually there are four parathyroid glands; occasionally there are three or five. Anatomically, they are arranged in pairs, the superior pair on the posterior surface of the thyroid gland intimately related to the recurrent laryngeal nerves, the inferior pair closer to the lower pole of the thyroid gland. The position of the glands and their number is variable and locating them at operation can be difficult.

The parathyroid glands secrete parathormone (PTH), which plays a vital role in calcium metabolism by mobilising calcium from the bones, reducing renal calcium excretion and promoting renal phosphate excretion. The secretion of PTH is inversely related to the circulating calcium level.

Overproduction of parathormone can be classified into three groups depending on the cause:

● primary hyperparathyroidism
● secondary hyperparathyroidism
● tertiary hyperparathyroidism.

Primary hyperparathyroidism

This is an autonomous production of PTH by the parathyroid glands, which is not inhibited by the prevailing circulating calcium level. It is caused, in order of frequency, by:

1. a single parathyroid adenoma
2. generalised parathyroid hyperplasia
3. multiple parathyroid adenomas
4. parathyroid carcinoma.

Clinical features

Today, most patients with hyperparathyroidism are discovered accidentally while they are asymptomatic during routine biochemical screening that includes a serum calcium determination.

Hitherto, many patients presented with a complex of symptoms caused by long-standing hyperparathyroidism:

- muscle weakness and arthralgia
- peptic ulcer disease
- abdominal pain and constipation
- renal calculi
- psychiatric disorders
- hypertension.

Diagnosis

The diagnosis is confirmed with biochemical tests:

- a high serum calcium level coupled with a low serum phosphate level is highly suggestive of hyperparathyroidism
- an elevated serum parathormone level coupled with a raised serum calcium level completes the diagnosis.

In long-standing disease there may be several radiological changes:

- subperiosteal bone resorption in the phalanges
- generalised skeletal demineralisation
- renal calculi or nephrocalcinosis.

Differential diagnosis. There are many conditions associated with an elevated serum calcium level. The most important are:

- metastatic cancer
- milk-alkali syndrome
- sarcoidosis.

Treatment

In a fit patient, surgery is the treatment of choice even when the disease is asymptomatic. Parathyroid exploration is a demanding operation as the glands may be difficult to locate.

An attempt should be made to identify all four glands, which usually are red/brown in colour. An adenomatous gland is usually enlarged and the diagnosis must be confirmed by frozen section analysis. Multiple adenomas should be removed and the normal glands left undisturbed. If the glands are hyperplastic, a 'three and one half' parathyroidectomy is performed leaving a fragment of one gland to act as functioning parathyroid tissue.

After surgery, a careful check on the serum calcium must be maintained as the circulating calcium levels can drop precipitously and cause hypocalcaemic tetany. Oral or intravenous calcium supplements may be needed.

Secondary hyperparathyroidism

This develops as a result of some of the complex metabolic changes associated with chronic renal failure, which tend to produce a low serum calcium level and an elevated serum phosphate level. As patients with chronic renal failure now live longer as a result of dialysis and renal transplantation, secondary hyperparathyroidism is becoming more common.

Unlike primary hyperparathyroidism, the primary treatment is medical, aimed at reducing circulating serum phosphate levels and boosting the dietary intake of calcium. The condition usually resolves after transplantation.

Tertiary hyperparathyroidism

In this infrequent condition, the parathyroid glands develop autonomous function in patients who have had long-standing secondary hyperparathyroidism. It is often only detected after a successful renal transplantation, where patients develop a persistent hypercalcaemia. Surgical removal is indicated.

7.5 Adrenal gland disease

Patients with adrenal disease rarely present for surgery because of an abdominal mass arising from one or other of the adrenal glands. Instead, oversecretion of adrenal medullary or cortical hormones leads to a variety of complex syndromes that can be resolved by surgical removal of the diseased adrenal gland.

There are three surgically treatable disorders:

- phaeochromocytoma
- primary hyperaldosteronism
- Cushing's syndrome and Cushing's disease.

Phaeochromocytoma

A phaeochromocytoma is a benign red/brown tumour that arises from the chromaffin cells in the adrenal medulla. It affects both sexes, usually in early adult life. Phaeochromocytomas produce an excess of catecholamines (noradrenaline and adrenaline) either intermittently or continuously. 10% are bilateral, 10% are malignant and 10% are extra adrenal in position.

Clinical features

Patients present in two ways:

- dramatically, in a hypertensive crisis with sweating, palpitations, severe headache and occasionally a myocardial infarction or cerebrovascular accident
- insidiously, with diastolic hypertension.

Classically, the hypertensive attacks can be provoked by exercise, straining or abdominal palpation, all of which lead to the release of a pulse of catecholamines.

Diagnosis

As approximately 1 in 1000 of all newly diagnosed hypertensive patients have an underlying phaeochromocytoma, some physicians recommend that all young hypertensive patients should be screened for this disease.

Metabolite levels. The key diagnostic test is based on the detection of an elevated VMA (*vanillylmandelic acid*, a catecholamine metabolite) or elevated catecholamine levels in a 24-hour urine collection.

Tumour localisation. CT scanning or magnetic resonance imaging (MRI) are the best means of identifying the tumour.

Pharmacological tests. These were designed to provoke a hypertensive episode by causing catecholamine release; as they are dangerous they are no longer used.

Treatment

Because surgical manipulation of any adrenal gland bearing a phaeochromocytoma is likely to provoke massive catecholamine release, these patients require careful preoperative preparation and perioperative care in order to prevent wild and potentially fatal fluctuations in heart rate and blood pressure.

Usually, alpha-adrenergic blockade (phenoxybenzamine) is started some time before surgery, with agents such as nitroprusside and propranolol being used to control the blood pressure and heart rate during the operation.

Because the tumours can be bilateral and are occasionally situated in chromaffin tissue remote from the adrenal gland, most phaeochromocytomas are removed via a transabdominal approach.

Prognosis

Surgery is usually curative, although a mild hypertension may persist. Untreated, most patients with phaeochromocytoma will ultimately die during a hypertensive crisis

Primary hyperaldosteronism (Conn's syndrome)

The primary function of aldosterone (a mineralocorticoid) is to maintain the circulating intravascular volume. This is achieved by promoting renal sodium reabsorption in exchange for renal potassium loss. In normal individuals, the secretion of aldosterone is

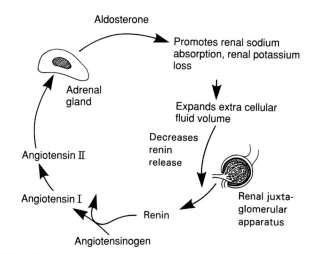

Fig. 47
Renin–angiotensin mechanism.

closely regulated by the renin–angiotensin mechanism (Fig. 47).

Most cases of primary hyperaldosteronism are caused by unilateral adrenal cortical adenomas. A few cases are caused by bilateral adrenal cortical hyperplasia. It is important to differentiate these preoperatively as hypertension caused by adrenal cortical hyperplasia does not always respond to adrenalectomy and these patients are better treated medically.

Clinical features

These are very non-specific. The diagnosis is usually suspected based on biochemical tests that show an unexplained hypokalaemia in a hypertensive patient. Vague headaches, muscle weakness and fatigue are the most common complaints.

Diagnosis

Establishing the diagnosis is a complex and time-consuming task. Three tests are often used in combination to detect inappropriately elevated aldosterone levels in the face of suppressed plasma renin levels.

Aldosterone secretion test. Failure to suppress endogenous aldosterone secretion after exogenous mineralocorticoid administration or intravenous saline infusion is indicative.

Renin stimulation test. Circulating aldosterone levels increase in response to renin infusion in patients with adrenocortical hyperplasia; those with a solitary adenoma do not show the increase.

Tumour localisation. A CT scan or MRI scan may identify an adrenal tumour. Adrenal vein sampling can be used to measure angiotensin levels and help differentiate small unilateral tumours (not detected on scanning) from bilateral hyperplasia.

Treatment

Bilateral hyperplasia is best treated medically using large doses of spironolactone, which acts as an aldosterone antagonist. A unilateral adrenalectomy is the treatment of choice for an adrenal adenoma. As these tumours are usually unilateral and small they can often be removed via a posterior retroperitoneal approach.

Cushing's syndrome and Cushing's disease

Cushing's syndrome is caused by an excess secretion of glucocorticoids (cortisone and corticosterone) by the adrenal cortex. There are three main causes:

- secondary to increased adrenocortical stimulation by ACTH (adrenocorticotrophic hormone) produced by a basophil pituitary adenoma (75% of cases); these patients have bilateral adrenocortical hyperplasia

- adrenocortical tumours (20% of cases), most of which are benign adenomas; carcinomas are rare

- ectopic sites of ACTH production (usually cancers) (5%).

In each case, it is important to be certain of the precise cause, as the management of each group is different.

Clinical features

Cushing's syndrome is at least 10 times more common in women than in men. One or more of the following features will be present:

- truncal obesity, moon face, buffalo hump
- abdominal striae, hirsutism
- menstrual disturbance
- psychological disturbance.

Many of these patients will be mildly hypertensive or diabetic.

Diagnosis

The two key questions are:

1. Is there excess glucocorticoid secretion?
2. If so, is it pituitary dependent?

A combination of tests are required to provide the answer. Excess glucocorticoid secretion is proved if:

- the normal diurnal variation of ACTH and cortisol secretion, with plasma levels peaking in the early morning and reaching a nadir in the evening, is lost
- 24-hour urinary cortisol excretion levels are elevated
- the administration of dexamethasone, a potent synthetic glucocorticoid, does not suppress endogenous corticosteroid production (dexamethasone suppression test).

These tests collectively will confirm the diagnosis of Cushing's syndrome. It remains to determine whether or not this is secondary to excess pituitary ACTH secretion (Cushing's disease). This is confirmed by:

- plasma ACTH measurements using radioimmunoassay; high ACTH levels are diagnostic of pituitary tumours, low levels are diagnostic of adrenal adenomas
- CT or MRI scanning of the adrenal glands and pituitary fossa, which will localise the adenoma in most cases.

Treatment

There are two surgical options:

- pituitary ablation
- adrenalectomy.

Pituitary ablation. ACTH-secreting pituitary tumours can be removed by neurosurgeons using microsurgical techniques. Currently, the favoured approach is through the sphenoid bone and the operation is termed a trans-sphenoidal hypophysectomy. In patients who are unfit for surgery, pituitary ablation can be performed by external beam irradiation.

Adrenalectomy. Patients with Cushing's syndrome are often obese, prone to infection and heal poorly. As a result, transabdominal bilateral adrenalectomy for Cushing's disease has been relegated to second place and is only considered when attempts at pituitary ablation have failed. Adrenalectomy is the only option for those patients with a hypersecreting adrenal adenoma or carcinoma.

Multiple endocrine adenomatosis (MEN). Parathyroid hyperplasia is occasionally associated with a familial tendency to develop multiple functioning endocrine adenomas known as multiple endocrine adenomatoses. Occasionally a carcinoma will develop. The two commonest combinations are:

MEN Type 1 syndrome. Parathyroid hyperplasia or adenoma; pituitary chromophobe adenoma; pancreatic islet cell adenoma.

MEN Type 2 syndrome. Parathyroid hyperplasia or adenoma; medullary thyroid carcinoma; phaeochromocytoma.

Patients present either with clinical features caused by the secretions of these functioning adenomas or with a mass in the abdomen or neck caused by the growing tumour. The individual tumours may grow synchronously or metachronously. Treatment is complex but is usually directed at removing the adenoma if this is technically possible.

Self-assessment: questions

Multiple choice questions

1. In patients with fibrocystic breast disease:
   a. Axillary lymphadenopathy is common
   b. The incidence peaks between 35–45 years of age
   c. Symptoms are worse after menstruation
   d. Gamma-linoleic acid can improve symptoms
   e. The incidence of breast cancer is doubled

2. The following points relate to mammography:
   a. All patients over 35 years of age with a nipple discharge need a mammogram
   b. All patients with fibrocystic breast disease need mammography
   c. Stellate lesions on mammography require biopsy
   d. Areas of microcalcification on mammography require biopsy
   e. It can detect cancers up to 2 years before they become palpable

3. Gynaecomastia:
   a. Is usually drug-induced
   b. Resolves spontaneously in most cases
   c. Is more common in patients over 25 years of age
   d. Can be bilateral
   e. Is occasionally caused by hypothyroidism

4. A bloodstained nipple discharge is associated with:
   a. Mammary duct ectasia
   b. An intraduct papilloma
   c. A fibroadenoma
   d. Paget's disease of the breast
   e. Breast carcinoma

5. Breast cancer is more common in women:
   a. With a family history of breast cancer
   b. Who have undergone bilateral oophorectomy
   c. Who have had endometrial cancer
   d. Who smoke
   e. Who have had a late first pregnancy

6. In Paget's disease of the breast:
   a. There is usually an underlying intraduct papilloma
   b. Itching is an early symptom
   c. An underlying breast mass is a common feature
   d. The diagnosis is made primarily on mammography
   e. Radiotherapy is the primary treatment

7. In the treatment of advanced breast cancer:
   a. Painful bone metastases respond best to chemotherapy
   b. 60% of patients are expected to live 5 years
   c. Mastectomy still has a role to play
   d. Oestrogen receptor status may influence management
   e. Adrenalectomy will help postmenopausal patients

8. The following points relate to goitres:
   a. They often cause hoarseness
   b. Stridor is an indication for thyroidectomy
   c. Diffuse goitres are associated with iodine deficiency
   d. Hot nodules are rarely malignant
   e. Most patients with multinodular goitres are euthyroid

9. In thyroid cancer:
   a. Papillary tumours spread mainly to the bones
   b. A preceding multinodular goitre is common
   c. A thyroid isotope scan is likely to show a cold area
   d. Radioiodine is the treatment of choice for secondary deposits from follicular cancers
   e. Cervical lymphadenopathy is more frequent with papillary cancers

10. The following statements relate to radioiodine therapy:
    a. Recurrent thyrotoxicosis is uncommon
    b. Agranulocytosis is a significant side effect
    c. Post-treatment hypothyroidism is infrequent
    d. It is the treatment of choice for recurrent thyrotoxicosis
    e. It should be avoided in childhood thyrotoxicosis

11. In primary hyperparathyroidism:
    a. A single parathyroid adenoma is the most likely cause
    b. Renal phosphate excretion is increased
    c. Most patients have radiological evidence of sub-periosteal bone resorption in the phalanges
    d. Chronic renal failure is uncommon
    e. Most patients will complain of polyuria and polydypsia

12. A phaeochromocytoma:
    a. Usually presents early in adult life
    b. Is diagnosed by an elevated serum vanillyl mandelic acid level (VMA)
    c. Is caused by adrenal cortical hyperplasia
    d. May be a cause of stroke
    e. Can be bilateral

13. A patient with Conn's syndrome:
    a. Is usually hyperkalaemic
    b. May present with hypertension
    c. Can be treated medically with spironolactone

d. Has an elevated plasma renin
e. Usually has an underlying adrenal cortical adenoma

14. A patient with Cushing's syndrome:
   a. Will occasionally have a visual field defect
   b. Is more likely to be male
   c. Will have a low evening serum cortisol level
   d. May be diabetic
   e. May have an associated thyroid cancer

Case histories

Case history 1

A 48-year-old woman presents with a 2 cm painless lump in the right breast that she detected during self-examination.

1. What features on physical examination would make you suspect the lump was malignant?
2. How would you confirm the diagnosis?
3. What treatment options would you recommend?

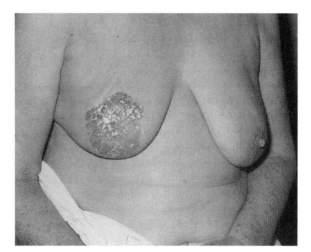
Photograph 1

Case history 2

A 36-year-old woman presents with a swelling in the right side of the neck. In addition she tells you she has lost 1 stone in weight in the last 3 months. When you examine her she appears to have a 5 cm nodule in the right lobe of her thyroid gland. Also you notice she has a fine tremor and a resting pulse rate of 110/minute.

1. What is the most likely diagnosis?
2. What investigations would you perform?
3. How would you treat this patient?

Photograph questions

Photograph 1

1. What is the most likely diagnosis?
2. What tests would you use to confirm the diagnosis?
3. What is the most appropriate treatment?

Photograph 2

1. What is this examination and what features does it show?
2. What is the most likely diagnosis?
3. How would you confirm the diagnosis?

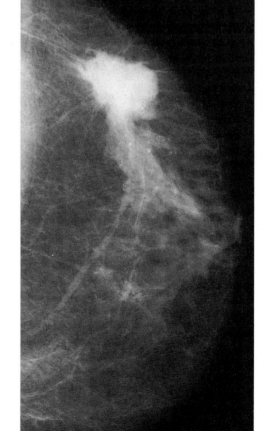
Photograph 2

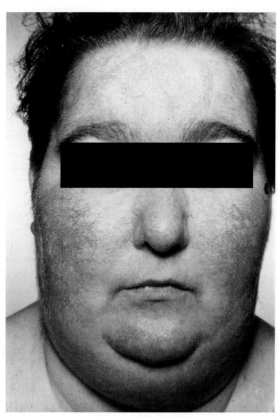

Photograph 3

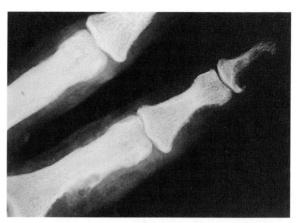

Photograph 4

Photograph 4

1. What abnormalities are present on this X-ray?
2. What is the most likely cause?
3. How would you confirm the diagnosis?

Photograph 3

1. What abnormal features can you identify?
2. What is the most likely diagnosis?
3. What other abnormal clinical features would you look for?

Self-assessment: answers

Multiple choice answers

1. a. **False.** Axillary lymphadenopathy is uncommon. Its presence should raise the suspicion of malignancy.
   b. **True.** The incidence of benign breast disease diminishes after the menopause.
   c. **False.** Symptoms are often worse premenstrually, especially in patients with cyclical breast pain.
   d. **True.** Gamma-linoleic acid (evening primrose oil) is useful; the mechanism is unknown.
   e. **False.** The incidence of breast cancer is the same in patients with or without benign breast disease.

2. a. **True.** These patients may have an underlying cancer.
   b. **False.** Often these patients are young with radiodense breasts. Mammography is best reserved for those patients over 35 years of age who have a localised area of nodularity or tenderness.
   c. **True.** A stellate lesion on radiography may be an invasive carcinoma.
   d. **True.** Any area of microcalcification needs to be excised to exclude a cancer.
   e. **True.** Breast cancers may remain impalpable for up to 2 years. It is this group of tumours that are detected by mammographic screening programmes, enabling earlier treatment.

3. a. **False.** Gynaecomastia is usually a physiological change at puberty. Drug-induced gynaecomastia is the second most common cause.
   b. **True.** Surgical treatment should be reserved for the few cases that do not resolve within 2 years.
   c. **False.** The peak incidence is around puberty.
   d. **True.**
   e. **False.** Gynaecomastia is associated with hyperthyroidism.

4. a. **False.** The discharge associated with duct ectasia is yellow/green in colour.
   b. **True.**
   c. **False.** Fibroadenomas are not associated with nipple discharge.
   d. **True.** An itching, excoriated bleeding nipple is the hallmark of Paget's disease.
   e. **True.** A bloodstained nipple discharge is related to an underlying breast cancer until proven otherwise.

5. a. **True.** The risk is doubled in patients with a first-degree relative (mother, sister or daughter) who develops cancer before the age of 50 years.
   b. **False.** Oophorectomy, particularly in young

women (under 35 years of age), reduces the risk of breast cancer.
   c. **True.** Endometrial and ovarian cancer appear to increase the risk of breast cancer.
   d. **False.** There is no link between smoking and breast cancer.
   e. **True.** A late first pregnancy, early menarche and late menopause are all associated with an increased risk.

6. a. **False.** There is usually an underlying intraduct breast carcinoma.
   b. **True.** Itching and scaling of the nipple are usually the first signs of Paget's disease.
   c. **False.** In the early stages of the disease, the underlying breast cancer is usually impalpable.
   d. **False.** Nipple biopsy is the key diagnostic test. Microscopic examination will reveal large round Paget cells with clear cytoplasm and hyperchromatic nuclei.
   e. **False.** The lesion should be treated as a breast cancer.

7. a. **False.** Radiotherapy is the treatment of choice for a painful bone metastasis.
   b. **False.** By definition these patients have Stage 3 and Stage 4 cancers, with a 40% and 10% 5-year survival, respectively.
   c. **True.** Mastectomy coupled with radiotherapy is probably the best way to deal with a locally extensive but resectable cancer that untreated may fungate or become attached to the chest wall.
   d. **True.** Oestrogen receptor-positive patients are more likely to respond to hormonal manipulation.
   e. **False.** Adrenalectomy is of most use in premenopausal patients.

8. a. **False.** Hoarseness suggests infiltration of the larynx or recurrent laryngeal nerves by thyroid malignancy.
   b. **True.** Stridor or dysphagia are an indication for thyroidectomy.
   c. **False.** A diffuse goitre is more likely to be physiological in origin during pregnancy or puberty. Iodine-deficient goitres are usually multinodular.
   d. **True.** Hot nodules are caused by areas of thyroid overactivity. Malignancy is associated with cold nodules.
   e. **True.** Hyperthyroidism uncommonly develops in a multinodular goitre.

9. a. **False.** Bone metastases arising from thyroid

cancer are usually associated with follicular tumours.
  b. **False.** Cancers infrequently develop in a multinodular goitre.
  c. **True.** Cold areas on scanning are caused by either malignancy or simple cysts.
  d. **True.** Follicular tumours avidly take up radioiodine, which destroys the deposits.
  e. **True.** Papillary cancers metastasise most often to the cervical lymph glands.

10. a. **False.** Radioiodine treatment is highly effective.
  b. **False.** Agranulocytosis is a side effect of antithyroid drug treatment with agents such as carbimazole.
  c. **False.** Many patients require thyroid hormone replacement after treatment. The incidence increases with time.
  d. **True.** Surgery for recurrent thyrotoxicosis can be difficult and risks damage to the recurrent laryngeal nerves and parathyroid glands. Radioiodine or antithyroid drugs are the treatment of choice.
  e. **True.** Although there is no increased risk of malignancy, almost all children treated with radioiodine will eventually become hypothyroid. For this reason, children should not have radioiodine treatment.

11. a. **True.** Of all cases of primary hyperparathyroidism, 90% are caused by a single adenoma.
  b. **True.** Parathormone inhibits renal reabsorption of phosphate.
  c. **False.** Subperiosteal bone resorption is a late sign in long-standing disease.
  d. **True.** Chronic renal failure is more usually the cause of secondary hyperparathyroidism.
  e. **False.** Most patients are diagnosed when asymptomatic, on routine biochemical screening.

12. a. **True.**
  b. **False.** The biochemical diagnosis is made on an analysis of a 24-hour urine collection for VMA which is a urinary metabolite of catecholamines.
  c. **False.** A phaeochromocytoma is a tumour of the adrenal medulla.
  d. **True.** A phaeochromocytoma can present dramatically as a hypertensive crisis that precipitates a stroke.
  e. **True.** Although unilateral disease is more common.

13. a. **False.** Conn's syndrome is characterised by hypokalaemia.
  b. **True.** Hypertension and hypokalaemia are frequently the cause for the investigation of hyperaldosteronism.

  c. **True.** Patients with a mild variant of the disease or those unfit or unsuitable for surgery can be maintained in the long term on an aldosterone antagonist such as spironolactone.
  d. **False.** Patients with primary hyperaldosteronism have a low plasma renin. A high renin level is characteristic of secondary hyperaldosteronism caused by hepatic or renal disease.
  e. **True.** 80% of patients with primary hyperaldosteronism have a solitary adrenal cortical adenoma. The remainder are associated with bilateral adrenal cortical hyperplasia.

14. a. **True.** Visual field defects are likely to develop as the pituitary adenoma enlarges and compresses the optic chiasm, classically causing a bitemporal hemianopia.
  b. **False.** Cushing's syndrome is 10 times more common in women than in men.
  c. **False.** Serum cortisol levels are normally at their lowest in the evening. Loss of this circadian rhythm with a high evening cortisol (and ACTH) are in keeping with a diagnosis of Cushing's syndrome.
  d. **True.** Glucose intolerance and fasting hyperglycaemia are common in Cushing's syndrome.
  e. **False.** Adrenal medullary tumours (phaeochromocytoma) are linked with medullary thyroid cancers in patients with multiple endocrine adenomatosis in MEN Type 2 syndrome.

Case history answers
Case history 1

1. The following features on inspection of the breast would be suspicious of an underlying malignancy:
  - a unilaterally indrawn nipple
  - skin tethering or peau d'orange changes (subcutaneous oedema).

The most important features on palpation would be:
  - an irregular hard mass
  - signs of tethering to either skin or underlying pectoral muscles or both
  - a bloodstained nipple discharge
  - axillary or supraclavicular lymphadenopathy.

2. Mammography and fine needle aspiration cytology would be the initial steps. In the unlikely event that a firm tissue diagnosis is not obtained, the diagnosis could be confirmed by an excisional biopsy of the lump under general anaesthetic. Once the diagnosis of malignancy is confirmed, the patient should be screened for metastases; the key steps being:

  - chest X-ray
  - liver scan (ultrasound or isotope)
  - isotope bone scan.

3. The main treatment options, assuming there is no evidence of distant disease spread, are a total mastectomy plus axillary clearance or a segmental mastectomy conserving the breast but widely excising the lesion together with an axillary gland clearance. The second treatment option would need to be followed by a course of postoperative radiotherapy to the remaining breast tissue.

   The choice of operation would be determined by the size and site of the tumour relative to the breast and would also take into account the patient's wishes about conservation of the breast.

Case history 2

1. A toxic nodule in a multinodular goitre.
2. From the history and clinical findings, the patient could be thyrotoxic. Thyroid function tests should be carried out, namely T_4, T_3 and thyroid-stimulating hormone level (TSH). An elevated serum T_4 (or T_3) with a suppressed TSH level would confirm the diagnosis.

   A thyroid isotope scan would confirm that the palpable nodule is functional (a hot nodule) and an X-ray of her thoracic inlet would check for tracheal deviation or a mediastinal component to the thyroid gland.
3. There are three possible treatment options for this thyrotoxic patient. They are:
   - antithyroid drugs
   - radioiodine treatment
   - surgical resection: thyroidectomy.

Antithyroid drugs are of most use in small diffuse goitres. The presence of a large nodule in the thyroid gland would be a relative contraindication to this treatment. Radioiodine therapy would probably be effective but is better reserved for patients who are over 40 years of age or who are unfit for surgery. A thyroidectomy is probably the best option for a young patient with a toxic thyroid nodule. The operation of choice would be a subtotal thyroidectomy, excising the majority of both lobes of the thyroid gland, leaving a rim of thyroid tissue to protect and conserve the parathyroid glands and the recurrent laryngeal nerves.

Photograph answers

Photograph 1

1. Paget's disease of the nipple.
2. Biopsy of the nipple together with mammography to identify any associated underlying breast cancer.
3. Total mastectomy and axillary clearance is the best treatment option in order to deal with the underlying ductal carcinoma.

Photograph 2

1. This is a mammogram. The radiograph shows a stellate lesion with puckering and irregularity of the adjacent breast tissue.
2. Breast cancer.
3. By fine needle aspiration cytology.

Photograph 3

1. This patient has a steroid or a 'moon face'.
2. This could be secondary to exogenous steroid administration or Cushing's syndrome or disease.
3. Hirsutism, abdominal striae, central abdominal obesity (buffalo hump), menstrual irregularities and hypertension might be present in any combination.

Photograph 4

1. This X-ray shows areas of subperiosteal bone resorption in the phalanges.
2. Primary hyperparathyroidism is the most common cause.
3. The diagnosis would be confirmed by demonstrating elevated serum calcium levels in the presence of an elevated serum parathormone level.

Cardiothoracic surgery

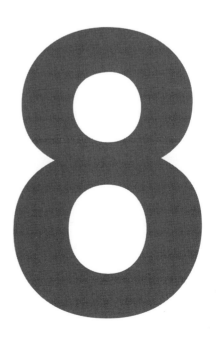

8.1 Cardiac surgery

Ischaemic heart disease

Medical treatment for coronary attacks (aspirin, beta-blockers, angiotensin-converting enzyme (ACE) inhibitors and angioplasty) has reduced the immediate coronary death rate. Consequently, there is an increasing requirement for bypass surgery.

The main factors contributing to atheromatous disease are:

- smoking
- hypertension
- diabetes
- hyperlipidaemia
- family history of ischaemic heart disease.

Pathology

Atheromatous plaques narrow the coronary artery lumen. A 40% reduction in cross-sectional diameter has a significant effect on blood flow. Localised, proximal coronary atheroma is amenable to bypass surgery. Disease that is diffusely spread along the coronary artery is not. Sometimes the intima and inner media of an artery obstructed by diffuse atheroma may be removed (coronary endarterectomy).

Classification of coronary artery disease

There are three coronary vessel systems, each based on one of the major coronary arteries:

- the right coronary artery
- the left anterior descending coronary artery
- the circumflex coronary artery (Fig. 48).

Patients are put into categories according to the number of diseased vessel systems. Patients with disease in the initial segment of the left coronary artery (Fig. 48) are referred to as having left main stem disease. These categories have prognostic implications for survival without surgery (Table 13).

Assessment

Preoperative evaluation is based on the anatomical extent of coronary disease demonstrated by angiography (Fig. 49) and the assessment of left ventricular function by echocardiography, and/or left ventricular angiography combined with intracardiac pressure measurement.

Table 13. Survival without coronary artery surgery

Diseased vessels	Annual mortality (%)
1 vessel	2
2 vessel	4–6
3 vessel	8–11
Left 'main stem'	9–11

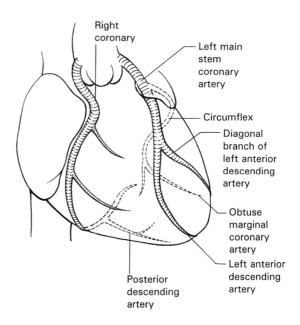

Fig. 48
Coronary vessel systems.

Selection for surgery

Elective surgery is advised for patients not adequately controlled by medical therapy and for those with main stem or three vessel disease. Urgent surgery is indicated in patients with crescendo (preinfarctional) angina and when a major vessel is in jeopardy after failed angioplasty.

Surgery

Coronary artery grafts are created from isolated segments of reversed long or short saphenous vein placed between the coronary artery and the ascending aorta (Fig. 50) or by using an internal mammary artery that remains attached proximally to the subclavian artery. Multiple grafts from both sources are often required. In patients with varicose veins or previous vein surgery, coronary artery bypass can still be achieved using a

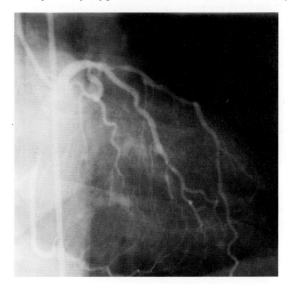

Fig. 49
Coronary angiogram: left coronary injection showing multiple stenoses.

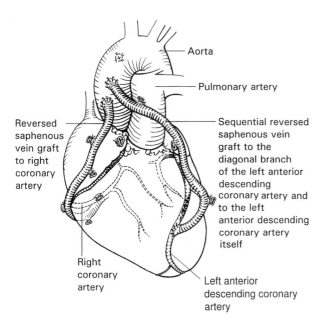

Fig. 50
Coronary artery bypass grafts.

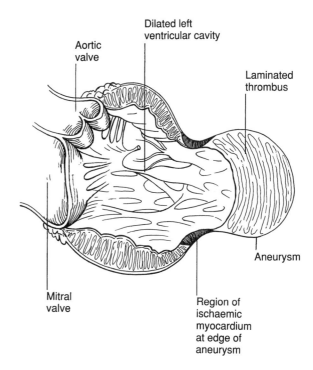

Fig. 51
Ventricular aneurysm.

combination of both internal mammary arteries, the short saphenous veins and occasionally the right gastroepiploic or radial arteries.

Results

Operative mortality after elective revascularisation is less than 2%. Emergency revascularisation following recent myocardial infarction or failed angioplasty has a higher mortality (6%). Up to 3% of patients will have a perioperative cerebrovascular accident. 80% of patients are symptom free at 1 year; the rest are significantly improved. Some degree of angina recurs in 5% of patients per year.

Surgery for the complications of ischaemic heart disease

Left ventricular aneurysm

Healing of a myocardial infarction may be accompanied by stretching of the scar, which assumes a sack-like shape (Fig. 51) termed a 'ventricular aneurysm'. The aneurysm usually contains a laminated thrombus, which may cause systemic embolisation. Left ventricular function is impaired and long-term survival is poor, with 80% of patients dying within 5 years.

Clinical features

Patients present with impaired exercise tolerance, left ventricular failure and dysrhythmias.

Diagnosis

Investigations:

- ECG: persistent ST segment elevation
- chest X-ray: enlarged cardiac silhouette

- echocardiography: confirms aneurysm, thrombus
- cardiac catheterisation: demonstrates concurrent coronary artery disease, the aneurysm and raised left ventricular end diastolic pressure.

Management

Management can be by:

- medical therapy: ACE inhibitors, diuretics
- surgery: excision of aneurysm, coronary artery bypass graft.

Postinfarction ventricular septal defect (VSD)

Postinfarction ventricular septal defect (VSD) is rare. The VSD results from necrosis of a portion of the interventricular septum involved in the myocardial infarction. Blood shunts from the left to the right ventricle, reducing the systemic cardiac output but increasing the right ventricular output; this causes pulmonary congestion and right heart failure.

Clinical features

A loud pansystolic precordial murmur is usual. There are few other features until cardiac decompensation develops.

Diagnosis

Investigations:

- echocardiography: demonstrates a dilated right ventricle with trans-septal blood flow
- cardiac catheterisation: measures the systemic arterial, venous and pulmonary arterial oxygen

139

saturation; this enables the size of shunt to be calculated

- LV angiography: confirms the location of the VSD
- coronary angiography: demonstrates concurrent coronary artery disease.

Management

Urgent closure with a synthetic patch is indicated if the pulmonary blood flow is more than twice the systemic blood flow. Results are poor if the patient has recently had a major infarct. If repair can be delayed to 4 weeks after the original infarction, the VSD margins become replaced with fibrous tissue and surgical repair is easier.

Mitral valve incompetence

Rupture of a papillary muscle can be an acute complication of myocardial infarction. Acute pulmonary oedema develops and urgent valve replacement is required. Mitral reflux may also result from chronic papillary muscle ischaemia.

Myocardial failure

Severe myocardial ischaemia can result in myocardial fibrosis and progressive cardiac failure. Cardiac transplantation is an option in patients who would not benefit from revascularisation.

Valvular heart disease

Heart valve implants

There are two types of heart valve substitutes:

- prosthetic devices
- homografts.

Prosthetic devices

Prosthetic valves have inherent limitations:

- risk of endocarditic infection
- relative obstruction to blood flow (compared with the human valve)
- haemolysis (caused by turbulence).

There are two main types.

Biological prosthesis. This is constructed from porcine aortic valves or from bovine pericardium. The tissue is preserved in glutaraldehyde and mounted on a frame with a dacron sewing ring (Fig. 52). The main advantages are:

- anticoagulation is not required
- the valves are silent.

The main disadvantages are:

- valve failure 6–14 years after implantation
- the potential need to replace the valve.

A bioprosthesis is the implant of choice in women who intend to have a family, as the teratogenic risks of war-

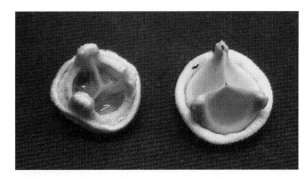

Fig. 52
Biological valve prosthesis.

farin and the need for heparinisation during pregnancy are avoided. They are also useful in the elderly or in others in whom anticoagulation is contraindicated.

Mechanical prosthesis. This is made from synthetic materials. The first design, a ball-in-cage valve, is still in use. Single or double leaflet flap valves are alternatives (Fig. 53). The main advantages are:

- it is unlikely to need replacing
- it is less obstructive to blood flow.

The main disadvantages are:

- it is audible
- it requires life-long anticoagulation
- haemolysis.

Mechanical valves are now the device of choice for most patients.

Homografts

Cadaveric human aortic valve tissue preserved in antibiotic solution can be used for aortic valve replacement.

The main advantages are:

- excellent haemodynamics
- no anticoagulation required.

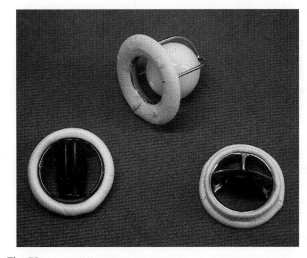

Fig. 53
Mechanical valve prosthesis.

The main disadvantages are:

- it still wears out (over a longer period)
- theoretical risk of virus contamination
- harvesting difficulties and short storage time.

Homografts are not commonly used because of significant problems with harvesting and storage.

Acquired disease

Valvular heart disease is decreasing in the UK because of the virtual abolition of rheumatic heart disease. The few rheumatic cases that remain are seen in late middle-aged or elderly patients. In developing countries where rheumatic valvular disease predominates, all ages are afflicted. In the UK, aortic valve replacement for calcific stenosis of a congenitally bicuspid aortic valve is becoming more common in elderly patients.

Diseased cardiac valves restrict blood flow (stenosis) or fail to seal correctly (incompetence, regurgitation or reflux). Some valves exhibit stenosis and reflux ('mixed' valve disease). Abnormal heart valves are susceptible to subacute bacterial endocarditis (SBE) and patients require prophylactic antibiotic cover at the time of any surgical or dental intervention. Acute valve replacement surgery may be needed if valve destruction from SBE causes sudden cardiac decompensation.

Aortic stenosis

This may be congenital or acquired (rheumatic valve disease). The most common cause in the adult is calcification of a bicuspid aortic valve. It is characterised by fatigue, syncope, an ejection systolic murmur radiating to the neck and a slow rising pulse.

Diagnosis
Investigation involves:

- ECG
  — sinus rhythm (occasionally atrial fibrillation)
  — left ventricular hypertrophy, ST depression in V leads
- chest X-ray: large left ventricle, dilated ascending aorta
- echocardiography
  — hypertrophic stiff left ventricle
  — restricted valve opening
- cardiac catheterisation: gradient of oxygen saturation across the aortic valve.

Management
Valve replacement is required for all significant stenoses. Valvotomy (division of the fused valve commissures) or resection of an obstructing membrane is appropriate in some children.

Aortic regurgitation

Abnormal valve leaflets and a dilated aortic valve ring are the chief causes of aortic regurgitation. The condition is often asymptomatic. Clinical features are a collapsing pulse, cardiac apex deviation to the left and a diastolic murmur at the left sternal edge.

Diagnosis
Investigation involves:

- ECG: sinus rhythm, eventual left ventricular hypertrophy
- chest X-ray: normal or dilated left ventricle
- echocardiography: dilated left ventricle, regurgitant aortic blood flow
- cardiac catheterisation: free aortic reflux, left ventricular dilatation.

Management
Aortic valve replacement is indicated when there is evidence of cardiac decompensation. Patients with dilatation of the ascending aorta may require replacement of the ascending aorta and aortic valve with a combined prosthesis into which the coronary arteries are reimplanted.

Mitral stenosis

This is usually caused by rheumatic heart disease. Patients have a history of rheumatic fever and embolism, exertional dyspnoea, orthopnoea, episodes of acute pulmonary oedema and right heart failure. Most patients have atrial fibrillation and a mid-diastolic murmur. There is a risk of embolisation of a left atrial clot.

Diagnosis
Investigation involves:

- ECG: atrial fibrillation, right ventricular hypertrophy
- chest X-ray: upper lobe blood diversion, small left ventricle, large pulmonary artery and left atrial appendage
- echocardiography: restricted valve opening
- cardiac catheterisation: elevated pulmonary artery and capillary wedge pressure.

Management
Medical therapy. Drugs used are digoxin, diuretics and warfarin (to reduce the risk of embolisation).

Surgery. This is indicated when pulmonary hypertension becomes marked. Balloon valvuloplasty or open mitral valve commissurotomy are options in occasional patients with mobile non-calcified valves. Mitral valve replacement is necessary for mixed valve disease and/or valvular calcification.

Mitral regurgitation

Mitral regurgitation is caused by:

- rheumatic fever
- annular dilatation from cardiomyopathy

- chordal rupture, papillary muscle dysfunction
- infective endocarditis.

Patients are dyspnoeic, orthopnoeic and fatigue easily. The cardiac apex is deviated laterally with a pansystolic murmur radiating to the apex.

Diagnosis

Investigation involves:

- ECG: atrial fibrillation, right ventricular hypertrophy
- chest X-ray: enlarged heart
- echocardiography: dilated, hyperactive left ventricle
- cardiac catheterisation: high left atrial pressure with regurgitation of contrast medium.

Management

Surgery is indicated in patients with progressive left ventricular dilatation. Results are better with earlier intervention. Mitral valve replacement is usual but valve repair and reconstruction is sometimes possible.

Tricuspid regurgitation

Tricuspid regurgitation is caused by:

- right ventricular dilatation secondary to pulmonary hypertension or myocardial infarction
- bacterial endocarditis
- rheumatic heart disease.

Patients have an elevated venous pressure with hepatomegaly, which is sometimes pulsatile. There is a pansystolic murmur at the right sternal edge.

Diagnosis

A chest X-ray will show an enlarged right atrium.

Management

Diuretic therapy is helpful. Surgical correction is only appropriate for cases secondary to mitral valve disease. Tricuspid regurgitation is dealt with by reconstructing the dilated valve annulus (ring). Valve replacement is rare.

Pericardial diseases

Tamponade occurs when there is sufficient intrapericardial fluid to decrease cardiac output. The pericardial fluid prevents the heart from filling in diastole by compressing the cardiac chambers and by occluding the venous return.

The main causes are:

- blood: knife wounds, cardiac surgery, aortic dissection
- fluid: uraemia, malignancy, connective tissue disease.

Clinical features

Acute tamponade. This is characterised by a reduced cardiac output, decreased blood pressure, narrow pulse pressure, elevated venous pressure and muffled heart sounds.

Chronic tamponade. This is similar but shows less marked changes: refractory 'right heart failure'.

Diagnosis

Investigation involves:

- chest X-ray: no specific features in acute cases, smoothly enlarged pericardial contours in chronic cases
- echocardiography: small compressed active heart with surrounding fluid.

Treatment

Acute tamponade. Temporary relief may be obtained by pericardial aspiration, but definitive open surgical drainage is mandatory.

Chronic tamponade. Some respond to aspiration but an operation is required if fluid reaccumulates. Continuing pericardial drainage is provided by creating a pericardial 'window' into the pleural cavity or through the diaphragm into the peritoneum.

Constrictive pericarditis

In this condition, impaired diastolic cardiac filling and constriction of the great vessels is produced by a thickened parietal pericardium, an inelastic visceral pericardium and obliteration of the pericardial space. Previous tuberculosis, pyogenic infection, cardiac surgery and connective tissue disorders are the principle causes.

Clinical features

Chronic fatigue, exertional dyspnoea, a low fixed cardiac output, raised jugular venous pressure and refractory peripheral oedema all suggest this diagnosis.

Diagnosis

Investigation includes:

- ECG: low voltage complexes
- chest X-ray: pericardial calcification (previous TB)
- echocardiography: restricted heart within a thickened pericardium.

Treatment

Pericardectomy, performed through a median sternotomy, is the treatment of choice.

8.2 Aortic disease

Aortic aneurysm

An aortic aneurysm is a localised dilatation of the aorta that is either tubular (fusiform) or saccular (Fig. 54).

The main causes are:

- hypertension
- atheroma
- syphilis
- cystic medical necrosis (Marfan's syndrome).

The aneurysm is often an asymptomatic finding on a chest X-ray. It may cause chronic back pain or present acutely after a leak that causes collapse or a haemothorax.

Diagnosis

Investigation includes:

- chest X-ray: the aneurysm is usually visible; there may be a haemothorax
- CT scan with i.v. contrast enhancement: confirms extent
- aortogram: defines arterial anatomy and relationships.

Management

In view of the risk of rupture and death, surgery is advised in all patients unless advanced age or coexisting medical conditions make survival unlikely. Aneurysms are treated by local resection and reconstruction with a dacron tube graft (Fig. 55).

Aneurysms of the ascending aorta are repaired with the aid of cardiopulmonary bypass to sustain body perfusion. Aneurysms of the aortic arch require interruption of the cerebral circulation; cardiopulmonary bypass is used to achieve total body cooling, which allows hypothermic circulatory arrest during the operation. Descending aorta aneurysms are repaired using left heart bypass or a local diversionary shunt. Operations on the descending aorta are associated with a risk of paraplegia (2–5%) resulting from inadequate perfusion of the spinal cord.

Aortic dissection

A tear in the aortic intima usually located just above the aortic valve or adjacent to the left subclavian artery allows blood to enter the media and create a false passage along the media layer. The false lumen spirals around the aorta (Fig. 56) and can occlude branches of the aorta, including the carotid and coronary arteries, causing a stroke or a myocardial infarction. The false lumen may burst into the pericardial cavity causing tamponade or into the left pleural cavity with exsanguination.

The main causes are:

- hypertension
- atheroma
- cystic medial necrosis.

Clinical features

Classically, patients will complain of a severe 'tearing'

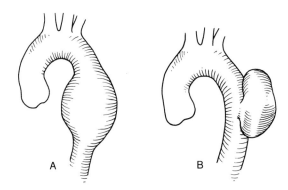

Fig. 54
Thoracic aortic aneurysm. **A.** Tubular. **B.** Saccular.

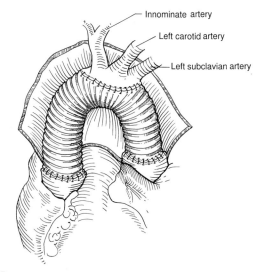

Innominate artery
Left carotid artery
Left subclavian artery

Fig. 55
Dacron tube graft replacement of ascending aorta arch and proximal descending aorta for thoracic aortic aneurysm.

acute chest pain that may radiate to the back. They may be hypotensive with variably absent pulses.

Diagnosis

Investigation includes:

- ECG: to exclude a myocardial infarction, which can accompany dissection
- chest X-ray: widened mediastinum and/or left pleural effusion
- CT scan with i.v. contrast: confirms double aortic lumen
- aortography: demonstrates luminal connections.

Management

Immediate surgery and graft replacement are required to control a dissection involving the ascending aorta and/or aortic arch. Surgery is performed using cardiopulmonary bypass. It may be necessary to replace the aortic valve and reimplant the coronary arteries and/or replace the aortic arch. If the dissection only involves the descending aorta, surgical and conservative management (controlling hypertension) are equally effective. Conservative treatment is favoured unless there is bleeding into the left chest or the vascular branches to the abdominal organs have been compromised. The sur-

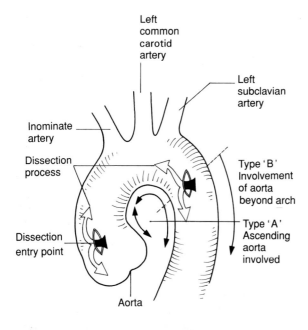

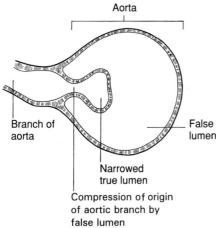

Fig. 56
Aortic dissection.

gical technique is similar to that used for a descending aortic aneurysm (see p. 143).

Traumatic aortic rupture

This occurs at the junction of the descending aorta and the aortic arch. It is a deceleration injury that accompanies a major accident, e.g. a road traffic accident or a major fall. The disruption is caused by a transverse shearing force created at the junction of the relatively mobile aortic arch and the fixed descending thoracic aorta. The intimal and medial layers rupture and aortic integrity depends upon the adventitia. There are usually associated multiple injuries. If the diagnosis is missed, patients die from massive haemorrhage or they develop a false aneurysm.

Clinical features
There is a history of severe major injury. General examination is dominated by other concurrent injuries. It is *essential* to have a high index of suspicion.

Diagnosis
Investigations of use are:

- chest X-ray: wide mediastinum
- aortogram: shows intimal separation.

Treatment
Operation is undertaken through a left thoracotomy using a local shunt or left heart bypass to allow resection of the damaged area and tube graft repair. There is a risk of paraplegia.

8.3 Congenital heart disease

Although congenital heart disease is customarily regarded as referring to diseases presenting in early life, a variety of defects may not require attention until later life.

Classification
Congenital heart defects are divided into two groups: those with and those without central cyanosis. Some conditions start acyanotic and later become cyanotic. This occurs with conditions causing large shunts of blood from the left to the right side of the heart. The massive increase in pulmonary blood flow eventually causes pulmonary hypertension. As the pulmonary artery pressure exceeds the systemic pressure, the shunt of blood reverses and produces cyanosis (Eisenmenger syndrome).

Atrial septal defect

Left to right shunting of blood occurs at the atrial level, increasing the right ventricular work and causing right ventricular hypertrophy and pulmonary congestion. Emboli ejected from the right ventricle may lodge in the systemic circulation because of paradoxical embolisation across the defect.

Clinical features
Atrial septal defect is often asymptomatic. Exertional dyspnoea and progressive pulmonary hypertension develop in adulthood. Examination reveals a right ventricular heave, widely fixed split second heart sound and a pulmonary ejection flow murmur.

Treatment
The defect is repaired with a patch of pericardium or dacron.

Ventricular septal defect

Ventricular septal defects (VSDs) mostly occur in the membranous septum (Fig. 57). Small defects close spontaneously. Significant left to right shunting occurs across larger defects with consequent pulmonary congestion.

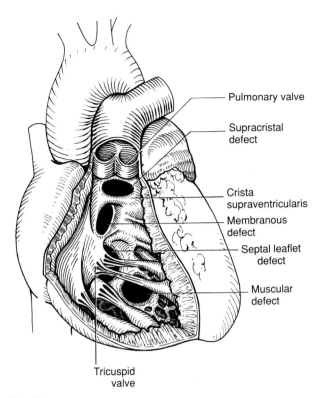

Fig. 57
Ventricular septal defect.

(labels: Pulmonary valve; Supracristal defect; Crista supraventricularis; Membranous defect; Septal leaflet defect; Muscular defect; Tricuspid valve)

Clinical features

Infants with large defects may present with frequent chest infections. Others are often asymptomatic. A pansystolic murmur is audible, maximal at the left sternal edge. The second heart sound may be loud.

Diagnosis

Investigation involves:

- ECG: biventricular enlargement
- chest X-ray: pulmonary plethora
- echocardiography: demonstrates the defect.

Treatment

Asymptomatic defects are kept under observation. Early operation is preferred for large defects to prevent irreversible pulmonary hypertension. Isolated VSDs are closed with a dacron patch.

Patent ductus arteriosus

This defect results from a failure of the ductus arteriosus to close after birth. It can cause the pulmonary blood flow and pressure to significantly increase, leading to pulmonary congestion and hypertension. Growth is often retarded and there is a continuous 'machinery' type murmur.

Diagnosis

Investigation includes:

- chest X-ray: pulmonary congestion
- echocardiography: excludes concurrent intracardiac defect.

Treatment

In premature children, the duct may close with indomethacin infusion, but clipping or division through a left thoracotomy is often needed. Endovascular passage of an occluding umbrella is an option in older children.

Aortic coarctation

Coarctation is a narrowing of the thoracic aorta usually at the level of the ligamentum arteriosum. It causes upper body hypertension and may lead to heart failure in infancy, although children and young adults can be asymptomatic. Extensive chest wall collaterals develop as a means of delivering blood around the obstruction into the distal aorta.

Clinical features

The femoral pulses are absent or weak and delayed. Upper limb hypertension is present. A systolic murmur may be audible over the back.

Diagnosis

Investigation includes:

- ECG: left ventricular hypertrophy
- chest X-ray: enlarged left ventricle, reduced aortic knuckle, rib 'notching' resulting from the enlarged and tortuous intercostal arteries eroding the ribs.

Treatment

Open surgical correction is required. In infants, an onlay patch graft is created from the left subclavian artery. A dacron bypass graft is used in older children and adults. The proximal hypertension does not resolve in adult cases.

Tetralogy of Fallot

This complex defect (Fig. 58) is the most common cause of cyanotic congenital heart disease. It is characterised by:

- a high ventricular septal defect
- an aorta that overlies the septum
- right ventricular outflow obstruction
- right ventricular hypertrophy.

The obstruction to right ventricular outflow causes right to left shunting across the ventricular septal defect and, consequently, cyanosis.

Clinical features

The clinical features depend upon the severity of the right ventricular outflow obstruction. This may not be significant when the child is at rest but may be precipitated by adrenergic events. Consequently, the child may become blue and faint during feeding or crying.

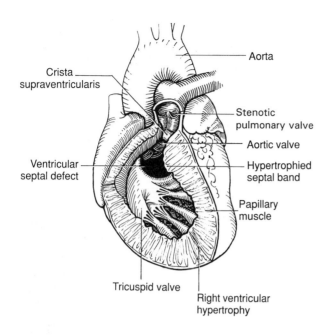

Fig. 58
Tetralogy of Fallot.

Diagnosis

Investigation involves:

- ECG: right ventricular hypertrophy
- chest X-ray: small pulmonary artery
- echocardiography: demonstrates anatomy
- cardiac catheterisation: demonstrates pulmonary artery size.

Treatment

Correction is achieved by closing the ventricular septal defect with a patch, resecting the right ventricular muscle bands, which contribute to the outflow obstruction, and enlarging the right ventricular outflow tract, usually with a patch graft. In children unfit for this procedure, a shunt from the subclavian artery to the pulmonary artery will increase pulmonary blood flow and buy 'time', allowing the child to grow with a view to definitive correction at a later date.

8.4 Thoracic surgery

Bronchogenic carcinoma

Bronchogenic carcinoma is the most common cause of cancer death in males (second most common in females) in the UK. It usually presents after the fifth decade. Cigarette smoking is the dominant risk factor. Exposure to asbestos, radioactive dusts, bichromates and nickel ore is also important.

Tumours may be central (at the hilum) or peripheral (coin lesions, Fig. 59). Cavitation is not uncommon and invasion of adjacent structures (chest wall, pericardium, trachea, phrenic nerve and superior vena cava) can occur (Fig. 60).

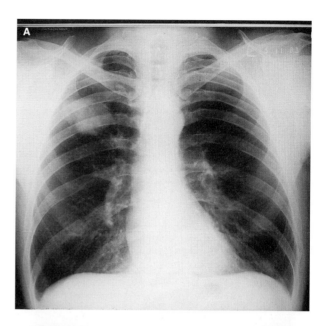

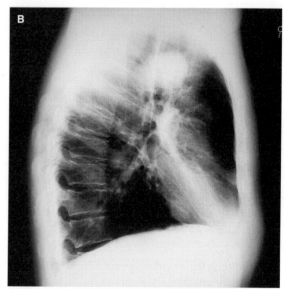

Fig. 59
A. Pulmonary coin lesion. 4 cm mass in right upper zone. **B.** The same lesion as top seen on lateral view which shows the lesion to be in the apical segment of the upper lobe.

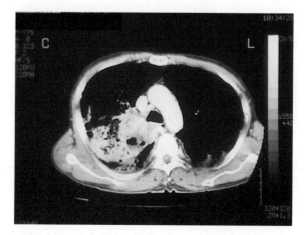

Fig. 60
Advanced bronchogenic carcinoma. CT scan of thorax. Right hilar mass invading mediastinum. There is collapse and cavitation of the lung parenchyma distal to the tumour.

The main cell types are:

- squamous: 45%
- small cell: 25%
- adenocarcinoma: 15%
- large cell: 15%.

Approximately 70% are inoperable at presentation. Lymphatic spread is via intrapulmonary nodes to the hilar nodes and finally to the mediastinal nodes. Eventually the scalene nodes may be involved. Distant haematogenous spread is to the brain, adrenals, liver and bones.

Clinical features

Cough, haemoptysis and pneumonia are typical, with occasional chest pain. Often the tumour is an asymptomatic finding on a chest X-ray. Weight loss and tiredness are common.

Examination may be normal or reveal clubbing, signs of consolidation or collapse (Fig. 61) or a pleural effusion.

The following features indicate inoperability:

- scalene lymphadenopathy
- hepatomegaly
- superior vena caval obstruction
- Horner's syndrome (sympathetic chain involvement).

Diagnosis

Investigation involves:

- chest X-ray
  — peripheral opacity/cavity or hilar mass
  — consolidation or collapse
- CT scan
  — identifies mass plus any mediastinal lymphadenopathy
  — images any liver metastases
- sputum cytology: may reveal carcinoma cells
- fine needle aspiration: may confirm tissue diagnosis
- bronchoscopy
  — used to assess operability
  — may provide tissue diagnosis
- mediastinoscopy: used to exclude/confirm involvement of mediastinal nodes.

Treatment

Resection is indicated in all fit patients with localised non-small cell cancer. Detailed assessment of cardiac and respiratory function is essential. Arterial blood gas estimation is helpful because CO_2 retention is an absolute contraindication to surgery in view of the risk of postoperative respiratory failure. Overall, approximately 30% of patients presenting with a bronchogenic carcinoma are suitable for surgery. Resection (lobectomy or pneumonectomy) is performed through a posterolateral thoracotomy. Radiotherapy is reserved for inoperable or unfit patients.

The treatment of small cell cancer is controversial.

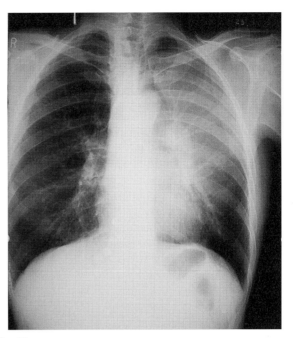

Fig. 61
Collapse/consolidation of left upper lobe associated with a bronchial neoplasm.

Surgery is probably best for early tumours but is less likely to benefit advanced lesions. These tumours often respond well initially to chemotherapy.

Postoperative radiotherapy does not enhance survival but reduces local recurrence. Postoperative chemotherapy improves survival in patients with very advanced local disease.

Prognosis

The overall operative mortality is 5%. Survival varies according to cell type (squamous > adeno > large cell > undifferentiated > small cell), blood vessel invasion and disease stage (based on a TNM system) (see p. 122). One third of resected patients will be alive 5 years later.

Pulmonary infection

Bronchiectasis

This condition is characterised by dilatations of the bronchial tree containing infected pools of secretion. Bronchiectasis usually results from childhood pneumonia or chronic bronchial obstruction, e.g. after foreign body inhalation.

Clinical features. There is a history of a chronic productive cough with frequent exacerbations. Intermittent haemoptysis can be severe. One third of patients have finger clubbing.

Diagnosis:

- bronchoscopy: excludes chronic obstruction
- bronchography: outlines bronchiectatic areas with a contrast medium
- CT scan of thorax: most common method of delineating disease.

Treatment. Conservative treatment with postural drainage and antibiotics for acute episodes or to control infection in winter is the rule. Surgery is indicated if disease is localised to one lobe or to control massive haemorrhage.

Lung abscess

This condition usually complicates pneumonia but may follow infection of a pulmonary cyst or bulla or may follow central necrosis in a bronchogenic cancer or pulmonary infarct. In cases with a pneumonic origin, the initial cause is often aspiration in patients who are unable to protect their airway. It is a feature of debilitated or unconscious patients and after inhalation of gastric contents during anaesthesia.

Clinical features. Symptoms include cough, fever, haemoptysis.

Diagnosis:

- chest X-ray: cavity with an air fluid level (Fig. 62)
- bronchoscopy: excludes an underlying carcinoma.

Treatment. Broad-spectrum antibiotic therapy is the cornerstone of treatment. Resection is indicated if there is an associated carcinoma or severe haemorrhage.

Interstitial lung disease

A variety of diseases can cause widespread pulmonary shadowing:

- pneumoconioses
- miliary TB
- lymphangitis carcinomatosis
- fibrosing alveolitis
- allergic alveolitis
- connective tissue disease, e.g. sarcoidosis
- drug toxicities.

These conditions can be difficult to distinguish on the basis of clinical findings and radiological appearances.

Diagnosis

Surgical biopsy (for histology and culture) is the investigation of choice. This can be performed thoracoscopically using minimal access surgical techniques.

Treatment

Any provoking allergens (e.g. birds) should be removed. Steroid therapy helps; an infective process requires antibiotic therapy. Occasionally an infiltrative malignant process is discovered.

Pneumothorax

Air in the pleural space is termed a pneumothorax. A pneumothorax is spontaneous if it is caused by an air leak with no external cause, iatrogenic after instrumentation of the chest or traumatic following chest trauma. Air may arise from an internal air leak from some part of the respiratory system (closed pneumoth-

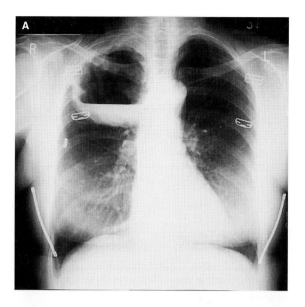

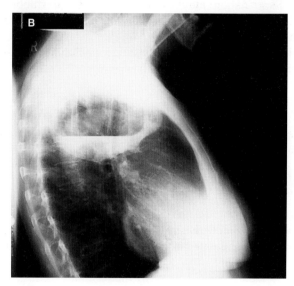

Fig. 62
Lung abscess. **A.** PA view lung abscess right upper zone.
B. Lateral view shows abscess is in the upper lobe.

orax) or from the oesophagus. A pneumothorax may also result from a communication between the pleural cavity and the outside atmosphere through a defect in the chest wall (open pneumothorax). The intrapleural pressure remains constant and mediastinal shift does not occur. A tension pneumothorax develops when the pleural air in a closed pneumothorax is under sufficient pressure to deviate the mediastinum to the opposite side and compress the ipsilateral lung (Fig. 63). This results from a valve-like effect at the leakage site, where each successive breath increases the intrapleural pressure.

Spontaneous pneumothorax

This occurs in two quite different groups of patients:

Primary pneumothorax. This typically affects young, tall, asthenic individuals, males more often than

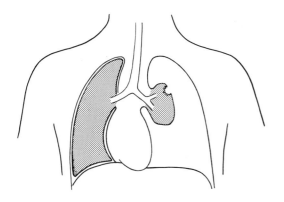

Fig. 63
Left tension pneumothorax.

females. The lung looks normal and has small apical air blisters. The prognosis is excellent.

Secondary pneumothorax. This usually develops in elderly patients with a background of bronchitis and emphysema. The air leak stems from a large air sac or bulla in the lung. Mortality is high because of poor lung function, slow healing and the risk of pneumonia.

Clinical features
Sudden onset of dyspnoea with hyper-resonance and reduced breath sounds are the hallmark of a pneumothorax. In a tension pneumothorax dyspnoea is severe; patients may be cyanosed with tracheal deviation and reduced blood pressure and pulse volume.

Diagnosis
Investigation by chest X-ray will show pneumothorax and any bullous lung disease and emphysema in the other lung.

Treatment
Unless the pneumothorax occupies less than one third of the periphery of the lung on a chest X-ray or is loculated, an intercostal drain which is connected to an underwater seal drain should be inserted. This should be sited at the lateral border of pectoralis major. This location is safer as it avoids the risk of damage to the internal mammary artery and is cosmetically more acceptable in a young woman.

A patient with a tension pneumothorax may not be able to wait for a confirmatory X-ray and should have a wide-bore needle placed into the pleural cavity as a first aid measure to relieve the intrapleural pressure. Patients with minute pneumothoraces can be treated conservatively.

In most cases lung re-expansion occurs within 24–48 hours, and provided that there is no ongoing leak the drain can be removed. Surgery is indicated for:

- recurrent unilateral pneumothorax
- bilateral pneumothorax
- continued air leak
- any occupation where pneumothorax would be a hazard.

Operative management is based on securing any air blisters or bullae and achieving pleural fusion (pleurodesis) using chemicals or abrasion techniques or by stripping the parietal pleura (pleurectomy).

Pleural effusion

A pleural effusion may be a transudate (protein content < 3 g/dl) or an exudate (protein content > 3 g/dl). Transudates are usually bilateral and relate to underlying cardiac, renal or hepatic disease. Exudates are associated with malignancy, pneumonia, connective tissue disease, tuberculosis, pancreatitis and ovarian tumours.

Clinical features
Any features suggesting any of these underlying causes should be sought from the history and examination. The classic features of a pleural effusion are dullness to percussion with reduced or absent breath sounds.

Diagnosis
Investigation includes:

- fluid biochemistry: the amylase content is diagnostic in a pancreatitis-related effusion
- culture and microscopy: identifies infection and sometimes malignant cells
- chest X-ray: a postdrainage film may reveal an underlying tumour
- sputum cytology
- bronchoscopy: ⎫
- pleural biopsy ⎬ may provide a tissue diagnosis

Treatment
The effusion should be drained for diagnostic and therapeutic reasons. If the preceding investigations are negative, thoracoscopy is indicated and any pleural or pulmonary abnormalities are biopsied.

If biopsies confirm malignancy, a sclerosing agent can be inserted via a chest drain to prevent reaccumulation of the effusion.

Pleural empyema

An empyema is an intrapleural collection of pus, usually a consequence of pneumonia. Other causes are lung abscess, a complication of thoracic surgery or the sequel to chest drainage.

Clinical features
A swinging fever and weight loss with a preceding history of pneumonia characterise empyema. A large empyema may be associated with breathlessness.

Diagnosis
Investigations involve:

- chest X-ray: a basal effusion may be present
- aspiration: is diagnostic, pus should be cultured.

Treatment

A recent empyema with thin pus (usually postpneumonic) may be drained fully using an intercostal tube and underwater seal drain. More often, the diagnosis is delayed and follows several courses of antibiotic therapy, resulting in a densely fibrous capsule around the empyema with little prospect of the underlying lung re-expanding. In a young fit patient the empyema cavity is excised and the fibrous tissue removed from the underlying lung (decortication) through a thoracotomy. This allows the lung to re-expand. Tube drainage may be all that is possible in the elderly unfit patient.

Thoracic trauma

Rib fractures

A moderate impact injury will cause a simple fracture of one or several ribs. Double fractures of ribs create a free floating or flail segment which moves paradoxically with respiration (Fig. 64). This effect can tip elderly patients into respiratory failure. Fractures of the 9th–11th ribs are often associated with splenic or renal injury. Fractures of the first rib denote a high energy injury and may be associated with a neurovascular injury. Bilateral rib fractures imply a major transmediastinal force, which can be associated with injuries to the heart, great vessels and trachea.

Pulmonary injury

Pulmonary contusion is associated with all rib injuries. If contusion is extensive, the lung becomes consolidated causing impaired blood and gas exchange. A penetrating pulmonary injury (even by fractured rib ends) may produce a haemopneumothorax. Massive rates of air loss suggest a bronchial injury.

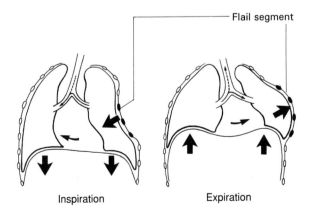

Fig. 64
Flail segment. Movement of the mediastinum and paradoxical motion of the flail segment in a patient with flail chest injury.

Treatment

Treatment depends on the severity of the injury:

- uncomplicated rib fractures
  - oral analgesia with or without intercostal nerve block
  - physiotherapy
  - monitor arterial saturation, blood gases
- flail segment, major chest injury
  - as for uncomplicated injury
  - may need positive pressure ventilation
- penetrating injury (e.g. stab wound)
  - intercostal drainage and observation
  - thoracotomy if bleeding > 150 ml/hour or > 1 litre initially (bleeding is usually from chest wall vessels)
- major airway injury
  - immediate thoracotomy and repair.

Cardiovascular injury

Great vessel injury. This is usually associated with a transmediastinal or a deceleration injury. The aorta and subclavian vessels are most often affected. Injury to the subclavian vessels and brachial plexus can follow fractures to the first rib. Decreased pulse pressure and perfusion are evident in the affected limb with a soft tissue swelling in the supraclavicular area. There may be sensorimotor abnormalities.

Cardiac injury. This should be considered in blunt sternal fractures or penetrating anterior chest wounds. Sternal fractures are often the sequel to a seat-belt injury. Myocardial contusion may be present. Clinical features are similar to right ventricular infarction, with reduced cardiac output and elevated venous pressure. All patients with a fractured sternum should be admitted for observation. The management of any underlying myocardial contusion is supportive as with myocardial infarction. Penetrating wounds cause cardiac tamponade (see p. 142).

Diaphragmatic rupture

Abdominal squash injuries lead to a sudden bursting pressure that may cause diaphragmatic rupture. The patient complains of dyspnoea, air entry is decreased and bowel sounds may be audible in the chest.

Diagnosis
Investigation involves:
- chest X-ray: may show bowel loops in chest
- ultrasound: may confirm diagnosis.

Treatment
Repair is undertaken via a thoracotomy; associated injuries to the viscera should be sought. Sometimes the diagnosis is missed and patients present years later with symptoms referable to bowel herniation into the chest (Fig. 65).

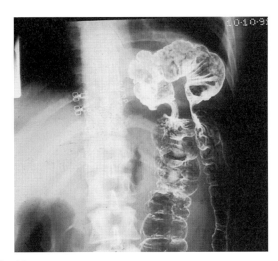

Fig. 65
Traumatic diaphragmatic hernia.

Self-assessment: questions

Multiple choice questions

1. Factors contributing to the development of coronary artery disease include:
   a. Hypertension
   b. Family history of ischaemic heart disease
   c. Diabetes mellitus
   d. Hyperlipidaemia
   e. Smoking

2. Coronary artery bypass surgery improves survival in:
   a. Severely symptomatic patients
   b. Patients with three vessel coronary artery disease
   c. Patients with a strong family history of coronary artery disease
   d. Patients with impaired ventricular function
   e. Patients with left main stem disease

3. Coronary artery bypass may be performed using:
   a. Internal mammary artery
   b. Synthetic small calibre graft
   c. Long saphenous vein
   d. Short saphenous vein
   e. Right gastroepiploic artery

4. The following are complications of ischaemic heart disease:
   a. Left ventricular aneurysm
   b. Mitral stenosis
   c. Ventricular septal defect
   d. Aortic incompetence
   e. Cardiomyopathy

5. Mechanical heart valves:
   a. Require anticoagulation
   b. Are liable to infection
   c. Last for about 6–14 years
   d. Are most commonly implanted in the UK for rheumatic heart valve disease
   e. Are relatively obstructive to blood flow

6. Causes of thoracic aortic aneurysm include:
   a. Hypertension
   b. Atheroma
   c. Syphilis
   d. Age
   e. Marfan's syndrome

7. Atrial septal defect:
   a. Causes increased pulmonary blood flow
   b. Characteristically causes cyanosis
   c. Is associated with a pulmonary ejection flow murmur and a fixed split second heart sound
   d. Is a complication of myocardial infarction
   e. Can be associated with mitral regurgitation

8. Bronchial carcinoma:
   a. Histologically is most commonly a small cell carcinoma
   b. Spreads via the bloodstream to the brain, adrenals and bone
   c. Is often an asymptomatic finding on a chest X-ray
   d. Is always associated with clubbing
   e. May have a normal chest X-ray

9. In the management of bronchial carcinoma:
   a. Surgery is only suitable for patients with malignant disease confined to the ipsilateral lung
   b. Lung resection is only feasible if FEV_1 (forced expiratory volume in 1 second) > 1 litre
   c. Radiotherapy produces better results
   d. Survival after surgical resection depends on tumour size and node status
   e. A small cell carcinoma is always best managed by chemotherapy

10. Spontaneous pneumothorax:
    a. Occurs in two different patient age groups
    b. Can cause mediastinal deviation and compression of the contralateral lung
    c. If suspected, a confirmatory chest X-ray should always be taken prior to treatment
    d. Is best managed by immediate pleurectomy
    e. Is usually associated with structural abnormalities of the lung

11. In patients with pleural effusion:
    a. Surgically relevant cases are usually unilateral
    b. A sample of pleural fluid should be sent for culture and microscopy
    c. An intercostal drain should be inserted
    d. Sclerosants are useful in malignant cases
    e. Surgical exploration and biopsy may be necessary

12. An empyema:
    a. Is an intrapleural collection of pus
    b. Tends to occur at the apex of the chest
    c. Commonly follows an episode of pneumonia
    d. Is always pulmonary in origin
    e. Is best managed by decortication in all cases

13. In patients with multiple rib fractures:
    a. An associated pneumothorax should be excluded
    b. Pulmonary contusion always occurs
    c. Splenic and renal injuries may be present
    d. Artificial ventilation may be required
    e. Surgical repair of ribs is helpful

Case histories

Case history 1

A 57-year-old male patient with a 3-year history of chronic stable angina presents with worsening symptoms despite maximal medical therapy. An exercise ECG demonstrates widespread ischaemic changes at a low exercise level. Cardiac catheterisation reveals significant stenoses in the right coronary artery, the left anterior descending coronary artery and the circumflex coronary artery, with good distal vessels and good left ventricular function. Surgery is discussed with the patient.

1. What probability of relief of symptoms could he be offered?
2. Would he derive any survival benefit from surgery?
3. What risks would he face with surgery?
4. What likely combination of conduits would be used to construct his coronary artery grafts?

Case history 2

A 73-year-old previously fit male patient is admitted to hospital through the casualty department having sustained a syncopal episode. He has a past history of a 'murmur' noted at medical examination many years ago. On examination, he has recovered completely but you find a slow rising pulse and an apex beat that is deviated to the left. A loud ejection systolic murmur is audible, best heard in the second right interspace and radiating to the neck.

1. What is the probable diagnosis?
2. What would be the likely results of a chest X-ray and ECG?
3. What other investigations would be relevant?
4. What treatment would you recommend?
5. What risks would you quote to the patient?

Case history 3

A 64-year-old woman is brought to the casualty department having collapsed with severe chest pain radiating through to her back. There is a past history of hypertension. She complains of weakness in the left limbs and a cold right arm. On examination she is sweaty, distressed and has a tachycardia of 115/min. Her right radial pulse is very weak and the right arm blood pressure is 80/60 compared with the left arm pressure, which is 160/60. An early diastolic murmur is audible.

1. What is the most likely diagnosis?

2. Why does she have reduced pulse pressure in the right arm and left-sided neurological symptoms?
3. What investigations would you order?
4. Why might she have an aortic diastolic murmur?
5. What are the treatment options for this condition and which would apply in this case?

Case history 4

An 18-year-old motorcyclist is admitted to the casualty department following a road traffic accident in which he was thrown from his bike. On examination he is semiconscious but moving all limbs and has shallow respiration. His pulse is 100/min of moderate volume and his blood pressure is 95/60 mmHg. He is tender over the left chest and pelvis. There is an obvious compound fracture of the left lower leg. Chest X-ray shows multiple rib fractures, a widened mediastinum, left pleural fluid and a right pneumothorax. Skull films show no fracture. Pelvic films show a left fractured pubic ramus. His leg X-ray confirms fractured left tibia and fibula.

1. What intrathoracic injury would you suspect?
2. How would you investigate this?
3. Would you wish to perform any procedure prior to further investigation?
4. What therapy is appropriate if the investigation is positive?
5. What warning should be given to the patient's family?

Case history 5

An 18-year-old male is admitted collapsed to the casualty department having been stabbed in the anterior left 5th interspace adjacent to the left sternal edge. On examination he smells strongly of alcohol and is drowsy, irritable and uncooperative. He has shallow respiration at a rate of 20/min. He has a tachycardia of 130/min with very low pulse volume and a blood pressure of 70/60 mmHg. His venous pressure is elevated to his ear lobes.

1. What is the likely diagnosis?
2. What form of treatment is required?

Case history 6

A 64-year-old male patient complains of cough, haemoptysis and weight loss. He has noticed some joint aches over the preceding weeks. He has a history of smoking 25 cigarettes per day for 40 years and has mild stable angina for which he has occasional nitrate therapy. He admits to long-standing mild shortness of breath on exertion. On examination he is clubbed and has slightly swollen fingers, but there are no other findings. A posteroanterior (PA) chest X-ray shows a 6 cm mass in the right upper zone, confirmed on a lateral film to lie in the upper lobe.

1. What is the presumptive diagnosis?
2. What is the likely cause of his joint symptoms?
3. What further radiological investigation would you order and why?
4. What diagnostic procedures could you try?
5. If surgery is to be considered, what further assessment procedures would be necessary?

Case history 7

A 69-year-old female patient is admitted to the medical unit with pneumonia. She has been a lifelong smoker and has mild bronchitis but is otherwise independent and fit. Her chest X-ray shows shrinkage and consolidation of the entire left lung. Her systemic symptoms improve with antibiotic therapy and she is mobile but not breathless when up and about in the hospital. Her chest X-ray remains unchanged and her respiratory function tests show an FEV_1 of 1 litre as against a predicted value of 1.6 litres for her size and age. Her gas transfer tests are approximately 66% of the predicted value.

1. What is bronchoscopy likely to show?
2. What possible choice of therapy would be available?
3. Would her respiratory function tests influence your decision?
4. What would you advise her regarding further tests prior to therapy?
5. What would you say to her regarding her survival prospects?

Case history 8

A 19-year-old male student is admitted to the casualty department as an emergency. He is acutely short of breath and has difficulty speaking. He experienced sudden onset of right chest pain whilst he was bending over to pick up a book and rapidly developed severe difficulty with breathing and felt faint. A friend called an ambulance. There is a past history of a small left spontaneous pneumothorax treated by observation alone 2 years ago. On examination he is tachypnoeic, centrally cyanosed and in distress. His pulse is 120/min and his blood pressure 85/60 mmHg. His trachea and apex beat are displaced to the left and his right chest is hyper-resonant with absent breath sounds.

1. What condition do you diagnose?
2. What immediate action should you take?
3. What subsequent actions should you take?
4. What long-term treatment should be considered and what would you advise as the optimum treatment?
5. How would you explain this emergency?

Case history 9

A 66-year-old female was initially admitted to a medical unit some 3 weeks previously with a right lower lobe pneumonia. This was treated with intravenous antibiotics and her symptoms resolved over several days, but a right basal effusion was noted to evolve. This appeared to be reducing and aspiration 3 days after her admission had revealed only straw-coloured fluid. She was discharged to convalescence but readmitted 3 days ago with a spiking fever and general malaise. She had been off her food for a week and her condition was generally deteriorating. She had a neutrophil leucocytosis. Her chest film shows a large posterobasal collection in the right pleural cavity. Repeat aspiration revealed frank pus.

1. What is the diagnosis?
2. What are the possible causes and how might you separate them?
3. What initial treatment is necessary?
4. What long-term management would be appropriate in her case?

Essay questions

1. Discuss the surgical management of angina.
2. Discuss the pathophysiology, diagnosis and management of aortic dissection.
3. Discuss the surgical management of bronchogenic carcinoma.

Viva questions

1. What factors predispose to coronary artery disease?
2. What possible grafts can be used for coronary artery bypass surgery?
3. Which groups of patients will have statistically improved survival with coronary surgery?
4. What cardiac complications of myocardial infarction may require surgery?
5. What is a dissection of the aorta?
6. What is the 'Eisenmenger syndrome'?
7. What serious risk accompanies operations on the descending thoracic aorta?
8. What are the anatomical features of tetralogy of Fallot?
9. What clinical manifestations would suggest inoperable bronchogenic carcinoma?
10. What cell types are found in bronchogenic carcinoma and what is their relative frequency?
11. What determines the outcome of surgery for bronchogenic carcinoma?
12. How would you manage a patient with a pneumothorax?
13. Why might a patient develop a lung abscess?
14. What is an empyema and how do you treat it?

Picture questions

Photograph 1

> This 44-year-old male presented to his general practitioner with headaches and was found to have severe hypertension (blood pressure (180/120 mmHg) and reduced and delayed femoral pulses.

1. What abnormality is seen on this chest X-ray (Photograph 1)?
2. What is the diagnosis?
3. What form of treatment is required?
4. Will this cure his hypertension?

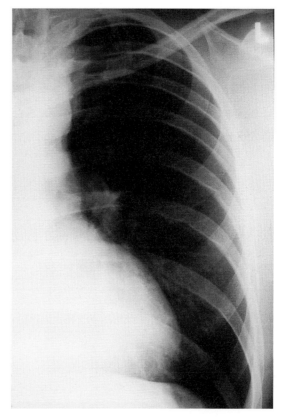

Photograph 1

Photograph 2

> This 57-year-old male presented to his GP with a history of abdominal distension and ankle swelling. On examination, he was found to have a low volume pulse with the jugular venous pressure (JVP) elevated to 8 cm. Heart sounds were quiet with no murmurs. The liver was enlarged by five finger breadths and ascites was present.

1. What feature is evident on the chest X-ray (Photograph 2)?
2. What diagnosis do you suspect?
3. What is the likely aetiology of this condition?

4. What are the mechanisms causing the clinical features?
5. What surgical intervention is required?

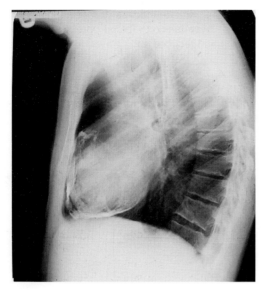

Photograph 2

Photograph 3

> This 58-year-old man was involved in a road traffic accident and sustained blunt trauma to his upper abdomen. He complains of shortness of breath.

1. What abnormality is evident on this chest X-ray (Photograph 3)?
2. What is the diagnosis?
3. What other organ injury may exist?
4. What treatment is required?

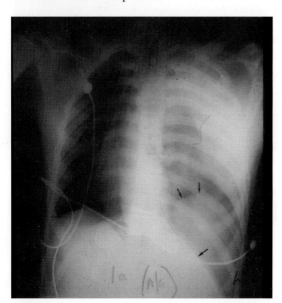

Photograph 3

Photograph 4

> This 24-year-old male was admitted to the casualty department with acute left chest pain and severe shortness of breath.

1. What abnormality is seen on the chest X-ray (Photograph 4)?
2. What immediate treatment is necessary?
3. What long-term treatment is required?

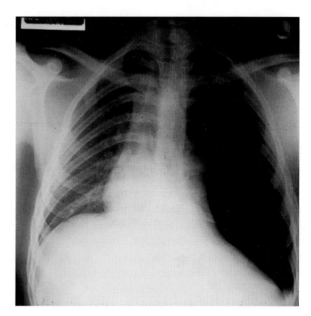

Photograph 4

Self-assessment: answers

Multiple choice answers

1.a–e. **True.** This is a list of the most important risk factors for coronary artery disease.

2. a. **False.** Although patients with severe symptoms require urgent bypass surgery, the effect on survival is determined by the pattern of disease present.
   b. **True.** Three vessel disease is an index of extensive disease.
   c. **False**. The effect on survival is determined by the pattern of disease present.
   d. **True**. Survival is improved particularly if left ventricular function is impaired before surgery.
   e. **True.** Left main stem disease is an index of extensive disease.

3. a, c–e. **True.** This is a list of the most frequently used coronary artery grafts.
   b. **False**. Artificial grafts do not remain patent.

4. a. **True.** A left ventricular aneurysm is caused by ischaemic damage to the myocardium, which leads to healing by fibrosis and scarring. The scar stretches to form a saccular aneurysm.
   b. **False.** Rupture of a papillary muscle may follow infarction. This would cause mitral reflux or regurgitation rather than stenosis.
   c. **True.** A ventricular septal defect may result from full thickness necrosis of the interventricular septum after infarction.
   d. **False.** The aortic valve is not affected by myocardial ischaemia.
   e. **True.** This is an occasional complication of acute myocardial infarction.

5. a. **True.** Because they are made from synthetic materials.
   b. **True.** Endocarditic infection is always a potential risk. Antibiotic prophylaxis is essential in patients undergoing invasive surgical or dental procedures.
   c. **False.** Mechanical heart valves should last indefinitely; bioprosthetic valves have a lifespan of 6–14 years.
   d. **False.** Because of the fall in incidence of rheumatic fever, surgery for rheumatic valve disease is no longer the most common reason for valve replacement. Its place has been taken by bicuspid calcific aortic stenosis.
   e. **True.** Compared with a human valve, all prosthetic valves restrict blood flow.

6. a. **True.**
   b. **True.**
   c. **True.**
   d. **False.** Age is not causative, although advancing age is often associated with aneurysm development.
   e. **True.** a–c and e are the main causes of a thoracic aortic aneurysm.

7. a. **True.** The left to right shunt increases pulmonary blood flow.
   b. **False.** Atrial septal defects only rarely cause cyanosis, usually late in adult life, when long-standing pulmonary hypertension may cause shunt reversal as the pulmonary artery pressure begins to exceed the systemic pressure (Eisenmenger syndrome).
   c. **True.** These are classic features of an atrial septal defect.
   d. **False.** A ventricular septal defect is a complication of myocardial infarction.
   e. **True.**

8. a. **False.** Squamous cell carcinoma is the most common type.
   b. **True.** Together with the liver these are the most common sites of haematogenous spread.
   c. **True.** A routine chest X-ray may reveal the disease unexpectedly.
   d. **False.** Clubbing is not always present and may result from other causes.
   e. **True.** Occasionally the chest X-ray may be clear; the diagnosis being made on bronchoscopy or sputum cytology.

9. a. **True.** Contralateral malignant disease represents metastatic disease therefore surgery will be contraindicated.
   b. **False.** The minimum acceptable FEV_1 varies according to the patient's predicted value, pulmonary gas transfer and the extent of functioning lung to be removed.
   c. **False.** The results of radiotherapy are not as good as those of surgery.
   d. **True.** Along with histological type, these are the key factors that predict outcome.
   e. **False.** Most cases of small cell carcinoma present at an advanced age and are managed by chemotherapy. The few that are caught at an early stage are better resected.

10.a. **True.** Primary pneumothorax affects young patients with grossly normal lungs apart from apical air blisters. Secondary pneumothorax occurs in an elderly age group with underlying lung disease and usually large bullae.
   b. **True.** This is the hallmark of a tension pneumothorax.

c. **False**. In patients with a tension pneumothorax, any delay (as in waiting for an X-ray) may cause death from cardiorespiratory embarrassment. Urgent chest drainage may be needed. The decision to X-ray or not depends on the clinical assessment of severity.

d. **False**. Surgery is reserved for young patients with recurrent or bilateral tension pneumothorax or those whose occupation makes pneumothorax especially dangerous.

e. **True**. Usually apical air blebs or bullae.

11.a. **True**. Bilateral effusions are usually medical in origin, e.g. cardiac failure, uraemia.

b. **True**. This is a key analytical step.

c. **True**. Intercostal drainage provides symptomatic relief and a large volume of fluid for analysis. A postdrainage chest X-ray may reveal previously hidden underlying pathology.

d. **True**. They may prevent reaccumulation of a malignant effusion.

e. **True**. Surgical exploration is normally achieved by 'thoracoscopy'. Occasionally a minithoracotomy is needed to obtain a pleural biopsy.

12.a. **True**. The pus collects within the pleural space.

b. **False**. An empyema develops as a basal or posteromedial collection under the influence of gravity.

c. **True**. Pneumonia or a lung abscess are the most common underlying causes of empyema.

d. **False**. Although most are pulmonary in origin, other important causes include oesophageal leak, subphrenic and liver abscess, surgery and repeated pleural aspiration.

e. **False**. This is the procedure of choice in a young fit patient. In others, tube drainage may be adequate.

13.a. **True**. The fractured rib ends may puncture the lung parenchyma and cause an air leak.

b. **True**. Contusion is inevitable if the injury force is sufficient to cause multiple rib fracture.

c. **True**. The spleen is an anterior relation to the left rib cage. Injuries of sufficient force to cause multiple rib fractures may also be sufficient to produce major visceral injury.

d. **True**. Patients with a large flail segment or deteriorating gas exchange may require positive pressure ventilation.

e. **False**. Surgical repair of rib fractures has been abandoned in favour of ventilation.

Case history answers

Case history 1

1. He would have an 80% chance of being symptom free at 1 year and a 15–20% chance of residual but improved symptoms. He should be told that symptoms recur thereafter at about 5% per year.

2. This patient has triple vessel disease and would be likely to gain a survival advantage with surgery.

3. He should be told that there would be an operative mortality of 2% and a risk of cerebrovascular accident of up to 3%. As with all surgical patients, the possibility of wound infection and postoperative pulmonary infection exists. Deep venous thrombosis is remarkably infrequent after coronary artery surgery and is an insignificant risk. Many patients experience considerable discomfort from the leg vein donor site, sometimes added to by injury to the saphenous nerve, which causes numbness on the medial aspect of the lower leg and front of the foot.

4. Unless there were contraindications, it would be customary for him to have an internal mammary graft to the left anterior descending coronary artery and saphenous vein grafts to the right and circumflex coronaries.

Case history 2

1. He is likely to have had a syncopal episode associated with severe aortic stenosis. This results from a dysrhythmic episode. One would have to consider a cerebrovascular accident, but this would be ruled out as he had no lasting disability. A transient ischaemic episode would be a possibility, although unlikely as some residual cerebral disturbance usually persists for a few hours after the event.

2. The chest X-ray would show an enlarged ventricular outline and might show valvular calcification. The ECG would probably be in sinus rhythm, with evidence of left ventricular hypertrophy and strain.

3. Echocardiography and cardiac catheterisation should be performed. Echocardiography would provide an estimate of the aortic valve gradient on Doppler. Cardiac catheterisation would quantify the gradient and demonstrate the presence of any concurrent coronary artery disease.

4. Aortic valve replacement should be undertaken urgently in any patient with significant aortic stenosis and syncope.

5. Operative mortality would be about 4% and the risk of cerebrovascular accident should be discussed.

Case history 3

1. Aortic dissection should be considered in any patient with a history of collapse and acute chest pain radiating to the back. The principle differential diagnosis is myocardial infarction. Other possibilities would include a leaking aortic aneurysm, oesophageal rupture and thoracic vertebral collapse.

2. In this patient, the false lumen of the dissection process has closed down the brachiocephalic artery,

the first of the three aortic arch vessels, and has, therefore, interrupted flow into the right subclavian artery and right common carotid artery. This manifests as decreased arm perfusion and contralateral weakness resulting from decreased cerebral perfusion.

3. She should have an urgent contrast-enhanced CT scan to confirm the diagnosis. This investigation may also allow the radiologist to comment on the dissection entry site. Aortography will usually demonstrate this and also which femoral artery is connected to the true aortic lumen. This is important information as the patient will have to be perfused retrogradely via a femoral artery during surgical repair.

4. This patient probably has damage extending into the aortic root. Separation of the aortic wall layers often occurs at this level.

5. Treatment is principally determined by which section of the aorta is involved. In this case, surgery is required to replace the entry point and the damaged proximal aorta. It is likely that this patient would need replacement of the ascending aorta and aortic arch and possibly also the aortic valve.

Case history 4

1. With the nature of the accident and the combination of thoracic rib cage injury, widened mediastinum and left pleural effusion, ruptured thoracic aorta must be suspected.
2. Aortography is the investigation of choice.
3. The pneumothorax is an immediately life-threatening condition and an intercostal drain should be inserted prior to embarking on further investigation.
4. Urgent left thoracotomy and synthetic graft replacement of the ruptured portion of the aorta.
5. They would have to be aware that (apart from the risk of death if the aorta ruptures completely prior to the completion of surgery) there is a 5% risk of paraplegia associated with this procedure.

Case history 5

1. Cardiac tamponade.
2. Emergency surgery is required to drain the pericardial collection and to allow the cardiac injury to be repaired. If surgical facilities or expertise are not immediately available, the tamponade may be transiently improved by aspirating the pericardium (pericardiocentesis). This is not always a good option because the heart may be further damaged by the manoeuvre. Also, it does not remove pericardial clots and fresh bleeding will continue to occur.

Case history 6

1. Bronchogenic carcinoma.

2. Hypertrophic pulmonary osteoarthropathy.
3. Contrast-enhanced CT scan. This would establish that there were no lesions in the other lung and would screen the liver and adrenal glands for metastatic disease. Any enlarged mediastinal glands would also be detected.
4. Sputum cytology, bronchoscopy and fine needle aspiration.
5. If there is any abnormality in plasma calcium, phosphate or alkaline phosphatase, a bone scan should be arranged. A liver ultrasound scan is a useful complement to the initial CT. Mediastinoscopy would be needed to confirm the mediastinal glands are free of disease. Preoperative respiratory function tests, arterial blood gas estimation and cardiac assessment by ECG and echocardiography would be helpful in determining his ability to tolerate surgery.

Case history 7

1. She must have a lesion obstructing the left main bronchus as neither lobe is aerated. This could result from inspissated secretions or even a foreign body but is most likely caused by a tumour.
2. Secretions or a foreign body would be removed. A tumour would have to be further staged with consideration towards either radiotherapy or surgery.
3. No, the left lung is totally non-functional at present so her respiratory function tests are largely irrelevant. She will still have a small residual right to left shunt through the left lung and pneumonectomy would, therefore, actually improve her respiratory status.
4. She will need a mediastinoscopy, screening for metastatic disease and assessment of her cardiac status to enable a decision to be made.
5. Radiotherapy would be palliative and would probably provide a survival of 8–12 months at best. If the lesion can be removed surgically, survival would depend upon tumour stage and final cell type. (Cell type in the tumour mass does not always correlate with that reported in a biopsy.)

Case history 8

1. Tension right pneumothorax.
2. One or two large calibre intravenous cannulae (14 gauge or below) should be inserted into the right chest to depressurise the tension element of the pneumothorax.
3. He requires an intercostal drain and a chest film to verify re-expansion of the right lung.
4. He should have a procedure to achieve pleurodesis of the right lung. There are two reasons for this. First, this was a tension pneumothorax which is life-threatening and, second, he has had a contralateral pneumothorax which would make pleurodesis

desirable in any event. A right pleurectomy would be the procedure with the highest long-term success rate and this would allow the lung to be inspected for blebs or bullae that could be ligated at the same time.

5. The right lung has leaked air through a flap valve mechanism probably in an apical bleb. This process allows air to be pumped into the right pleural cavity causing the lung to be totally flattened and the mediastinum to be displaced to the left. The left lung becomes compressed and cardiac output is reduced as the great vessels become distorted.

Case history 9

1. Empyema.
2. This is most likely to be postpneumonic but it could result from contamination of her right basal effusion at the time of the initial aspiration. Some clue would be obtained from the organism grown from the empyema; for example, staphylococci are a frequent contaminant (unless the original pneumonia was staphylococcal in origin). Sometimes a mixed culture of organisms will be obtained.
3. She should have a chest drain inserted into the collection to provide drainage and relieve her toxic symptoms.
4. Rib resection and open tube drainage would be the likely long-term management in someone of her age.

Essay answers

1. Between 400–700 coronary artery bypass grafts are required per million population. As greater efforts are made to prevent myocardial infarction, this need may increase even further. The long-term needs may also increase as the long-term efficacy of angioplasty, currently an alternative to surgical intervention, is unknown.

Coronary angiography is used to define the surgical anatomy and identify significant lesions that are amenable to surgery (usually > 70% luminal constriction). The ideal lesion is a tight proximal stenosis with good calibre distal vessels. Diffuse coronary disease is not suitable for surgery. Very poor ventricular function is a relative contraindication for surgery.

Surgery is appropriate for patients with severe symptoms, those unresponsive to maximal medical therapy and patients with three vessel and left main stem disease.

The operation is carried out during cardiopulmonary bypass usually with long saphenous vein grafts being used as conduits. The internal mammary artery is used for bypass to the left anterior descending coronary artery whenever possible.

The operative mortality is in the region of 2% with a perioperative CVA (cerebrovascular accident) rate of 3%. Approximately 80% of patients will experience complete relief of angina; most of the remainder will notice some improvement. Angina recurs at a rate of 5% per year. The graft patency of the internal mammary grafts exceeds that of the long saphenous vein grafts.

2. **Pathophysiology.** Aortic dissection is associated with hypertension, Marfan's disease (cystic medial necrosis) and atheroma. The split occurs in the intima, which allows blood to track along the media creating a false passage. The entry point of the split is usually just above the aortic valve or at the beginning of the descending aorta. The spiral pattern of dissection occludes branches of the aorta, causing stroke, myocardial infarction, mesenteric ischaemia or a pulseless limb. The dissection can rupture into the left pleural space or the pericardium.

Diagnosis. Patients have a history of severe chest and/or back pain. On examination, peripheral pulses may be missing and there is a differential blood pressure in the arms. A contrast CT scan shows a double aortic lumen; aortography is helpful in defining the entry point and connections to the femoral vessels.

Management. Usually, urgent surgery is required to control the dissection. A graft is implanted during cardiopulmonary bypass. If the dissection only involves the descending aorta and is without complication, conservative management by controlling the patient's hypertension will be equally effective.

3. All patients must undergo a thorough preoperative evaluation to assess their suitability for surgery. Evidence of advanced disease (e.g. Horner's syndrome, hoarseness, scalene lymphadenopathy) should be sought on a general clinical examination. All patients should be screened for metastatic disease (e.g. by liver ultrasound and CT scan) and a bronchoscopy should be performed to determine the endobronchial extent of the disease and to obtain a tissue diagnosis.

Mediastinoscopy is important to exclude the presence of involved mediastinal nodes, which would preclude a resection. The general fitness of the patient should also be assessed, paying particular attention to concurrent ischaemic heart disease (ECG; cardiac echo) and the patient's respiratory function (arterial blood gases; pulmonary function tests).

Surgery is usually performed through a posterolateral thoracotomy. A lobectomy, bilobectomy or pneumonectomy is performed. Occasionally if pulmonary function is limited, a local wedge resection can be undertaken.

The main immediate postoperative problems are pulmonary embolus, pneumonia, myocardial infarction, cerebrovascular accident (CVA) or a cardiac arrhythmia such as atrial fibrillation. Occasionally, an air leak will persist. Overall the perioperative mortality rate is 5%.

Survival depends on the cellular type of the tumour, the stage of disease at the time of resection and the presence or absence of blood vessel invasion.

Viva answers

The key points to remember when answering these viva questions are:
1. Hypertension, diabetes, hyperlipidaemia, family history, smoking history.
2. Long and short saphenous veins, internal mammary artery, right gastroepiploic artery, radial artery.
3. Patients with three vessel disease and left main stem disease.
4. Left ventricular aneurysm, mitral reflux, ventricular septal defect, ischaemic cardiomyopathy.
5. Creation of a false passage in the media of the aorta by blood entering through a split in the intima.
6. Reversal of a left to right shunt because of pulmonary hypertension.
7. Paraplegia.
8. High ventricular septal defect, overriding aorta, pulmonary stenosis, right ventricular hypertrophy.
9. Scalene lymphadenopathy, Horner's syndrome, superior vena caval obstruction, hoarseness, medial aspect arm pain and hepatomegaly: all these suggest inoperability in patients with bronchogenic carcinoma.
10. The cell types and relative frequency are: squamous 45%, adenocarcinoma 15%, large cell 15%, small cell 25%.
11. Cell type, tumour stage (size, node status), DNA characteristics, blood vessel invasion are the most important determinants of outcome.
12. Intercostal drainage for all but a tiny asymptomatic pneumothorax, which may be observed; immediate needle decompression of a tension pneumothorax; pleurodesis for tension, recurrent or bilateral pneumothoraces.
13. Usually secondary to a pneumonia; occasionally complicates a pulmonary cyst or bulla. The pneumonia is often caused by aspiration and is seen in debilitated or unconscious patients (drunks, epileptics, anaesthetised patients).
14. A collection of pus in the pleural cavity; treatment is by intercostal drainage followed by either open tube drainage (elderly and very unfit patients) or decortication (younger patients).

Picture answers

Photograph 1

1. The chest X-ray shows rib notching.
2. Coarctation of the aorta.
3. Left thoracotomy and construction of a bypass graft to take blood around the coarctation.
4. No. The bypass graft will result in a lower blood pressure but the patient will remain hypertensive. The response to drug therapy is much better after bypass of the coarctation.

Photograph 2

1. Pericardial calcification.
2. Chronic constrictive pericarditis.
3. Tuberculosis; less likely causes include rheumatoid arthritis and haemopericardium.
4. Constriction of venous inflow at the junction between the pericardium and the great veins; thickened, inelastic visceral pericardium and rigid shrunken parietal pericardium preventing diastolic filling of the heart.
5. Pericardectomy.

Photograph 3

1. Opacification of the left chest with air fluid levels suggestive of bowel loops.
2. Ruptured diaphragm.
3. Spleen (which was also ruptured in this case).
4. Thoracotomy, splenectomy if necessary, and repair of the diaphragm.

Photograph 4

1. Tension left pneumothorax.
2. Insertion of a chest drain; a large calibre i.v. cannula may be required to relieve the tension while this is being prepared.
3. Left pleurodesis probably by pleurectomy with ligation of any pulmonary blebs.

Neurosurgery

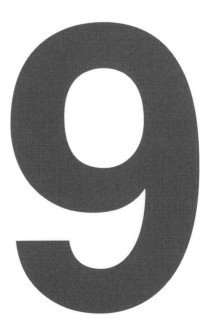

9.1 **Head injury**

Epidemiology and causes

Head injury is common. In the UK, of the one million who attend hospital annually, 100 000 are admitted and 10 000 of these are transferred to neurosurgical units.

There are three categories depending on the seriousness of the injury:

- mild head injury not requiring hospital admission
- moderate head injury requiring hospital admission
- severe head injury requiring transfer to a neurosurgical unit.

Most moderate and severe head injuries result from road accidents (50%), falls (30%) and assaults (10%). Many minor head injuries result from accidents in sport and play.

Pathology of traumatic brain damage

There are two types of brain damage after head injury:

- primary brain damage occurring at the time of injury
- secondary brain damage as a result of later events.

A good result after serious head injury often depends upon preventing secondary brain damage by prompt recognition and treatment of complications.

Primary brain damage: 'impact injury'

There is a wide spectrum of severity in primary brain damage, from mild concussion to instant death. Mechanical deceleration forces act on the brain at the moment of impact, disrupting neurones and the cerebral microcirculation.

The severity of primary brain damage is assessed by measuring the conscious level. There may be focal neurological signs, depending on the exact pattern of damage throughout the brain.

The management of primary brain damage is to prevent complications while any recovery takes place by:

- maintaining cerebral perfusion and oxygenation
- preventing or treating raised intracranial pressure.

Secondary brain damage: 'second insult'

Secondary brain damage occurs any time after injury, when events reduce cerebral blood supply (and oxygen supply) to the injured neurones. The main causes are:

- extracranial
  - hypoxia and hypercarbia (e.g. blocked airway, inadequate ventilation)
  - shock (e.g. blood loss from other injuries)
- intracranial
  - intracranial haematoma
  - epileptic seizures (if prolonged or repeated)

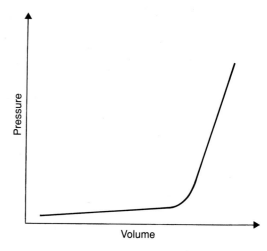

Fig. 66
Intracranial pressure–volume relationship.

  - meningitis / brain abscess (after a penetrating injury).

All these complications cause brain swelling and a rise in intracranial pressure (ICP), which aggravates existing damage to the neurones. Neurotoxic molecules such as free radicals and neurotransmitters do further damage.

Raised intracranial pressure

There is little spare room within the skull and the cranial contents are not easily compressed. A small increase in intracranial volume can be accommodated with little rise in ICP, but if the volume goes on increasing (e.g. because of haematoma or brain swelling) then the ICP rises steeply (Fig. 66). This in turn decreases cerebral blood flow and oxygen supply. Whether the resulting damage to neurones is reversible or not depends on the severity and duration of the high ICP, so prompt diagnosis and correction are vital.

Clinical assessment of the head-injured patient

History

Some history may be available from the patient or a witness. Ambulance crew are an invaluable source of information about the time and circumstances of injury (e.g. pattern of vehicle damage, height of fall, type of weapon) and whether the patient has improved or deteriorated since the injury. It is extremely important to know how much neurological function the patient had immediately following the injury and to use this as a baseline for the Glasgow Coma Scale (see below).

Priorities in assessment and treatment

Standard protocols are used in the initial assessment of every seriously injured patient, to identify and treat life-threatening problems. The priorities are:

A — airway (with cervical spine control)
B — breathing

Table 14 Glasgow Coma Scale and score

	Extent of response	Point scale
Eye opening response	Spontaneous	4
	To speech	3
	To pain	2
	No response	1
Best motor response	Obeys commands	6
	Localises painful stimuli	5
	Withdraws from painful stimuli	4
	Spastic flexion	3
	Extension	2
	No response	1
Best verbal response	Orientated	5
	Confused	4
	Inappropriate words	3
	Incomprehensible sounds	2
	No response	1
Minimum score		3
Maximum score		15

C — circulation (with haemorrhage control)
D — dysfunction (of the nervous system)
E — exposure and identification of injuries.

Assessing conscious level
The Glasgow Coma Scale (Table 14) is used throughout the world. Conscious level is based on three independent variables:

- eye opening response
- best motor response in the upper limbs
- best verbal response.

The 'score' for each of the three variables (see Table 14) can be added to yield a coma score between 3–15. Measurements of conscious level should be made as soon as possible after injury, repeated often and charted to monitor the trend. Changes in conscious level are the most sensitive index of a patient's progress. A falling score warns of continuing neurological damage.

Focal neurological signs
Focal neurological signs reflect damage to specific areas of the brain. The most common are:

- asymmetry of pupil size or response to light stimulus
- asymmetry of motor response between left and right limbs.

A dilated pupil indicates damage on the same side of the brain. Unilateral limb weakness (hemiparesis) indicates damage on the opposite side of the brain. Receptive or expressive dysphasia indicates damage to the speech centre in the fronto-temporal area of the dominant cerebral hemisphere (usually the left).

Radiological assessment

This takes second place to the recognition and correction of life-threatening injuries and complications. Only stable patients should be sent to the X-ray department or CT suite.

Skull films
Figure 67 shows the classification of skull fractures. A fracture greatly increases the risk of intracranial haematoma or infection. Every patient found to have a skull fracture (5%) should be admitted to hospital. Skull films are indicated:

- after a road traffic accident, fall from a height, or assault with a weapon
- if the patient has been unconscious
- if the conscious level is abnormal at hospital
- if there are focal neurological signs
- if the skull has been penetrated (obvious depressed fracture, cerebrospinal fluid (CSF) leak
- if there is marked bruising or scalp lacerations.

Computed tomographic (CT) scan
This can detect haematomas, contusions, brain swelling, skull injury or evidence of penetration. The decision to scan a head-injured patient closely parallels the indications for referral to a neurosurgeon (see p. 166).

Early management and transfer

Careful monitoring of a patient's vital signs is important. Shock is almost never caused by the head injury,

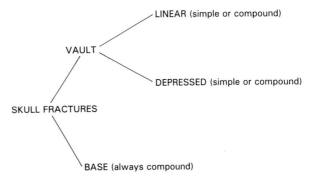

Fig. 67
Classification of skull fractures.

but blood loss elsewhere may have been overlooked and should be sought and treated.

Unexpected neurological deterioration

Common reasons for unexpected deterioration are hypoxia, hypercarbia, shock or a fit. It is essential to check that:

- the airway is clear
- the patient is breathing adequately and has high flow oxygen
- the patient is not shocked.

If the patient has had a fit, the airway should be protected until the fit stops. Anticonvulsants are given only if the fit is prolonged or repeated. Intravenous or rectal diazepam will abort a fit. Intravenous phenytoin prevents further fits.

If these complications are all excluded, or if focal neurological signs develop, the deterioration is probably caused by a critical degree of brain compression by an intracranial haematoma. The patient should be intubated and ventilated and urgently referred to a neurosurgical unit. Mannitol, an osmotic diuretic, can be given to control raised ICP (after neurosurgical consultation). Steroids have no place in the management of acute head injury.

Referral to a neurosurgeon

Late referral for neurosurgical investigation and treatment still causes avoidable death and disability because complications like a haematoma are missed and treatment is delayed. Widely agreed guidelines for neurosurgical referral are:

- immediate (after initial assessment and resuscitation)
  — any altered level of consciousness if there is a skull fracture
  — coma persisting after resuscitation, even without a fracture
  — unexplained neurological deterioration
- urgent (within 6–8 hours of admission)
  — confusion that persists
  — compound depressed skull fracture
  — suspected CSF leak from nose or ear.

Safe transfer to the neurosurgeon

Transfer can be a time of great danger. The patient must be resuscitated and stabilised before the journey begins, monitored during transfer and accompanied by an escort able to deal with any problems en route (e.g. airway obstruction, respiratory arrest, fits). A doctor must accompany every patient with a serious head injury during transfer.

Neurosurgical management

The role of the neurosurgeon is to deal with complications of head injury that threaten life or the quality of

survival. These include intracranial haematomas, contusions, brain swelling and penetrating brain injuries.

Haematomas and contusions

There are three types of post-traumatic intracranial haematoma. All are diagnosed by CT scan:

- extradural
- subdural
- intracerebral.

An **extradural haematoma** forms when a skull fracture tears a dural artery. Usually conscious level is altered from the start because of associated primary brain damage, but some patients have a 'lucid interval' before the conscious level starts to fall — sometimes dramatically. The expanding haematoma compresses and distorts the brain, raises ICP and impairs cerebral perfusion. As the conscious level falls, focal signs develop: a dilating pupil on the same side as the haematoma and weakness of the contralateral limbs. Without timely surgery, signs of brainstem compression or 'coning' develop (rising blood pressure, falling pulse rate and slowing respiration). If the haematoma is not promptly removed, the patient dies or suffers permanent brain damage. With early surgical intervention, 90% of patients will survive and most recover well.

A **subdural haematoma** results from a tear of a vein draining blood from the brain surface to a venous sinus. Conscious level is almost always abnormal from the time of injury because of associated primary brain damage. A large subdural haematoma causes a clinical picture similar to that of an extradural haematoma and treatment is equally urgent.

Intracerebral haematomas and cerebral contusions are most common in the frontal and temporal lobes. They vary in size and clinical importance. Large intracerebral haematomas and contusions cause the same signs of progressive brain compression as extradural and subdural haematomas, and surgical evacuation is essential.

A large haematoma or area of contused brain ('burst lobe') is evacuated through a craniotomy — a large hole cut in the overlying skull and hinged back as a flap. Small haematomas and contusions can be left alone if the patient is well, but if in doubt the ICP can be measured by implanting an intracranial pressure transducer.

Diffuse brain swelling

The treatment is mainly supportive and pharmacological:

- control blood gases by ventilation (avoid hypoxia, hypercarbia)
- reduce brain water by diuretics (e.g. mannitol)
- reduce cerebral metabolic rate using drugs (e.g. the anaesthetic agent propofol).

Neuroprotective drugs may be introduced soon to inactivate toxic molecules or block unnecessary depolarisation by neurotransmitters.

Penetrating injuries

Three clinical types can be distinguished:

- compound depressed fracture of skull vault
- fracture of skull base
- penetration of cranium by a missile or sharp object.

Compound depressed fractures usually result from a direct blow from a blunt object. The main complications are epilepsy and intracranial infection. Epilepsy is more likely if there is underlying dural laceration or cortical contusion. Treatment of the injury includes surgical wound toilet, elevation of bone fragments and repair of any underlying dural tears under antibiotic cover.

Skull base fractures form a pathway for endogenous pathogens like pneumococci to enter the brain and cause infection. A CSF leak may develop from the nose or ear. Antipneumococcal antibiotics are usually given until the leak stops. Some patients need surgical repair of the leak.

Brain penetration by a sharp weapon or a missile such as a bullet or bomb fragment is uncommon in the UK but common in many countries. Basic surgical principles are applied: surgical wound toilet, removal of devitalised tissue, broad-spectrum antibiotic therapy.

Outcome, recovery and disability

After a severe head injury:

- one-third make a good recovery
- one-third survive with disabilities
- one-third die.

The prognosis depends on the initial injury (primary brain damage), the amount of any secondary brain damage and the age of the patient (older patients fare worse).

The biology of recovery

Patients with a mild head injury recover quickly. Recovery after severe brain damage is slow and can continue over months or years, especially in children. Injured brain neurones have limited potential for repair but can sometimes reform synapses with other neurones to re-establish functional circuits. Recovery is best seen in parts of the brain concerned with learning and memory because these neurones are normally in a constantly dynamic state. For similar reasons children tend to make a better recovery.

Disabilities

Common disabilities include:

- Physical
  — headache and facial pain
  — limb weakness
  — poor hand function
  — impaired balance/vision/hearing
  — seizures

- mental
  — personality change
  — depression
  — loss of short-term memory
  — poor concentration
  — learning problems
  — communication problems (expressive or receptive).

The Glasgow Outcome Scale (Table 15) measures outcome in broad categories, but a more detailed assessment by physiotherapists, occupational therapists, speech therapists, psychologists, etc. can identify specific physical and mental deficits needing correction. Good motivation and a supportive family are invaluable. Neurological rehabilitation is complex and some patients need the intensive multidisciplinary approach of special rehabilitation units.

Table 15. Glasgow outcome scale

Outcome	Characteristics
Good recovery	Normal social/family life; can return to work; may have minor deficits
Moderate disability	Independent but disabled; can feed/wash/dress; can use public transport; may be able to work
Severe disability	Dependent for some daily activities
Persistent vegetative state	Non-functioning cerebral cortex; some preserved function in deep hemisphere centres and brainstem
Death	

9.2 Subarachnoid haemorrhage

Classification of cerebrovascular disease

Cerebrovascular accidents (CVAs) are common and like all degenerative diseases occur more often in middle or old age. Prevention is better than any attempt to repair the damage caused. Cigarette smoking, poorly controlled hypertension, fat-rich diet, obesity and too little exercise all increase the risk of CVA.

Arterial occlusion (by thrombosis or embolism) causes 80% of CVAs and usually affects vessels chronically narrowed by atheroma. Haemorrhage from rupture of a vessel weakened by atheroma or a congenital anomaly causes the remaining 20%. The treatment of most CVAs is medical rather than surgical, but in some cases the neurosurgeon can intervene to remove an intracranial haematoma or prevent a further bleed, especially after a subarachnoid haemorrhage.

Subarachnoid haemorrhage

Aetiology and pathogenesis

Subarachnoid haemorrhage (SAH) means bleeding into

the subarachnoid space and, therefore, into the CSF. Bleeding can spread into the ventricles or the brain; the clinical effects of which can outweigh those of the SAH itself.

The amount of escaped blood varies, but even small volumes cause profound symptoms. At first, the CSF is uniformly bloodstained but after some days it becomes yellowish (xanthochromic) as the blood starts to break down. These breakdown products can cause spasm of the cerebral microcirculation and aggravate the clinical picture.

Although head injury commonly causes SAH, by convention the term refers only to cases where the subarachnoid bleeding results from other causes including:

- cerebral aneurysm   80%
- arteriovenous malformation (AVM)
- dural fistulae   10%
- vascular tumours
- no identifiable cause ('cryptogenic')   10%

Aneurysms form where smooth muscle in the arterial wall is congenitally deficient — often where vessels branch. Most occur at well-defined sites at or near the circle of Willis; 10% are multiple. The hydrostatic pressure within the lumen gradually bulges the thin arterial wall out to form a blister-like saccular or 'berry' aneurysm, which can reach > 1 cm diameter before diagnosis — usually after it ruptures causing an SAH. Once ruptured, an aneurysm is liable to rebleed unless treated.

An arteriovenous malformation (AVM) is a tangle of abnormal blood vessels in the brain containing fistulous connections between arteries and veins. The veins become dilated, tortuous and friable as blood at arterial pressure is shunted into them. Dural fistulae are closely related to AVMs. They are partly formed from vessels in the dura.

Clinical features

The onset of SAH is dramatic and unexpected. Headache is severe and sudden, occipital at first but radiating quickly over the top of the head to the frontal area. Most patients also have neck pain, nausea, photophobia and vomiting, caused by escaped blood irritating the meninges. Some have an epileptic fit at the time of the bleed. In 50% of patients, the conscious level is affected and the extent depends on the severity of the bleed. SAH is an important cause of sudden death.

Neck stiffness is the most consistent finding on physical examination. Some patients are febrile. Focal neurological signs such as hemiparesis or pupillary asymmetry indicate that the bleeding has caused a focal haematoma in the brain; retinal or sub-hyaloid haemorrhages may be evident. The most severe cases show signs of brainstem compression: bradycardia, rising hypertension and irregular respiration.

Differential diagnosis

Sometimes a patient is found collapsed, unable to give a history and with altered consciousness, headache and neck stiffness. Apart from SAH, the two main alternative diagnoses are meningitis and other types of CVA. In other types of CVA (e.g. cerebral infarction), profound focal neurological deficits dominate the clinical picture. Acute bacterial meningitis usually has a less dramatic onset than SAH, but other diagnostic clues (high fever, skin rash) are not always present.

Diagnosis

The diagnosis is confirmed by:

CT or MRI (magnetic resonance imaging) brain scan. Either of these examinations carried out within 72 hours will confirm the bleed and can also show complications (brain swelling, hydrocephalus).

Lumbar puncture. A lumbar puncture is essential if CT or MRI is not available or if the scan is normal despite a good clinical history. Uniformly bloodstained or xanthochromic CSF confirms the diagnosis. Lumbar puncture carries risks if ICP is raised but must be done if bacterial meningitis is a possible diagnosis.

Cerebral angiography. This is used to show the detailed anatomy of the cerebral vessels and any abnormality (e.g. an aneurysm) causing the SAH.

Complications

These are common and include:

- recurrent SAH
- cerebral ischaemia
- hydrocephalus
- systemic complications.

Recurrent SAH. Ruptured aneurysms and AVMs tend to rebleed. The risk is highest initially and falls over the following weeks. A recurrent bleed can kill the patient or add to existing neurological deficits.

Cerebral ischaemia. Cerebral autoregulation malfunctions after SAH and cerebral perfusion can also fall if the patient dehydrates from vomiting or poor fluid intake. Breakdown products of subarachnoid blood can cause cerebral vasospasm and ischaemia, with infarction in severe cases. Vasospasm can be confirmed using transcranial Doppler ultrasound. The calcium channel-blocking drug nimodipine gives some protection, and other neuroprotective drugs are likely to emerge soon.

Hydrocephalus. Blood flow in the subarachnoid space and ventricles can impede the normal CSF flow, causing hydrocephalus and a rise in ICP. The CSF must then be diverted by an external drain or an internal shunt.

Systemic complications. SAH can cause subendocardial ischaemia, which can progress to myocardial infarction. Cardiac ischaemia and disturbance in the electrical rhythm is a cause of sudden death after SAH. Sodium loss in the renal tubule often lowers the serum sodium concentration severely, with harmful fluid shift into brain cells. This is treated by sodium supplements, not fluid deprivation.

Other clinical effects of aneurysms and arteriovenous malformations

A giant aneurysm (> 2 cm diameter) can act like a brain tumour and cause symptoms of raised ICP or focal deficits. Acute expansion of the aneurysm can cause a painful third nerve palsy (diplopia, dilated pupil and severe retroorbital pain). Urgent treatment is needed to avert aneurysm rupture.

An AVM can cause epilepsy by directly damaging adjacent brain tissue or by causing ischaemia. AVMs can 'steal' blood from the brain and cause progressive neurological symptoms such as hemiparesis or intellectual disturbance.

Treatment of aneurysms
The main risk is that a ruptured aneurysm will rebleed and the aim is to seal the aneurysm before this can happen. There are two treatment options.

Surgery. This is the usual treatment, using a special metal clip to isolate the aneurysm from the parent artery. The timing of this delicate operation is controversial, but most neurosurgeons operate within a few days of the bleed. There is a balance of risks, which depends on:

- age and general condition of the patient
- neurological status (conscious level, focal deficits)
- any complications (e.g. vasospasm)
- likelihood of technical difficulty.

Interventional radiology. This is the alternative treatment. A fine catheter is guided through the artery into the aneurysm and used to position tiny balloons or fine copper wire to induce thrombosis. This endovascular technique requires great skill and carries some risks. Some patients are treated conservatively because they are unfit, have neurological damage or refuse treatment. Advanced age is not in itself a bar to surgery.

Treatment of arteriovenous malformations
Patients with AVMs are younger and fitter than those with aneurysms, but the lesions are often more difficult to deal with on account of their size, position or complex arterial supply and venous drainage. Conservative management is more common than with aneurysms, especially if the AVM has not bled. The three options for active treatment are:

- surgery
- interventional radiology
- high-intensity ionising radiation (radiosurgery).

The aim of treatment is to destroy the lesion totally. Anything less leaves the patient liable to further bleeds. The likelihood of achieving a complete surgical removal must be set against the risk of causing harm by damaging brain tissue. Interventional radiology can obliterate even large AVMs by embolisation, either as a definitive procedure or as preparation for surgical removal. It is not without risk. With radiosurgery a highly focused beam of ionising radiation is directed onto the AVM, damaging its vessels and causing a slow obliteration over the next year or two.

Prognosis and outcome

SAH is an important cause of sudden death. Many survivors have significant neurological disabilities. The pattern of damage resembles that seen after a head injury and rehabilitation has the same aim — to identify and treat specific problems and restore as much brain function as possible.

9.3 Brain tumours

Classification

There are three types of tumour found in the brain:

- primary and benign (e.g. meningioma)
- primary and malignant (e.g. most gliomas)
- secondary and malignant (e.g. metastatic bronchial carcinoma).

Malignant primary brain tumours never spread outside the CNS, so even a malignant glioma does not metastasise.

The main types of brain tumour are:

Primary tumours:
- glioma: usually malignant
- meningioma: benign
- pituitary tumours: benign
- Schwannoma (neuroma):   benign
- developmental tumours: usually malignant.

Secondary tumours: these are malignant.

Clinical features

Most brain tumours are more common in the middle-aged or elderly. There are three types of clinical presentation:

- raised intracranial pressure (ICP)
- focal damage to affected areas of the brain
- epileptic fits.

The speed of onset of symptoms depends on the tumour type and rate of growth.

Raised intracranial pressure
Most patients with a brain tumour gradually develop a constant, pounding, generalised headache that steadily worsens, peaking in the early morning and waking the patient from sleep. Nausea and vomiting are common. Confusion, drowsiness and coma develop if the raised ICP is not relieved.

Focal brain symptoms
The pattern of focal brain damage depends on the location of the tumour:

- personality change: frontal lobes
- hemiparesis: motor cortex (opposite hemisphere)
- homonymous hemianopia: parietal/occipital lobe (opposite hemisphere)
- dysphasia: dominant temporal lobe
- ataxia: cerebellum or brainstem.

Epileptic fits

A first epileptic fit may be the catalyst that makes a patient seek help. Symptoms of raised ICP or focal brain damage extending back over weeks or months often emerge. Three types of fit occur:

- generalised (grand mal) convulsions
- focal seizures of limbs or face
- complex partial seizures.

Generalised fits involve tonic–clonic jerking movements of all limbs, loss of consciousness and incontinence of urine, and can threaten the airway. During focal seizures, the patient remains conscious and the fit can be followed by temporary paralysis of the affected limbs (Todd's palsy). Complex partial seizures are often caused by tumours deep within the cerebral hemispheres.

Diagnosis

Plain skull films. These rarely help. Occasionally they show focal calcification in a tumour, or skull erosion from chronically raised ICP.

CT scans. A CT scan enhanced by intravenous contrast is the investigation of choice. It will show tumour size, position, contour and internal structure, as well as peritumoral oedema, distortion of adjacent brain tissue and evidence of raised ICP.

Magnetic resonance imaging (MRI). This is an alternative to CT. Its superior resolution and multiplanar capability makes it the investigation of choice for tumours of the posterior fossa and skull base.

Angiography. Angiography can deliniate a tumour's blood supply and allow its interruption by embolisation as a prelude to surgery.

Surgical biopsy. The clinical features or scan appearances are sometimes diagnostic. If not, a surgical biopsy of the tumour allows the most appropriate treatment to be planned. Computer-guided techniques (stereotactic biopsy) allow precise positioning of the biopsy needle even into a very small tumour.

Treatment

There are four main treatment options, which can be combined for maximum effect:

- surgery
- radiotherapy
- chemotherapy (cytotoxic or endocrine)
- steroids.

The potential benefits of treatment must always be balanced against the possible risks.

Surgery

Surgery can cure a benign tumour and is the treatment of choice for meningiomas, acoustic Schwannomas and pituitary tumours. Cure rates can exceed 90%, but the surgery needed for some large tumours can be technically challenging and risky.

Surgery can palliate symptoms from an incurable tumour by improving the quality of life and extending survival. Severe headache can be relieved by excising the bulk of a large infiltrating tumour, or by draining a large fluid-filled tumour cavity. Operative damage is minimised in someone with limited life expectancy by stereotactic techniques, which allow the maximum resection without unnecessary sacrifice of brain tissue.

Radiotherapy

Radiotherapy is most effective in tumours made up of homogenous populations of rapidly dividing cells. Few will be cured, but radiotherapy provides useful palliation (with or without surgery). Its effectiveness can be increased by:

- surgical placement of radiation sources into the tumour (brachytherapy)
- using hyperbaric oxygen
- radiosurgery (the 'gamma knife').

Ionising radiation can damage normal tissue in the brain and elsewhere (radionecrosis). Doses are given in multiple fractions over several weeks to minimise the systemic upset – important for the quality of life in patients with limited life expectancy. Special care is needed in the developing brain, and radiotherapy is seldom used for brain tumours in children less than 3 years of age.

Cytotoxic chemotherapy

These agents can be used to complement surgery and radiotherapy.

Endocrine therapy

Some brain tumours (e.g. meningiomas) express receptors for hormones like oestrogen on their cell surfaces. Receptor-blocking drugs can help to control cell multiplication in these tumours.

Steroids

Glucocorticoids reduce brain swelling around a tumour, which often contributes to symptoms, and can give remarkable relief of headache, drowsiness and focal neurological deficits within a day or two.

Specific types of brain tumour

Glioma

These are the most common primary CNS tumours.

They occur throughout the brain and spinal cord in all age groups. The main histological types are:

- astrocytoma (80%)
- oligodendroglioma
- ependymoma.

Gliomas cause gradually worsening symptoms of raised ICP, focal neurological damage or fits. They show a wide spectrum of biological and clinical behaviour. Low-grade tumours have few mitoses and grow slowly for years. High-grade tumours show rapid growth, killing the patient within months. Low-grade gliomas contain areas of more active growth, which eventually dominate the tumour and change its behaviour. The treatment and prognosis are guided by determining the grade of tumour obtained by biopsy.

Gliomas infiltrate adjacent brain early on. Even when the CT scan shows a well-defined tumour, glioma cells will already have migrated some distance and will cause recurrence. For this reason, the treatment of gliomas is palliative not curative. Surgery aims to debulk large tumours or drain a cyst; radiotherapy is used to shrink the tumour. Steroids are useful to alleviate the symptoms of raised ICP.

Apart from a few benign gliomas in children, most tumours recur after an interval dependent upon the histological grade. Further treatment is usually ineffective and attention turns to palliative symptomatic relief (headache, nausea, etc.) in terminal care.

Meningioma

These are benign, slow-growing, usually solitary tumours that arise in the dura mater inside the skull base, on the falx or tentorium, or overlying the convexity of the brain. Usually a meningioma is a solid mass, less often a sheet of tumour spreading over the dura (an 'en plaque' meningioma).

Meningiomas occur mainly after the age of 40 and more often in women. Symptoms of raised ICP and focal brain damage develop slowly, often so gradually they are attributed to illnesses like stroke or normal ageing. Tumours in eloquent areas like the motor cortex are diagnosed earlier. An epileptic fit can precipitate diagnosis.

A CT scan shows a well-defined mass enhancing evenly with intravenous contrast. MR scanning can define relationships with nearby major vessels. Cerebral angiography can show the tumour's blood supply and help in planning treatment.

Surgery is the treatment of choice. Even large meningiomas do not infiltrate surrounding brain tissue and a cure is theoretically possible. Difficult access or the involvement of major vessels or cranial nerves can make surgery risky. After surgery, 10% of meningiomas recur. Radiotherapy has little effect. Some meningiomas express oestrogen receptors on the cell surface and the anti-oestrogen tamoxifen can improve outcome.

The prognosis for most patients is good (90% cure; 10% risk of significant complications).

Pituitary adenomas

These are solitary, benign, slow-growing, non-infiltrating tumours of the glandular tissue of the anterior pituitary lobe. Microadenomas are confined to the gland and overproduce one of the anterior pituitary hormones, causing acromegaly (growth hormone), Cushing's syndrome (ACTH) or infertility and galactorrhoea (prolactin).

Large adenomas grow out of the pituitary fossa and compress the optic chiasm, causing progressive visual field loss (typically a bitemporal hemianopia). A few become big enough to compress the brain itself and cause frontal lobe symptoms or hydrocephalus. Although they do not secrete hormones, larger adenomas compress and damage the normal pituitary tissue and cause chronic hypopituitarism or acute haemorrhagic infarction and swelling of the pituitary gland (pituitary apoplexy).

Whatever the tumour size, the diagnosis is confirmed by CT or MR scan. Three treatment options exist:

- surgical excision (usually by the trans-sphenoidal route)
- radiotherapy
- hormone antagonist drugs (e.g. bromocriptine).

The prognosis is usually excellent, although a few pituitary adenomas will recur. Some patients will need long-term endocrine replacement therapy.

Secondary brain tumours

Cancers often metastasise to the brain via the bloodstream. Lung and breast are the most frequent primary sites, with relatively few from the gastrointestinal tract. Others arise from malignant melanoma, lymphoma, testicular tumours, and head and neck cancers (which reach the brain by eroding through the skull).

The clinical history is short and distinctive: headache, altered mental state and focal neurological features that worsen rapidly over a few days. Sometimes the underlying primary tumour is already known. Diagnosis is by CT or MR scan, which typically shows multiple small lesions in the white matter that often cause a considerable space-occupying effect because of surrounding oedema. If a single tumour is seen, the diagnosis may need biopsy confirmation.

Surgical decompression can be useful for a single metastasis at an accessible site (e.g. cerebellar hemisphere, frontal lobe) and stereotactic localisation can help locate the tumour with minimal disruption of brain tissue. In most cases, treatment is by radiotherapy or chemotherapy supported by steroids. Death ensues within a few months and good quality terminal care is important.

9.4 Spinal tumours

Classification

Tumours can arise within:
- the spinal cord
- the nerve roots, which emerge from the cord
- the bone of the veretebral column.

There are several types of spinal tumour:

Primary tumours:

- intramedullary (within cord): glioma
- extramedullary (outside cord): meningioma, neurofibroma.

Secondary tumours. These are extradural:

- carcinoma
- lymphoma
- malignant melanoma
- multiple myeloma.

Clinical features

Spinal tumours compress and damage the spinal cord and/or nerve roots, according to the site and nature of the tumour:

- cord compression causes myelopathy below that segment level (upper motor neurone lesion)
- root compression causes radiculopathy in the distribution of that root (lower motor neurone lesion).

A spinal tumour usually causes a developing myelopathy. Control of the lower limbs (and upper limbs too, if the tumour compresses the cervical spinal cord) is progressively lost. Tone and reflexes are increased in the affected limbs with extensor plantar responses, reflecting damage to the upper motor neurones of the spinal cord. Muscle power then decreases if the myelopathy is untreated, to the point of paralysis: paraplegia (the lower limbs) or tetraplegia (all four limbs). Sensation is disturbed and ultimately lost below the segmental level of cord compression. Proprioception (dorsal column sensation) is affected before deep pain and temperature (spino-thalamic) sensation. Sphincter control and sexual function are impaired and then lost.

Less often, a spinal tumour causes a developing radiculopathy, with progressive pain, weakness and sensory disturbance in the distribution of that nerve root. The pain often has a burning 'dysaesthetic' quality. Lower motor neurone damage is evident in the distribution of the affected root with reduced power, muscle bulk, sensation and reflexes.

These symptoms and signs can develop over days, weeks or months. Some patients with a spinal tumour show features of both a myelopathy and a radiculopathy.

Diagnosis

The differential diagnosis of a suspected cord or root compression includes:

Other causes of compression:

- spinal trauma
- disc prolapse
- spondylosis (bony degeneration)
- syringomyelia (cyst within cord)
- haematoma (spontaneous or traumatic)
- abscess.

Non-compressive disease:

- demyelination
- infection
- inflammation
- infarction
- degenerative cord syndromes.

Further investigations are always necessary to establish whether there is cord or root compression and the likely cause.

The most useful investigations are:

- plain films: bone erosion or destruction
- myelography: 'filling defect' or block of flow to contrast
- CT scan: shows relationship of tumour to cord and spinal column
- MR imaging: delineates tumour in great detail.

Treatment and prognosis

The main methods of treatment are surgery and radiotherapy (the choice depends on the type of tumour) with steroids as an adjunct. Chemotherapy is often more useful with spinal tumours than with brain tumours. Benefits and risks of any treatment must be individualised for each patient.

Survival depends on the tumour type. The prognosis for neurological improvement depends on the severity and duration of spinal cord or nerve root compression before treatment. Cord compression recovers less well than root compression.

Specific types of spinal tumour

Intramedullary tumours

Spinal gliomas behave like brain gliomas, growing with variable speed but infiltrating and surrounding the spinal cord early on. They can extend over many segments of the cord and even into the brainstem. They cause progressive myelopathy affecting the lower limbs and sphincters and (in a cervical glioma) the upper limbs as well. Pain is rare, but patients steadily lose power, sensation, coordination and sphincter control.

Other spinal tumours, motor neurone disease, vasculopathies and multiple sclerosis are the main differential diagnoses. MR imaging is the investigation of choice. Open biopsy guides management by differentiating slow-growing from fast-growing tumours.

Treatment is palliative. Surgical decompression is useful for low-grade tumours containing cysts or those with a good plane of cleavage from normal tissue. Radiotherapy can be used alone or in combination with surgery. Steroids have a useful palliative effect. Death is from damage to respiratory centres in the cervical cord or brainstem.

Extramedullary tumours

Meningiomas and neurofibromas (Schwannomas) are benign, slow-growing tumours that arise on a nerve root. They cause a radiculopathy in the distribution of that nerve root and, if large enough, compress the spinal cord and cause a myelopathy. Meningiomas and Schwannomas never infiltrate the cord or metastasise but can reach a large size and erode adjacent vertebrae. Although usually solitary, multiple neurofibromas arise on the spinal nerves in the hereditary condition of neurofibromatosis (von Recklinghausen's syndrome) and can become large enough to extend out of the spine into the neck, chest, or abdomen.

Symptoms develop slowly. The diagnosis is often delayed until an important function like hand coordination is affected. Plain films, myelography and CT scanning are all useful but the best investigation is MR imaging. Surgical excision of the tumour is usually curative, but there is a risk of increasing the neu-

rological deficit in large tumours that compress the cord.

Extradural tumours

Secondary tumour deposits reach the extradural space via the bloodstream or by direct extension from a vertebral focus. Most originate in carcinomas (lung, breast, prostate, kidney), malignant melanoma, lymphoma and multiple myeloma. They grow quickly, destroying bone and infiltrating paraspinal soft tissues. The features of spinal cord compression develop rapidly and can progress to a complete paraplegia within a few days. Investigation and treatment are urgent.

Diagnosis. Plain films show bone destruction, and myelography shows a partial or complete block to contrast flow at the tumour site. CT and MR scanning are of value in showing the extent of tumour spread within and outside the spine. A percutaneous biopsy under X-ray control can yield tissue for histology.

Treatment. There is an urgent need to shrink the tumour and decompress the cord. If bladder control is already lost, the window of opportunity for rescue is only 24 hours. Surgery, radiotherapy, chemotherapy and steroids are used alone or in combination.

Prognosis. Survival depends on the tumour type. Recovery of cord function depends upon the duration and extent of cord compression. Often the diagnosis is made too late to restore function.

Self-assessment: questions

Multiple choice questions

1. In the clinical management of head injury:
   a. The first priority in the management of an unconscious head injury is the assessment of pupil and limb responses
   b. A patient with a skull fracture who is fully conscious can safely be sent home from the accident department
   c. A patient in a coma after a head injury should be intubated and ventilated before transfer to a neurosurgical unit
   d. A patient who has had an epileptic fit after a head injury should be given 10 mg diazepam as quickly as possible
   e. Clinical signs of shock are unlikely to be caused by the head injury itself

2. A deteriorating level of consciousness in the accident department an hour after serious head injury:
   a. Is almost certainly caused by an expanding intracranial haematoma
   b. May reflect rising intracranial pressure
   c. Should routinely be treated with mannitol and steroids
   d. Is not significant unless the patient also develops focal neurological signs
   e. Automatically requires immediate transfer to the nearest CT scanner

3. The clinical features of a large left-sided acute extradural haematoma are likely to include:
   a. Left hemiparesis
   b. Dilated left pupil
   c. Left-sided skull fracture
   d. Deteriorating conscious level
   e. Tachycardia

4. The following statements about head injury are true:
   a. About one million patients are admitted to hospital in the UK each year because of head injury
   b. Fractures of the skull base are usually diagnosed on clinical rather than on radiological grounds
   c. Outcome from an acute intracranial haematoma is not related to the patient's preoperative conscious level
   d. The risk of post-traumatic epilepsy is increased by a depressed fracture with a dural tear and cortical contusion
   e. Personality change is common in survivors of severe head injury

5. The following are true of cerebrovascular accidents:
   a. They never occur in patients in their 20s
   b. They are more common in women than in men
   c. High blood pressure is an important risk factor
   d. Haemorrhages are more common than infarcts
   e. Damage to the brain can never recover

6. Clinical features of a diffuse subarachnoid haemorrhage include:
   a. A severe occipito-frontal headache
   b. Neck stiffness
   c. Constricted pupils
   d. Sudden onset of symptoms
   e. Repeated vomiting

7. Cerebral berry aneurysms:
   a. Are usually present at the time of birth
   b. Occur mainly where arteries bifurcate
   c. Are usually multiple
   d. Can only be treated by a surgical operation
   e. Can become large enough to compress nearby cranial nerves

8. Common complications of aneurysmal subarachnoid haemorrhage include:
   a. A further haemorrhage
   b. Congestive cardiac failure
   c. Salt-losing nephropathy
   d. Communicating hydrocephalus
   e. Cortical blindness

9. Presenting features of a glioma of the left temporal lobe may include:
   a. Progressive headache
   b. Weakness of the left hand
   c. Focal seizures of the right hand
   d. Expressive dysphasia
   e. Jaundice from liver secondaries

10. Intracranial meningiomas:
    a. Are usually multiple tumours
    b. Infiltrate the surrounding brain at an early stage
    c. Can present with an epileptic fit
    d. Are very radiosensitive
    e. Can usually be cured by surgical excision

11. The following are true of secondary brain tumours:
    a. The history is usually short and rapidly progressive
    b. The most common primary sites are lung, stomach and colon
    c. The CT scan often shows a great deal of oedema
    d. Surgery is never useful in their treatment
    e. Steroids may give dramatic symptomatic relief

12. Radiotherapy for brain tumours:
    a. Can cause brain damage unless the dose is carefully controlled

b. Is the ideal treatment for brain tumours in children under 3 years of age
c. Has its greatest effects with rapidly dividing tumours
d. Causes side effects that are well tolerated by most patients
e. Is ineffective in pituitary tumours

13. The clinical features of a myelopathy that has been rapidly progressive over 1 week are likely to include:
    a. Preservation of proprioceptive sensation
    b. Increased knee and ankle reflexes
    c. Sciatic pain
    d. Marked wasting of muscles of the lower limbs
    e. Loss of bladder control

14. Spinal cord compression from an extradural secondary tumour at the level of the fourth thoracic vertebra:
    a. Causes progressive weakness of all four limbs
    b. Is often associated with destructive changes in the adjacent bone
    c. Can lead to loss of bladder control within a few days
    d. Always requires surgical decompression
    e. Can be the first presentation of a bronchogenic carcinoma

15. A neurofibroma arising from the left eleventh thoracic nerve root:
    a. Is likely to cause symptoms that progress slowly
    b. May cause a band of pain around the left loin
    c. Can cause vertebral erosion that is visible on plain films
    d. Causes an extradural block to contrast flow on myelography
    e. Has a 10% chance of infiltrating the surrounding spinal cord tissue by the time of diagnosis

Case histories

Case history 1

A 10-year-old, previously well except for mild asthma, falls off his bicycle and strikes his head on a kerbstone. He is not unconscious but vomits shortly afterwards and returns home. About an hour later, significant headache develops but the child is neurologically normal. He vomits again and becomes a little restless and breathless.

1. The family's general practitioner is contacted by the parents; what would the most appropriate response be:
   a. to advise analgesics and wait and see

   b. to advise bed-rest and use of an inhaler
   c. to refer the patient directly to the accident and emergency department
   d. to make a routine house call later in the day?

An hour later the parents see the child shaking on the left side and he says his headache is getting worse. They bring him directly to the A & E department, where the following clinical signs are noted: slurred but coherent speech, eyes open to command only, normal upper and lower limb power, spasticity and brisk reflexes on the left, right pupil larger than the left but reactive to light.

2. These clinical signs are most likely the result of:
   a. concussion
   b. diffuse axonal injury to the brainstem
   c. right-sided traumatic intracranial haematoma?

3. Faced with these clinical features, the most appropriate response is to:
   a. X-ray the skull and admit him to the ward for overnight observation
   b. contact the neurosurgical team on call promptly?

Case history 2

A 55-year-old company executive collapses on the floor of his office and is at first unresponsive. Within a minute or two he starts to wake up and complains of severe headache and nausea. He is taken to hospital, where a history of recent overwork and much foreign travel on business is elicited. His blood pressure is 190/105 mmHg, there is mild neck stiffness, a temperature of 37.5°C and no focal neurological deficit.

1. The most likely clinical diagnosis is:
   a. a viral respiratory illness with mild meningitis
   b. a subarachnoid haemorrhage
   c. an acute hypertensive episode?

He is admitted to a medical ward for further investigation and treatment.

2. The most important aspect of this is:
   a. intravenous antihypertensive therapy
   b. an EEG
   c. an urgent brain scan
   d. throat swabs for viral culture?

Case history 3

A 64-year-old housewife with a long history of hypertension and mild depression has complained of frontal headaches over about 2 months that she feels are getting worse. Two paracetamol tablets no longer clear the headache which wakes her now most days. She visits her GP for advice. She denies any other symptoms. A neurological examination shows slightly brisker reflexes on the left side, but generalised examination is normal. It is not possible to obtain a good view of her optic fundi.

1. The most appropriate management at present is:
   a. reassurance and an arrangement to review her in a month
   b. a stronger (codeine-based) analgesic
   c. urgent referral for a specialist opinion in hospital?

A week later her husband telephones the GP about her. He is worried because she has become 'odd' in the last few days, forgetting about meals and once talking about her dead sister as if she was still alive. He thinks she is perhaps becoming depressed again and asks the GP to see her again. It is found that her right hand is a little weak but she seems unconcerned about this and her headache.

2. The most likely diagnosis at this stage is:
   a. a stroke affecting the left cerebral hemisphere
   b. a tumour of the left frontal lobe
   c. recurrence of her previous depressive illness?

The GP phones the local hospital and speaks to a consultant physician who agrees to admit her for tests later that week. However, that night he is called to see her as she has fallen out of bed and become very drowsy. He finds her lying on the bedroom floor, eye opening to speech and mumbling incoherently. Her right side is weak and there is twitching of the right side of the face. The left pupil is larger than the right, but both react to light. Her blood pressure is 200/130 mmHg. There is no external evidence of injury.

3. Emergency treatment at this stage should include:
   a. intravenous diazepam 10 mg stat
   b. administration of a rapidly acting antihypertensive drug
   c. basic airway care during transfer to hospital?

Short notes

Write short notes on:
1. the priorities in the initial assessment and resuscitation of a patient with a severe head injury
2. complications of skull vault fractures
3. common physical and mental deficits after severe head injury
4. the risk factors for stroke
5. the steps in diagnosing a ruptured cerebral aneurysm
6. the complications of aneurysmal subarachnoid haemorrhage
7. the clinical features of raised intracranial pressure
8. the factors that determine the optimum treatment for a fit 60-year-old woman found on CT scan to have a solitary tumour within the left temporal lobe
9. the clinical presentation of pituitary adenomas and microadenomas
10. the investigation of a patient with a midthoracic myelopathy that has developed over a week
11. the options for management of a T4 extradural tumour (seen by MR scan) in a 70-year-old, unable to walk or pass urine for 12–24 hours.

Self-assessment: answers

Multiple choice answers

1. a. **False.** Managing any seriously injured patient begins by identifying and correcting life-threatening problems of the airway, breathing and circulation, before neurological assessment.
   b. **False.** A patient with a skull fracture should always be admitted for observation, even if neurologically well, as a fracture is a powerful risk factor for an intracranial haematoma.
   c. **True.** An unconscious patient should be intubated and ventilated before being transferred out of the resuscitation room.
   d. **False.** Diazepam is a respiratory depressant and should only be given to a patient whose fit lasts more than a minute or two and then only in small increments with facilities available for respiratory support.
   e. **True.** Shock is almost never caused by the head injury itself, but by blood loss from extracranial injuries, which initially may be unrecognised.

2. a. **False.** Falling level of consciousness after head injury is a sensitive warning of continuing brain injury and must always be taken seriously. It can be caused by intracranial complications or by systemic injuries and complications that reduce cerebral perfusion and oxygenation.
   b. **True.** A rise in ICP is paralleled by a fall in conscious level in response to brain compression and reduced cerebral perfusion.
   c. **False.** Mannitol lowers raised ICP for less than an hour. Steroids carry no benefit (and possibly some detriment) in the management of acute head injury.
   d. **False.** It is dangerous to wait for focal neurological signs before acting.
   e. **False.** The patient should not be transferred to the CT scanner or neurosurgical unit until life-threatening problems have been excluded or corrected.

3. a. **False.** A right hemiparesis develops.
   b. **True.** The pupil of the left eye dilates because of compression of the oculomotor nerve.
   c. **True.** An extradural haematoma is almost always caused by an overlying skull fracture that lacerates a dural vessel.
   d. **True.**
   e. **False.** If the haematoma is not evacuated, brainstem compression causes a slowing of the pulse rate.

4. a. **False.** Most of the one million head-injured attenders at hospital in the UK each year do not need admission, but it is important to identify the 10% who do. This group are at risk of complications and prompt intervention is needed to minimise the harmful effects of these complications.
   b. **True.** Meningitis can result from neglect of the clinical signs of a radiologically invisible fracture of the skull base.
   c. **False.** The worse a patient's conscious level has become before removal of the intracranial haematoma the worse the outcome is likely to be.
   d. **True.** A depressed skull vault fracture carries a risk not only of infection but of epilepsy, especially if the underlying dura and brain are damaged.
   e. **True.** Survivors of severe head injury often show personality change, which can be marked.

5. a. **False.** Cerebrovascular accidents can occur in all age groups, although they are more common in the middle-aged and elderly.
   b. **True.** Women outnumber men about 6 : 4.
   c. **True.** Uncontrolled hypertension is the key risk factor, along with cigarette smoking, hyperlipidaemia, obesity, stress and diabetes.
   d. **False.** Infarcts are much more common (80%) than haemorrhages (20%).
   e. **False.** Infarcts and haemorrhages both cause neuronal death in an area of the brain. Damage to surrounding neurones can recover with time and supportive therapy, leading to recovery of function.

6. a. **True.** The usual history of a subarachnoid haemmorrhage involves the sudden onset of a severe generalised headache.
   b. **True.** The neck is usually stiff.
   c. **False.** Focal neurological signs can be present or absent, but the pupils are normal or dilated in this condition.
   d. **True.**
   e. **True.** The features of meningeal irritation (nausea, photophobia, repeated vomiting) usually accompany a subarachnoid haemorrhage.

7. a. **False.** The muscle abnormality is congenital, but the aneurysm itself almost always develops only in adult life.
   b. **True.** A cerebral aneurysm arises where an artery branches. Pressure from blood in the vessel balloons out the wall where the smooth muscle layer is weak.
   c. **False.** Most are single, but 10% are multiple.
   d. **False.** Options for management now include endovascular obliteration by radiological techniques as well as surgical treatment.

e. **True.** The most common nerve to be so affected is the oculomotor nerve, causing a dilated unreactive pupil on the same side as the aneurysm.

8. a. **True.** The main fear with a ruptured aneurysm is that it will rupture again. This risk is especially high in the early weeks after the initial bleed.
   b. **False.** A cardiac dysrhythmia is the most common cardiac complication.
   c. **True.** The salt-losing nephropathy can cause severe hyponatraemia.
   d. **True.** The hydrocephalus is usually of the communicating type, caused by clogging of the arachnoid villi by blood.
   e. **False.** Vasospasm induced by blood breakdown products in the subarachnoid space causes ischaemia, but rarely is the occipital cortex sufficiently affected to cause blindness.

9. a. **True.** The space-occupying effect of a glioma and its surrounding oedema steadily raises ICP and makes headache worse.
   b. **False.** A left-sided cerebral lesion will produce right-sided neurological signs.
   c. **True.**
   d. **True.** Focal damage is likely to affect the speech centre (causing expressive dysphasia).
   e. **False.** No matter how aggressive its behaviour within the brain, a glioma will not metastasise to other parts of the body.

10. a. **False.** A meningioma is usually solitary.
    b. **False.** Meningiomas do not infiltrate the surrounding brain.
    c. **True.** It grows steadily and the symptoms of raised ICP and focal brain damage are at first underestimated by the patient, often until a dramatic event, like a fit, takes place.
    d. **False.** Radiotherapy has little effect on such a slow-growing tumour.
    e. **True.** Even a large meningioma can usually be cured by surgical excision.

11. a. **True.** They grow quickly and cause symptoms quickly but this is often because of marked cerebral oedema rather than the size of the metastases themselves.
    b. **False.** Most cerebral metastases arise from carcinoma of the lung or breast — few are from gastrointestinal tumours.
    c. **True.**
    d. **False.** Palliative surgery can help to relieve troublesome pressure symptoms from a large and apparently solitary metastasis, even when the long-term outlook is poor.
    e. **True.** The patient's headache and other symptoms of raised ICP resolve rapidly with steroids.

12. a. **True.** The risk of radiation damage to normal tissue limits the dose that can be given.
    b. **False.** The risk is especially high in the developing brain, and radiotherapy is only justified in children under 3 years of age if it is a life-saving measure and no other treatment is effective.
    c. **True.** Radiotherapy is especially useful for fast-growing tumours.
    d. **True.** Systemic side effects on bone marrow, skin, hair and gut are usually well tolerated at the doses used.
    e. **False.** Even a pituitary tumour which grows slowly will shrink or cease growth after treatment.

13. a. **False.** Proprioception tends to be affected before deep pain sensation.
    b. **True.** This reflects signs of an upper motor neurone lesion below the level of cord compression.
    c. **False.** Radicular pain (e.g. sciatica) is not a feature of myelopathy.
    d. **False.** There is no wasting of muscles until the myelopathy has caused disuse atrophy.
    e. **True.** This also is a sign of an upper motor neurone lesion below the segmental level of cord compression.

14. a. **False.** The myelopathy caused by a tumour in this position causes motor and sensory loss in the lower limbs but not the upper limbs.
    b. **True.** Such tumours destroy bone extensively.
    c. **True.** Loss of sphincter control under these circumstances can be rapid.
    d. **False.** The extensive adjacent bone involvement often limits the value of surgery, especially in an elderly or frail patient. Radiotherapy and/or chemotherapy (with steroids) often provides equally effective palliation.
    e. **True.** The likeliest primary tumour is a carcinoma, hitherto undiagnosed.

15. a. **True.** A neurofibroma grows slowly.
    b. **True.** It arises on a spinal root in its intervertebral foramen and causes slowly worsening features of a radiculopathy in the distribution of that root, which in this case would include a sensory disturbance in the left loin.
    c. **True.** As it enlarges, erosion of the adjacent vertebra occurs and can be seen on plain films.
    d. **False.** They are intradural tumours, and the appearance of a filling defect on a myelogram distinguishes them from extradural tumours.
    e. **False.** Neurofibromas displace nervous tissue rather than infiltrating it and even when very large they remain well demarcated.

Case history answers

Case history 1

1. This boy initially seems fine after an apparently minor head injury, but his increasing headache and persistent vomiting are warnings that all is not well. These clinical features should always be taken seriously in a child who has had a head injury, and justify prompt referral to an accident department.
2. The boy deteriorated before arrival at hospital and may have had a focal epileptic seizure. The clinical findings at hospital — a mildly altered conscious level, focal limb weakness and pupil asymmetry — strongly suggest a right cerebral hemisphere expanding lesion, possibly an extradural haematoma.
3. This child is highly likely to deteriorate further, possibly with dramatic speed, and must be referred at once to a neurosurgical unit with a view to transfer. A skull X-ray will not influence the decision to transfer him for a CT scan and neurological assessment, which can be made on the clinical information already available.

Case history 2

1. The features of this man's sudden illness all strongly suggest an intracranial bleed, most likely an SAH. Viral infections start less abruptly, and stress-related hypertensive crises do not cause neck stiffness. These diagnoses could be entertained safely only after excluding an intracranial bleed. Investigation is urgent because management of the three conditions is very different.
2. Reducing the blood pressure with drugs (necessary in a hypertensive crisis) can be dangerous after an SAH, as cerebral autoregulation is impaired and the cerebral perfusion passively follows systemic blood pressure. The key investigation is a CT scan, which would almost certainly show free blood after an SAH. A lumbar puncture some hours after the bleed is almost as sensitive but carries a small risk of complications. When an SAH has been diagnosed by CT scan, a lumbar puncture becomes redundant. An EEG will not be able to confirm or refute any of the three diagnoses and viral cultures are slow and can add nothing to the immediate management of this case.

Case history 3

1. The headache has some features of raised ICP, and the focal neurological signs (unilateral brisk reflexes) in this woman should alert the GP to the possibility of an intracranial mass lesion. The GP should refer the patient urgently to a physician or (if available) a neurologist or neurosurgeon, with a view to investigation by CT scanning. Simply reassuring the patient or prescribing strong analgesics without referring the patient is not appropriate.
2. The new symptoms reported by the patient's husband the following week suggest a progressive change in personality and behaviour. While depression can cause such symptoms, their association with brisk right-sided reflexes and right-hand weakness points strongly to a focal lesion in the brain, most likely in the left frontal lobe. The gradual and progressive tempo of the illness suggests a tumour rather than a stroke, but urgent hospital investigation is needed.
3. The next day the illness has worsened dramatically. Although her husband describes a fall, the circumstances of this make it more likely to be the result rather than the cause of her deterioration. She may have been having focal seizures of right-sided limbs, but unless these lead to repeated or prolonged generalised convulsions intravenous diazepam is not indicated. Although she is hypertensive (and has a history of this), this may be a response to raised ICP, and antihypertensive medication may be dangerous and is contraindicated. She should go to hospital by ambulance after basic resuscitation.

Short notes answers

1. The priorities are the same in the initial assessment and resuscitation of any patient with a serious head injury: to identify and correct life-threatening problems first, and in the order they threaten life. The airway is always the top priority and is addressed simultaneously with stabilisation of the cervical spine by in-line immobilisation. Breathing is the next priority, then the circulation (with control of haemorrhage) and only at this point is attention paid to neurological dysfunction. The correct order of action is simple to remember by the first letters of the order of priorities: airway, breathing, circulation, dysfunction of the nervous system exposure.
2. The skull has a vault and a base. Fractures of the vault can be linear or depressed, and either can be compound (overlying wound) or simple (no wound). A linear fracture (whether simple or compound) implies that major energy transfer to the head occurred at the time of injury. It is an important risk factor for traumatic intracranial haematoma, and admission to hospital for a period of observation is mandatory even if the patient is well. Depressed fractures are caused by a direct blow to the head with a blunt object and are nearly always compound. They can be followed by delayed intracranial infection (meningitis, brain abscess, empyema) from indriven foreign bodies (hair, dirt, weapon fragments, etc.) if the wound is not surgically debrided.

3. Injury to the brain can resolve with time by complex healing and recovery processes or can be followed by symptoms and signs of brain damage. These can be primarily physical (epilepsy, headache and facial pain, focal limb weakness, cranial nerve palsies, disturbances of sight or hearing) or primarily mental (impaired memory and concentration, learning difficulties, personality change, mood swings, loss of energy and drive, loss of social inhibitions). Many patients have a complex mixture of both types of problem and there are often secondary social consequences (loss of employment, family disruption, alcohol abuse, antisocial or violent behaviour). Even patients who seem to do well after severe head injury often have a degree of impairment on careful assessment. Effective rehabilitation services can identify specific problems and reduce their impact on the patient and family.

4. Uncontrolled hypertension and cigarette smoking are the major risk factors for cardiac and vascular diseases, including stroke. Also important are obesity, hypercholesterolaemia, inadequate exercise, diabetes mellitus and alcohol abuse. Many of these are 'lifestyle' factors and can be controlled if the patient is willing to make the effort. The role of health professionals is to provide information and encouragement, and if necessary supportive medical treatment (e.g. antihypertensive drugs or anticoagulants; control of diabetes) or surgical treatment (e.g. carotid endarterectomy).

5. Two questions must be answered. Is it a subarachnoid haemorrhage (SAH)? If so, what is the cause? Clinical suspicion of an SAH (sudden severe headache, neck stiffness, evidence of meningeal irritation) is confirmed by CT scan or lumbar puncture. Both are sensitive ways to detect subarachnoid blood, but lumbar puncture can be normal in the first few hours and CT scans can be normal after the first few days. Lumbar puncture is contraindicated in an unconscious patient or one with focal deficits, which suggest a clot in the brain. Definitive diagnosis of the underlying aneurysm is by angiography of the carotid and vertebral circulations. This can be done by intra-arterial or intravenous injection, using conventional catheter techniques or magnetic resonance angiography.

6. A ruptured aneurysm can cause rapid death by the destructive effect of haemorrhage on the brain. Patients who survive the first bleed are still at risk of another one, and this risk is highest at first and falls exponentially over the subsequent days and weeks. Preventing a rebleed is the main aim of the treatment of aneurysms by surgery or endovascular obliteration. Cerebral ischaemia (even to the point of major infarction) can result from the vasospasm triggered by blood

breakdown products in the CSF. Blood can obstruct the normal circulation of CSF and cause communicating or, rarely, obstructive hydrocephalus. SAH can cause subendocardial ischaemia and trigger cardiac dysrhythmias (leading to sudden death) and also a salt-losing nephropathy (causing severe hyponatraemia).

7. Raised ICP causes headache with a number of characteristic features: it is bilateral and poorly localised, throbbing or 'bursting', constant and unremitting, progressively severe as time passes, worse in the morning and only temporarily alleviated by analgesics. Associated clinical features include nausea and vomiting, visual disturbances such as blurring, and clouding of consciousness. The optic disc margins may be blurred and the discs themselves swollen (papilloedema). The tempo of these symptoms and signs (over days, weeks and months) depends on how fast the tumour grows.

8. The issue is always the balance between potential benefits and risks of treatment. The scan may suggest the likely tumour type, but if not this can be established by biopsy, which carries a small risk of bleeding or brain swelling. With a slow-growing tumour, surgical excision offers the best chance of cure or a prolonged recurrence-free interval, at the risk of impairing quality of life from surgical damage. With a rapidly growing tumour, these risks are less worthwhile, and the lower risk of radiotherapy becomes a better option. However, if the tumour is particularly large, surgical decompression to reduce its size can make radiotherapy more effective.

9. Some pituitary adenomas secrete enormous quantities of one of the trophic anterior pituitary hormones and cause endocrine syndromes like acromegaly, infertility / galactorrhoea and Cushing's syndrome. Because of their endocrine effects, these tumours are diagnosed when only a few millimetres in diameter and confined to the pituitary gland (microadenomas). Non-secretory adenomas grow larger before they cause symptoms from the pressure they exert on other structures, e.g. the normal adjacent pituitary tissue (causing acute or chronic pituitary failure), the optic chiasm (visual field defects, classically bitemporal hemianopia) or even the frontal lobes (personality change) or ventricles (obstructive hydrocephalus).

10. The spinal cord compression has been rapid , and the diagnosis and treatment are urgent. The investigation of choice is MR imaging, but if this is not available a myelogram may show a block (complete or partial) to the flow of contrast. And an axial CT scan through that level can show the position of the tumour relative to the cord and the extent of any bony destruction and spread into the paraspinal tissues—valuable for planning

treatment. In selected cases, a needle can be guided into the tumour under X-ray control to remove tissue for biopsy and for a histological diagnosis.

11. An extradural tumour in this location is almost certain to be a metastasis from a carcinoma or other malignant tumour whose identity may already be known (or can be inferred at this stage from clinical examination or radiology). The key to managing this patient is to relieve the pressure on the spinal cord before irrevocable damage is done.

Surgery is the fastest and most direct approach but can be technically challenging and it may be only possible to remove part of the tumour (e.g. if it is all around the cord). Also, it is potentially hazardous in an elderly or unwell patient. Radiotherapy is safer but slower. Chemotherapy is useful only if the tumour is known to be chemosensitive. Steroids are a useful addition to whatever other treatment is proposed.

Plastic surgery

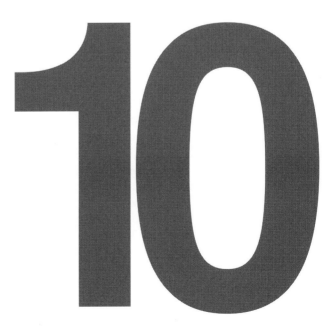

10.1 **Soft tissue trauma**

Soft tissue trauma is one of the most frequent causes for attendance at an accident and emergency department. Penetrating lacerations may be life-threatening if major vessels are injured (e.g. in the neck). Crush injuries may result in considerable morbidity and delayed healing. Recognition of the different categories of soft tissue injury is important because it reduces the risk of missing injuries to deep structures and it enables appropriate primary management to be instigated.

The five main types of soft tissue injury are:

- laceration
- crush injury
- degloving injury
- avulsion injury
- haematoma.

Laceration

Stab wounds are typical laceration wounds. The incision-like injury is usually caused by a sharp implement (knife or broken bottle). These wounds are often deep and penetrating with little surrounding bruising. Associated fractures are rare, but vascular or nerve injuries are common, especially in the head and neck. Tendons are frequently injured in the hand. Skin loss is rare.

Crush injury

Crush injuries are caused by a blunt force and are characterised by diffuse soft tissue damage. Compared with lacerations, bone and joint injuries are more frequent. The force behind the injury causes vessel and nerve compression. Bruising is often extensive. Complete division of neurovascular structures is uncommon. Skin devitalisation is seen more often than in a laceration injury.

Degloving injury

In degloving injuries, external forces shear the skin off the underlying tissues, usually in a tissue plane between the subcutaneous fat and deep fascia. This injury is most frequent in the limbs. Severe degloving injuries are classically associated with roller type machinery or where a vehicle tyre runs over a limb. Less severe though more common is the degloving injury seen in elderly patients who strike their legs against a low object such as a table or a bus platform. The skin is degloved between the fixed obstacle and the moving limb. In elderly patients with thin fragile skin, healing can be delayed and morbidity prolonged if the injury is not correctly recognised. These injuries can result in skin necrosis.

Avulsion injury

This implies tissue loss after injury and is a characteristic of human and animal bite wounds. Prominent parts of the face or limbs are often affected. Bite wounds are particularly prone to infection because of the large number of organisms in the mouth; they must be meticulously cleaned and debrided before repair. Broad-spectrum antibiotic treatment (flucloxacillin and metronidazole) is essential. These wounds present a formidable reconstructive challenge because of their complexity and location, frequently in cosmetically sensitive areas of the face. Occasionally, avulsed segments (particularly digits) can be reimplanted either as a free graft or by using microvascular techniques.

Haematoma

These are caused by a blunt force resulting in subcutaneous haemorrhage while the skin overlying the bleeding site remains intact. An expanding haematoma can devascularise the overlying skin and cause necrosis. Applying pressure dressings exacerbates the problem by further reducing the skin blood supply. Early diagnosis together with decompression and ligation or cautery of the injured vessels is the treatment of choice. Otherwise, skin necrosis will develop and a skin graft will be required.

Management in soft tissue trauma

Diagnosis

An accurate description of the nature of the injury is almost as important as the clinical examination of the wound. Many injuries, particularly if they are extensive, will be a combination of the various types of soft tissue injury listed above.

Complications

The most important complications following soft tissue trauma are:

- vessel, tendon and nerve injury
- foreign body inclusion
- skin loss and necrosis
- secondary infection.

Treatment

The key steps are:

1. careful assessment
2. thorough debridement
3. meticulous wound inspection under local or general anaesthesia to assess the extent of damage and to remove foreign bodies, e.g. glass fragments
4. primary repair of all severed structures unless the wound is grossly infected; skin graft as necessary

5. reassess tissue viability immediately and at 48 hours
6. antibiotic cover for all avulsion injuries and contaminated wounds.

10.2 Burns and skin grafts

The epidemiology of burns in the developed world has changed dramatically over the last 50 years. Legislation (e.g. outlawing inflammable children's nightwear) has reduced many types of burn injury. The most common burn injuries that remain are:

- scalds in children
- burns in elderly patients
- burns related to medical illness (e.g. following an epileptic fit)
- burns in alcoholics and drug addicts
- major disaster victims (e.g. Piper Alpha, Bradford football stadium, etc.).

Most burns are small (< 2% body surface area (BSA)) and can be dealt with in a casualty department. Burns > 10% in children (> 15% in adults) should be admitted for fluid resuscitation. Patients with suspected smoke inhalation should also be admitted.

Types of burn injury

Scald. A burn caused by wet heat, usually boiling water or steam.

Flame. A direct effect of burning gases on the skin. High temperatures damage skin proteins and cause deep burns with skin staining. Smoke inhalation injury is frequent.

Chemical. Caused by direct skin contact with chemicals (usually strong acid or alkali).

Electrical. Often causes a deep burn. The severity of damage depends on the tissue resistance (high in skin and bone), voltage and current. The electrical energy is transformed into heat energy. Low-voltage domestic burns often look small but are deep. High-voltage injuries can be fatal, causing cardiac arrhythmias and muscle spasm, which prevents the victim releasing himself from the current source.

Friction. Occurs when the body comes into contact with a rapidly moving surface (e.g. a tyre or belt drive). Often these wounds are deep and expose underlying fat or muscle.

Contact. Caused by direct conduction of heat from a hot surface to the skin, particularly when protective mechanisms are not functioning (e.g. an epileptic patient who falls into a fire following a seizure).

Inhalation. Lung and airway damage follows smoke inhalation. Several factors contribute, including effect of heat, hypoxia and toxic products in the smoke, plus secondary changes caused by pulmonary oedema and infection.

Burn depth

There are three categories of burn depth:

- superficial
- deep dermal
- full thickness.

Superficial burns. Damage is confined to the epidermis and the superficial dermal layers. Spontaneous healing occurs in 10–14 days as the epidermis regenerates from undamaged epidermal appendages in the dermis (hair follicles and sweat glands).

Deep dermal burns. Damage includes deeper layers of dermis. Only a few epidermal appendages remain. Although spontaneous healing occurs, it is often delayed 3–4 weeks and may result in a hypertrophic scar.

Full thickness burns. The epidermis and dermis are totally destroyed and spontaneous epithelialisation cannot occur. A very small full thickness burn will eventually heal as the wound contracts by epithelialisation from adjacent tissue.

Clinical features

Correct assessment of the burn depth and extent is the key to successful treatment:

Assessment of depth:

- superficial
  — moist blistered surface
  — sensitive to pin prick
- deep dermal
  — blistering
  — bright red
  — reduced pain sensitivity
  — cream coloured wound base
- full thickness
  — no blistering
  — dry, grey / white leathery
  — absent pain sensation.

Many burns are a combination of categories, e.g. a predominantly deep dermal injury is usually surrounded by a zone of superficial burn injury.

Assessment of extent. There are three commonly used methods of assessing the extent of a burn injury:

The rule of nine. This is the most common method of estimating burn surface area (BSA) (see Table 16). It is less accurate in young children because they have a proportionately larger surface area of the head compared with the trunk.

Lund and Browder charts. These provide a more detailed mapping system of a burn, again as a percentage BSA. Different charts are available for children and adults.

Palm of hand. The area of the patient's palm equates

Table 16. 'Rule of nine' method for estimating burn surface area

Area of body	Percentage of body surface area
Head/neck	9
Upper limb (each)	9
Front of trunk	18
Back of trunk	18
Lower limb (each)	18
Perineum	1

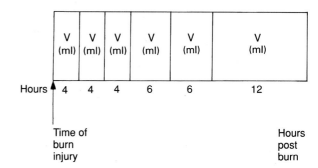

Fig. 68
Fluid resuscitation 'time' blocks following burn injury.

to a 1% BSA and can be used to estimate the extent of the burn.

Burn management

There are two phases to burn wound management:

- early
- subsequent/late.

Early management

Burns may be part of a multiple systemic injury to a patient; the initial assessment should follow the ATLS principles (see p. 72). There are three important components to the early management of burn injuries:

- fluid resuscitation
- wound management
  — open method
  — closed method

Fluid resuscitation
Fluid resuscitation by an intravenous route is required for burns of > 15% BSA in adults and > 10% BSA in children. Fluid resuscitation requirements (using plasma or a colloid substitute) are based on the Muir and Barclay formula (see Fig. 68). The volume of fluid required (V) for each 'block' of time is calculated from the following formula:

$$V = \frac{\text{weight of patient (kg)} \times \% \text{ BSA burn}}{2}$$

This calculation only forms a *basis* for resuscitation. The adequacy of resuscitation is monitored using hourly urine output and haematocrit as a guide and the infusion rate is adjusted accordingly. Baseline fluid maintenance therapy must be provided in addition for patients who are unable to take oral fluids.

Burn wound care
The main aim is to reduce the risk of infection until spontaneous healing occurs or the wound is ready for split skin grafting.
Open treatment. A dry eschar forms over burn wounds during the first few days after injury and acts as a biological barrier. This is particularly useful in burn wounds that are difficult to dress (e.g. face, perineum,

buttocks). The crust or eschar slowly separates from the wound margins after 7–10 days. In superficial burns, separation is complete by 14–21 days leaving a freshly epithelialised surface beneath. In deep burns, a granulating surface is left that requires skin grafting. Large burn wounds are treated by exposure. Patients are nursed in a warm room with clean filtered air (this forms the design basis for modern burns units).
Closed treatment. After cleaning the burn wound, a dressing is applied. Silver sulphadiazine has antibacterial properties and is particularly useful in burn wounds. If there is a lot of exudate, dressings are changed daily. The wound should be inspected at 5 days to re-evaluate the extent of the injury.

Hand burns can be treated by coating the affected areas with silver sulphadiazine and then applying a plastic bag around the hand and securing the bag at the wrist. Using this treatment, the patient can still use the affected hand to hold utensils, etc.

Subsequent/late management

After resuscitation has been completed, the burn should be reassessed. Unless the burn is superficial or a very small deep dermal/full thickness injury, skin grafting will probably be required.

Tangential excision
This technique, which is carried out 5–10 days after the injury, involves serial shaving of the burn wound until bleeding occurs from the wound surface:

- immediate bleeding indicates a superficial burn; these wounds are simply dressed until healing occurs
- a white pattern dermis on shaving indicates a deep dermal burn; these wounds are resurfaced with a split skin graft
- subcutaneous fat on shaving indicates a full thickness burn; these wounds are also resurfaced with a split skin graft.

Key points in major burn management

Analgesia. Use *i.v.* morphine or pethidine in sufficient amounts to relieve pain. Do *not* use subcutaneous or intramuscular routes as drugs will be poorly absorbed initially; later as resuscitation takes effect massive absorption of opiates may cause collapse.

Escharotomy. Use releasing incisions for deep circumferential burns to limbs. Otherwise as the tissues swell, dead skin that cannot expand will act as a tourniquet causing distal ischaemia.

Blood transfusion. Avoid in the first 24 hours after injury unless there is associated trauma. Transfusion exacerbates the haemoconcentration (and peripheral sludging) that follows plasma loss after a burn injury.

Admission to hospital. This should occur if:

- i.v. fluids are required
- burns are likely to need early grafting (e.g. eyelids, hands, etc.)
- burns affect difficult areas likely to need specialised nursing (e.g. perineum)
- non-accidental injury is suspected (e.g. in children).

Fluid resuscitation. Fluid needs should be calculated *from time of injury* and not from the time of hospital admission. Do not forget daily maintenance requirements.

Inhalation injury

This serious injury is usually associated with burns occurring in a confined space (e.g. in a house fire).

Clinical features
These include:

- burns to face and mouth
- black carbonaceous sputum
- ulcerated and oedematous oral mucosa
- wheezing and stridor.

Investigations
The degree of injury should be investigated by:

- measuring carboxyhaemoglobin level
- measuring arterial blood gases, monitoring arterial saturation
- obtaining a chest X-ray
- bronchoscopy (flexible).

A carboxyhaemoglobin level > 15%, 3 hours after injury or a $P_aO_2 < 10$ kPa when a patient is provided with 50% oxygen suggests inhalation injury.

Treatment
In the treatment of inhalation injuries:

- provide humidified oxygen via a face mask
- if stridor develops, intubate the patient
- use aggressive physiotherapy
- nurse in the head-up position
- bronchodilators may help, steroids probably will not
- ventilate patients whose P_aO_2 falls below 10 kPa

- consider therapeutic bronchoscopy to clear the airways
- use specific antibiotics after sputum culture.

Prognosis
Outcome after a severe inhalation injury is poor. Patients can die of bronchopneumonia and/or respiratory failure.

Late complications of burn injury

Hypertrophic scarring
Superficial burns heal with virtually no scarring. Many deep dermal and all full thickness burns will scar and some will become hypertrophic (thickened, red and uncomfortable), especially in children.

Treatment
Hypertrophic scarring can be reduced by:

- topical silicone gel
- compression garments: a specially manufactured lycra garment that compresses the scar during maturation (up to 12 months)
- steroid injection: used mainly in small raised scars.

Contractures
These develop where a scar extends longitudinally across a joint crease. They are particularly common in children, who should undergo follow-up until growth is complete. Surgical release may be necessary, resulting defects being repaired with skin grafts of flaps.

Unstable scar
Breakdown of a scar or graft can occur over bony prominences. Overgrafting or resurfacing with a more robust skin flap may be needed.

Alopecia
Deep scalp burns can cause alopecia. Scalp flaps, which are sometimes combined with tissue expansion, can usefully cover the areas with hair-bearing tissue.

Marjolin's ulcer
Squamous cell carcinoma can develop in an old scar (often from a burn). These develop many years after the original injury, often in elderly patients. Treatment is by excision and skin grafting.

10.3 Skin tumours

Skin cancer is increasing throughout the developing world. The number of cases of malignant melanoma is doubling every 10 years in the UK at present. Skin cancer is the most common cancer affecting mankind; there are three common types:

- basal cell carcinoma

- squamous cell carcinoma
- malignant melanoma.

Basal cell carcinoma

This is the most common type of skin cancer. It predominates in the elderly, especially on exposed parts of the body, particularly the face. These tumours generally grow extremely slowly over many years and only rarely metastasise.

Clinical features
Four types are recognised:

- cystic
- ulcerative
- multifocal, superficial
- sclerosing or morphoeic.

Most basal cell cancers occur on the head and neck. They are much less common on the limbs. They are especially common in fair-skinned people of northern European extraction who are exposed to long periods of sunlight. Basal cell carcinomas usually grow very slowly. Multiple lesions are sometimes found, representing a 'field change' in the skin. Occasionally basal cell cancers are pigmented and a malignant melanoma must be considered in the differential diagnosis.

Diagnosis
The diagnosis is based on the long history and the appearance of the lesion. Cystic tumours are well circumscribed, have a pearly smooth-domed appearance and small capillaries can be seen tracing across their surface. Ulcerative tumours are the classic basal cell cancer, with an ulcerated centre surrounded by a rolled margin. Multifocal and sclerosing tumours have ill-defined margins and great care is required to ensure they are completely excised.

Treatment
As these lesions rarely metastasise the main aim of surgery is to *ensure adequate local removal*. Careful sharp dissection is required with a gentle 'no touch' and 'non-crush' technique to prevent contamination and seeding of the surgical field. This is particularly important in ulcerated or fungating lesions.

Margin of excision. This varies with the type of lesion being excised. It is always helpful to draw a line around the outline of the lesion and a second line to demarcate the extent of the excision. Usually a margin of 2–3 mm is adequate for a cystic basal cell carcinoma. In multifocal or sclerosing tumours, great care must be taken to identify the interface between tumour and normal tissue. Under these circumstances magnification is often helpful. A wider margin of 5–6 mm or more (if the lesion is recurrent) should be measured out prior to excision. If there is any doubt about the adequacy of excision, especially in large deeply invasive recurrent basal cell cancers, frozen section examination at the time of operation is very helpful.

Overall, surgical treatment is usually preferred to other treatments because:

- it is a single-stage treatment
- it has a high cure rate
- it gives an opportunity to confirm the tissue diagnosis and adequacy of excision by histological examination.

Radiotherapy. Radiotherapy is an effective treatment in basal cell cancers. It is particularly useful for advanced tumours where underlying bone is involved. Radiotherapy is contraindicated in cancers that develop on limbs or for treating recurrence after previous radiotherapy. It should also be avoided in the treatment of lesions of the inner canthus, eyelids, tip of the nose and alar region, base of the ala nasi, external ear and auditory canal.

Topical cytotoxic therapy. A preparation of 5-fluorouracil (5-FU) is available as a cream that can be applied topically to these lesions (and to squamous cell cancers). It is applied once or twice per day for 3 to 4 weeks. Topical 5-FU is usually only effective in very early flat lesions. There is a high recurrence rate.

Squamous cell carcinoma

These cancers are also common in areas of the body exposed to sunlight for prolonged periods.

Clinical features
Squamous cell cancers are distributed usually on the head and neck. They occur on the limbs more often than basal cell cancers. These tumours grow more rapidly than basal cell cancers and can metastasise via the lymphatics to regional lymph nodes and via the bloodstream to distant sites, particularly lung and bone. They have an ulcerated surface and irregular margins. The lesions are often friable and bleed easily. Regional lymph nodes should always be examined, especially in large long-standing lesions.

Treatment
Surgical excision or radiotherapy is chosen based on the principles outlined for basal cell cancers.

Bowen's disease

This is a slow-growing, low-grade variant of a squamous carcinoma that develops intraepidermally. The lesion is well circumscribed, slightly raised, often pink/brown in colour with a scaly consistency. Multiple lesions occur on the limbs. Growth is very slow over many years but may progress to a frankly invasive squamous cell carcinoma.

Keratoacanthoma

This lesion is *not* a squamous cell carcinoma but is often mistaken for one. It can be very difficult to differentiate.

The history is of a rapidly growing exophytic lesion that characteristically has a large central keratin plug. The growth is self limiting and the lesion slowly regresses leaving virtually no scar. This rapid growth and aggressive appearance causes great alarm to the patient. A keratoacanthoma often cannot be differentiated from a squamous cell carcinoma on appearance alone. The diagnosis is usually made on the length of the history.

Treatment

Observation. The suspected keratoacanthoma can be observed for a period of *up to 6–8 weeks only*. If there is no sign of spontaneous regression excision is indicated.

Surgery. Excision may be needed followed by skin flap closure or grafting. It is essential that these lesions are sent for histological analysis.

Malignant melanoma

Malignant melanoma accounts for 11% of all UK skin cancers. Both incidence and death rates have risen significantly over recent years and this trend continues. Malignant melanoma is one of the few cancers to affect young adults; 22% of all melanomas occur in people under 40 years of age. The cancer is more common in females. The anatomical distribution differs between the sexes; melanomas are more common on the trunk in males and on the lower limb in females.

Several factors affect a given individual's risk of developing a melanoma:

- excessive exposure to the sun
- skin type
- change in an existing mole
- presence of a large number of naevi
- previous melanoma
- giant hairy naevi.

Up to 10% of melanomas are thought to be associated with inherited characteristics (dysplastic naevus syndrome). These moles are usually large (> 1 cm diameter) with irregular margins and often a variation in pigment density. There is a clear association between sunburn and melanoma.

There are four clinical types of melanoma:

- superficial spreading (50%)
- nodular (20–25%)
- lentigo maligna melanoma (15%)
- acral lentiginous (10%).

Malignant melanoma spreads via the regional lymphatics and bloodstream. Satellite lesions may be found in the skin. Liver, lung, brain and bone are the most frequent sites for metastases.

The prognosis is most accurately related to the thickness of the tumour (Breslow thickness, see Table 17).

Treatment

There is no consistently successful treatment for advanced melanoma. Long-term survival is poor for

Table 17 Breslow thickness and survival in patients with melanoma

Thickness of melanoma (mm)	5-year survival (%)
Less than 1.5	93
1.5–3.49	67
More than 3.5	37

thick lesions. An adequate surgical excision is the mainstay of treatment. For thick lesions, survival appears to remain the same irrespective of the margins of excision. The main thrust of management of this dangerous tumour is *prevention* and *early diagnosis*.

Prevention

Sunlight is the main aetiological risk factor linked with malignant melanoma. Studies have shown that the risk is significantly increased in:

- sunburn during childhood
- fair-skinned people who burn easily, tan poorly and who are exposed excessively to the sun.

These at-risk groups should avoid prolonged exposure to the sun (particularly between 11 a.m. and 3 p.m.). Sun beds and sun lamps should be avoided. Covering the skin with light clothing is effective; broad-brimmed hats afford similar protection for the head and neck. Sun screens are also helpful, filtering out ultraviolet radiation in the ultraviolet B range (the cause of blistering and burning). Sun screens are graded (by factor numbers) according to their ability to filter ultraviolet radiation, e.g. using a factor six sun screen a person can spend six times as long in the sun before getting burned. Ideally, nothing less than factor 15 should be used. Sun screens must be used liberally and reapplied every 2 hours if exposure to the sun continues.

Early diagnosis

Early signs of malignancy in a pigmented lesion include a change in size, alteration in pigment (particularly if the mole becomes unevenly pigmented), itching and notching of the margin. Later signs include bleeding and ulceration.

Treatment

Surgery. Complete excision is essential. Controversy exists with regard to the optimum margin of excision. As a guide, a margin of 1 cm for each millimetre Breslow thickness is appropriate. Incisional biopsies are to be condemned, as is an incomplete excision. Prophylactic lymph node dissection does not improve the prognosis.

Chemotherapy and radiotherapy. Various combinations of chemotherapeutic agents have been tried without notable success. Trials continue. Radiotherapy provides useful palliation, particularly for symptomatic bone metastases. The early results of immunotherapy have been encouraging.

Prognosis

The outcome is closely related to the thickness of the melanoma at the time of excision and is summarised in Table 17.

Self-assessment: questions

Multiple choice questions

1. The following statements relate to soft tissue injuries:

   a. Animal and human bite wounds are heavily contaminated

   b. Degloving injuries are best treated by simple suturing

   c. Crush injuries often result in devitalisation of soft tissues and fracture of bones

   d. Hand lacerations caused by broken glass or a knife are rarely associated with nerve or tendon injuries

   e. Haematomas should generally be evacuated urgently

2. Inhalation burn injury:

   a. Is often associated with burns on the face

   b. Can be difficult to diagnose in the early stages

   c. Can be rapidly fatal

   d. May need to be treated by early endotracheal intubation

   e. Is suggested by a carboxyhaemoglobin level of 5%

3. Basal cell carcinomas:

   a. Frequently occur on limbs

   b. Tend to be found in younger females

   c. Are very sensitive to radiotherapy

   d. Do not normally metastasise by lymphatic spread

   e. Generally grow slowly over many years

4. Squamous cell carcinomas of the skin:

   a. May arise in chronic scars (e.g. burns scars)

   b. Should be treated primarily with radiotherapy

   c. Tend to metastasise via the regional lymphatics

   d. Are more often seen in elderly than in young patients

   e. Often arise from a pre-existing mole

5. Malignant melanoma

   a. Is the most common malignant skin tumour

   b. In its early stages is indicated by bleeding and ulceration in a pre-existing mole

   c. Is continuing to show an increase in incidence

   d. Is particularly related to sunburn in childhood

   e. In its early stages, is best treated by radiotherapy

Case histories

Case history 1

A 19-year-old male was assaulted with a broken bottle as he came out of a pub. The laceration to the left cheek was in the form of an inverted 'C' (Fig. 69). The ambulance crew reported there had been excessive bleeding from the wound.

1. What type of soft tissue injury is this likely to be?
2. What is the correct management?
3. What structures may have been divided in this particular injury?
4. What long-term complications may develop as a result of this injury?

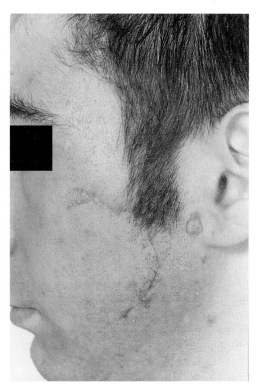

Fig. 69

Case history 2

A 37-year-old female was brought into the A & E department having been found in her home, which was on fire. On admission she was very distressed and appeared to be wheezing. Her weight was 65 kg and the burns were mainly confined to her trunk, face, right upper limb (including the hand) and her right thigh, affecting in total 35% of the body surface area excluding areas of erythema. The burn to the right arm was noted to be full thickness extending around the whole limb. The burn injury occurred at 9.30 p.m. and the patient was admitted to hospital at 11.30 p.m.

1. What are the important points in the *early* management of this patient?
2. What analgesia would you give? How would you administer the analgesia? Why?
3. Calculate the fluid replacement the patient will require and outline the initial fluid infusion regimen.
4. What type of fluid would you use?
5. What indices are the most important in helping you to assess the adequacy of fluid replacement?
6. How would you manage the burn to the right hand?

Case histories 3–6

Read the following four case histories. Look at the four skin tumours illustrated in Photographs 1–4. Match each tumour to one of the histories then answer the questions that follow each case history.

Case history 3

A 32-year-old female gives a history of a long-standing mole on her leg, which over a period of 6 months has changed in colour — becoming slightly darker. The mole has also begun to itch. She regularly holidays abroad in Spain and admits to being a 'sun worshipper'. On examination, she has an irregularly pigmented lesion measuring 1.5 cm in diameter on her leg. The margin has become irregular over the last 3 months.

1. What is the likely diagnosis?
2. What other areas of the body should you particularly examine?
3. What investigations would be appropriate?
4. What is the correct treatment?
5. The pathology report indicates that the lesion is 2.5 mm thick. What is the prognosis?
6. What advice would you give with regard to the prevention of further similar lesions appearing?

Case history 4

A 75-year-old retired soldier who has spent much of his time abroad in the tropics calls into your surgery for a routine hypertension check. Whilst recording his blood pressure you notice an ulcerating lesion on his arm, measuring approximately 6 cm in diameter and arising in an old scar from a war injury. The margin is irregular and friable (the patient usually keeps it covered with a dry dressing). There is also evidence of long-standing sun damage to the surrounding skin with multiple keratoses.

1. What is the differential diagnosis?
2. Where else should you examine?
3. What investigations would be appropriate?
4. How would you manage this patient?

Case history 5

A 62-year-old woman presents with a large crusted lesion on her face that has grown to its present size over a period of 3–4 weeks. She finds it very embarrassing as it is extremely prominent and unsightly. It is not painful. On examination it measures 3.0 cm in diameter, is raised and well circumscribed. There is no history of bleeding.

1. What is the differential diagnosis?
2. What else should your clinical examination include?
3. What advice would you give this patient, based on your diagnosis?

Case history 6

A 70-year-old woman comes to the surgery with a long-standing (several years) lesion that has been slowly increasing in size. It is not causing any symptoms but she is concerned because it is not 'going away'. On examination, a well-circumscribed lesion measuring 1.5 cm is noted on her cheek. It is circular in outline, ulcerated and has a raised margin. (Another similar lesion is noted incidentally near the inner canthus of her eye). Examination of the regional lymph nodes is normal.

1. What is the likely diagnosis?
2. What are the treatment options available for this patient and what would you recommend?
3. Is the lesion likely to metastasise to the regional lymph nodes or elsewhere in the body?

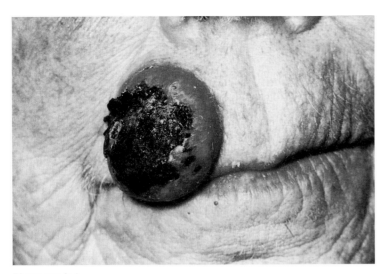

Photograph 1

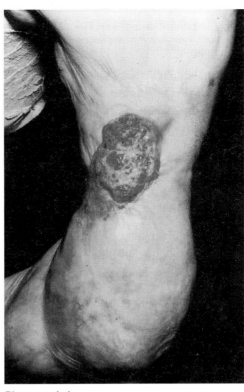

Photograph 4

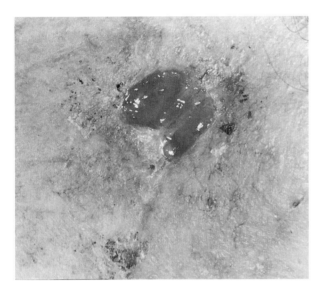

Photograph 2

Short notes

Write short notes on:
1. the classification and clinical features of burn injures of differing thicknesses
2. the measures a GP could take to help reduce the incidence of malignant melanoma in the area covered by his practice.

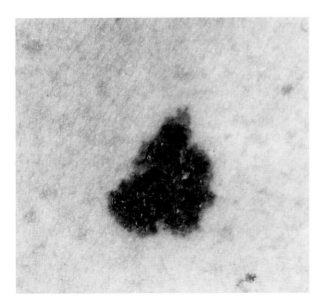

Photograph 3

Self-assessment: answers

Multiple choice answers

1. a. **True.** There are a massive number of organisms in the mouth. Broad-spectrum antibiotic cover is essential.
   b. **False.** Part or all of the degloved skin flap may be devascularised. The wound needs to be assessed carefully and any necrotic tissue debrided. A skin graft will almost certainly be needed.
   c. **True.** Diffuse soft tissue and bone and joint injuries are common following a crush injury.
   d. **False.** These wounds, which often appear small on the surface, tend to extend down to the bone with division of all intervening soft tissue structures. Careful clinical examination will help diagnose tendon, nerve or vascular injury. These wounds require careful exploration and repair.
   e. **True.** This will prevent an expanding haematoma devascularising the overlying skin.

2. a. **True.** Particularly if soot staining is noted around the mouth and lips.
   b. **True.** The history is important. Inhalation injury should be suspected after a burn that has occurred in a confined space. Always look for signs of burning to the face or evidence of difficulty with breathing.
   c. **True.** As oedema increases in the airway, respiration becomes progressively more difficult.
   d. **True.** Intervention and ventilation may be necessary in a severe inhalation injury.
   e. **False.** Although the carboxyhaemoglobin level is important, other investigations and signs and symptoms must be taken into account. A carboxyhaemoglobin level of 15% or greater suggests a significant inhalation injury.

3. a. **False.** They predominate on exposed parts of the body especially the face.
   b. **False.** Basal cell cancers are more common in the elderly.
   c. **True.** Radiotherapy is particularly useful for advanced tumours where underlying deep tissues such as bone are involved.
   d. **True.** They are slow-growing tumours spread by local direct invasion.
   e. **True.** They are slow-growing tumours that are spread by local direct invasion.

4. a. **True.** This variant is known as a Marjolin's ulcer.
   b. **False.** Squamous cell cancers do not always respond to radiotherapy. They often arise on limbs and extremities where radiotherapy is usually contraindicated.
   c. **True.** These tumours metastasise via the lymphatics to local lymph nodes and via the bloodstream to lungs and bone.

d. **True.** These tumours predominate in the elderly.
e. **False.** Squamous cell cancers develop de novo, usually in areas of the body exposed to strong sunlight.

5. a. **False.** Basal cell cancers are more common. Malignant melanoma accounts for approximately one in 10 of all skin cancers.
   b. **False.** Increase in size, alteration in pigmentation and itching are early signs. Bleeding and ulceration occur later.
   c. **True.** Incidence continues to increase.
   d. **True.** This is a high-risk period, even though the tumours do not develop until later in life.
   e. **False.** Adequate local excision is the treatment of choice. Radiotherapy is reserved for relieving painful bone metastases in patients with advanced disease.

Case history answers

Case history 1

1. This is a laceration caused by a sharp object (broken glass).
2. He has lost a significant amount of blood. Pulse and blood pressure should be checked to ensure he is not in shock. An intravenous infusion should be established and a full blood count obtained. The wound needs to be carefully explored in view of its extent, site and the chance that a major vascular structure may have been damaged in the depths of the wound. Exploration should be carried out under general anaesthetic. Local pressure with a bandage should control the haemorrhage until definitive exploration can be carried out.
3. The structures that could have been damaged include:
   - facial nerve branches
   - parotid duct
   - superficial temporal artery and vein
   - maxillary artery
   - infraorbital nerve
   - parotid duct.
4. The most serious complications following this injury are:
   - facial muscle weakness following nerve injury
   - hypertrophic scarring causing disfigurement
   - a salivary fistula from the parotid gland.

Case history 2

1. The most important points in the early management of this patient are:

a. check blood gases and obtain a chest X-ray as a smoke inhalation injury is suspected

b. provide adequate analgesia using morphine or pethidine

c. insert an i.v. cannula and catheterise the patient

d. consider an escharotomy for the circumferential wound to the right arm to prevent a 'torniquet effect' from the burn.

2. Intravenous morphine or pethidine would be the analgesics of choice. This route of administration is preferred because subcutaneous or intramuscular absorption in burn patients can be erratic leading to under- or overdosage.

3. The fluid requirements would be calculated according to the Muir and Barclay formula:

$$V = \frac{\text{Body weight (kg)} \times \% \text{ burn body surface area}}{2}$$

$$= \frac{65 \times 35}{2} = 1137.5 \text{ ml}$$

The fluid (V ml) must be given initially for three 4-hourly periods, commencing from the time of the burn. In this patient, the first 4 hours are from 9.30 p.m. to 1.30 a.m. Therefore, the projected hourly rate of infusion during this period would be 1137.5 ÷ 4, i.e. 285 ml/hour. However, on admission, 2 hours have already elapsed since the burn; therefore, the first fluid allocation of 1137.5 ml (for the first 4-hour period after the burn) has to be given in 2 hours (i.e. 11.30 p.m. to 1.30 a.m.). The infusion should run at 559 ml/hour (1137.5 ÷ 2), i.e. twice the rate first calculated. Thereafter, the standard rate of infusion, as calculated by the formula, is resumed but must be carefully monitored by the hourly urine output and haematocrit.

4. A colloid solution such as plasma protein substitute (PPS) is the most appropriate.

5. The key indices would be:
   - packed cell volume (PCV)
   - hourly urine output.

6. After initial cleaning, cover the fingers and hand with silver sulphadiazine cream and cover them with a plastic bag tied at the wrist. Later tangential excision and skin grafting would be required, 5–7 days after the burn.

Case histories 3–6

Photographs 1–4 relate to the case histories and diagnoses as below:

- Case history 3
  — malignant melanoma — Photograph 3
- Case history 4
  — squamous or basal cell carcinoma — Photograph 4
- Case history 5
  — keratoacanthoma or squamous cell carcinoma — Photograph 1

- Case history 6
  — basal cell carcinoma — Photograph 2.

Case history 3

1. Malignant melanoma; the patient presents with *early* symptoms of itching and colour change.'Notching' of the outline of the mole is also noted.

2. The surrounding skin should be examined to ensure there are no satellite nodules in the skin or subcutaneous tissues. The regional draining lymph nodes in the popliteal fossa and groin should also be examined, as should the liver for signs of hepatomegaly.

3. A chest X-ray and liver function tests.

4. *Complete* excision of the lesion is the key treatment. Partial biopsy should *not* be carried out. As this is quite a small lesion, it should be possible to close the resulting defect without a skin graft.

5. Half of the patients with a lesion of this thickness will die from recurrent disease within 5 years.

6. This patient is at a slightly higher risk than the general population of developing a further melanoma. She should be advised to avoid getting burned in the sun, to use a higher factor sun block (factor 15 or over) and to reapply this every few hours when out of doors, particularly in the middle of the day. Any remaining moles can be photographed as a base line should any change occur in them in the future.

Case history 4

1. This is either a squamous cell or a basal cell carcinoma. Sometimes these tumours can be difficult to distinguish.

2. The regional lymph glands in the axilla.

3. A chest X-ray.

4. The lesion will need to be excised, and because of its size and site a skin graft will be needed to repair the resulting defect. A diagnostic biopsy would be useful prior to formal excision.

Case history 5

1. Keratoacanthoma or squamous cell carcinoma are the most likely diagnoses.

2. The regional lymph nodes especially in the neck (submandibular, submental groups) and also the parotid nodes.

3. The most likely diagnosis given the short history and clinical examination is of a keratoacanthoma. If so, a spontaneous resolution can be expected but an expectant policy should only be pursued for a further 4 weeks or so. Thereafter, if there is no evidence of resolution, the lesion should be excised. At this site, a complex flap reconstruction will have to be carried out to minimise distortion of the lip.

Case history 6

1. A basal cell carcinoma is most likely.

2. The lesion could be treated by surgery or radiotherapy. The advantage of surgery is that histological analysis can be performed and the completeness of excision confirmed. Basal cell cancers are, however, sensitive to radiotherapy.

3. Only in exceptional circumstances do basal cell carcinomas metastasise to regional lymph glands.

Short notes answers

1. Burn injuries can be divided into three categories according to increasing severity:
   - superficial
   - deep dermal
   - full thickness.

   Superficial burns are characterised by blistering and an erythematous appearance. Sensation to pin prick is normal.

   Deep dermal burns are also blistered but the wound base is creamy white in colour. Pin prick sensation is reduced but *not* absent.

   Full thickness burns are not blistered and have a leathery grey/white appearance. Sensation to pain and pin prick is absent.

2. The most important education measures would be to raise public awareness of the risks, for example:
   - avoidance of sun lamps
   - avoidance of excessive exposure to sun light
   - appropriate use of barrier creams.

   It would also be important to educate the public regarding the warning signs of malignant change in pre-existing moles, such as:
   - increase in size
   - change in pigmentation
   - itching
   - bleeding and ulceration.

   A GP should also try to identify patients at particular risk:
   - those with multiple naevi
   - those with giant congenital naevi.

Transplantation

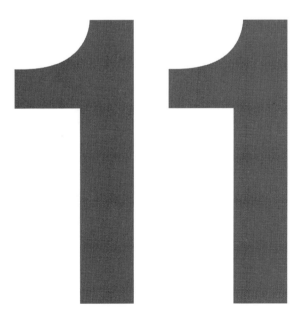

11.1 General principles

Although the technical barriers to whole organ transplantation were overcome at the beginning of the twentieth century, successful whole organ transplantation was impractical until the phenomenon of rejection was understood and reliable methods of immunosuppression had been developed. The modern era of transplantation really began in the 1960s with the first successful series of kidney transplants.

Currently, the most frequently performed transplants are:

- kidney
- liver
- heart
- lung.

Various terms and definitions are used in transplant technology. *Allotransplantation* means transplantation from a non-identical donor to a recipient of the same species (i.e. an allograft). Almost all human transplants are in this category. *Xenotransplantation*, transplanting between members of different species, is rare. *Grafts* which are implanted into a recipient are termed *orthotopic* if they occupy their normal anatomical site (e.g. liver transplants) or *heterotopic* if they occupy an ectopic site (e.g. renal transplants).

Rejection and immunosuppression

Early transplants inevitably failed because of a complex rejection process, which involved cellular immunity (T and B cell lymophocytes) and humoral immunity (circulating antibody) mechanisms.

The host response to the donor graft depends upon the tissue matching. The two most important compatibility systems are:

- ABO blood group
- HLA (human leucocyte antigen) Class I and Class II systems.

On the rare occasions when donor and recipient are identical twins, tissue matching will be perfect and there will be no antigenic difference and no rejection.

ABO blood group compatibility is essential. Placing a blood group B graft into a blood group O recipient, for example, will lead to immediate rejection because of

circulating (humoral) anti-group B antibodies in the recipient.

The HLA Class I and II antigen systems are extremely complex. Although close matching between donor and recipient confers a survival advantage of the graft in the recipient, such matching is not always possible because of the wide number of antigen permutations. It may be impossible to set up the perfect match between donor and recipient. Instead, it is necessary to settle for the best available match between a given donor and recipient.

The therapeutic goal of *immunosuppression* is to overide any response of the immune system to tissue histoincompatibility while at the same time to preserve the remaining functions of the recipient's immune system to protect against infection.

Three patterns of rejection are recognised:

- hyperacute
- acute
- chronic.

Hyperacute rejection. This occurs within minutes to hours after transplantation. The transplanted organ becomes swollen and tender and there is severe vascular damage, with thrombosis and endothelial damage. There is an abrupt cessation of graft function. This injury is mediated by circulating recipient antibodies and is usually caused by a major ABO or HLA system incompatibility.

Acute rejection. This develops within a few weeks/months of transplantation and is of rapid onset. The graft becomes tender and swollen and there is a deterioration in function. The rejection process is mediated by a combination of cellular and humoral (antibody) mechanisms. Biopsy of the graft will reveal a mixed cellular infiltrate (lymphocytes, monocytes and plasma cells) together with evidence of antibody-mediated vascular endothelial damage.

Chronic rejection. This begins months/years after transplantation. It is characterised by a progressive deterioration of the transplanted organ, with a mononuclear cellular infiltration on graft biopsy.

Methods of immunosuppression.

Drug therapy is the cornerstone of immunosuppression. The principal agents used are given in Table 18. A wide variety of combinations of these agents are used to combat rejection. Therapy is begun immediately following transplantation and continues indefinitely.

Table 18 Immunosuppressive drugs used in transplantation

	Action	Side effects
Cyclosporin A	Inhibits immunoactive leucocytes	Nephrotoxic, hepatotoxic
Azathioprine	Inhibits RNA and DNA synthesis	Bone marrow depression
Steroids	Inhibits inflammation	Growth retardation, hypertension, increased infection risk
Antilymphocyte globulin	Reduces lymphocyte numbers	
Antithymocyte globulin	Reduces thymocyte numbers	

11.2 Types of organ transplant

Renal transplantation

This is the most successful and frequent organ transplant. Most major medical centres in the UK have an established renal transplant programme and, nationwide, 3000 transplants are performed each year.

The main indication for transplantation is irreversible renal failure. The three most frequent causes are:

- chronic glomerulonephritis
- chronic pyelonephritis
- diabetic nephropathy.

Most patients who are on a transplant waiting list will require peritoneal or haemodialysis until a suitable kidney becomes available.

Donor sources
Kidneys for transplantation come from two sources:

- brain-dead donors (cadaveric transplants)
- living donors.

Most donor kidneys come from patients who have recently died in hospital, following either a stroke or a major head injury. Donors are accepted provided there is no evidence of active infection, extracerebral malignancy, hepatitis A, B or C infection or HIV infection.

Once brainstem death is confirmed and consent obtained, the kidneys are harvested as part of a multiple organ donation involving liver, kidneys, heart and lungs. Immediately the circulation is arrested, the intra-abdominal organs are perfused with a cold preservation fluid in order to minimise the period of warm ischaemic time and thus prevent organ degeneration. Most kidneys can be preserved for up to 24 hours.

Live donation is usually reserved for related donors who wish to help a family member with renal disease. Transplantation between unrelated individuals is less common and is fraught with ethical problems.

Transplant surgery
The kidney is transplanted into a heterotopic site in either the left or right iliac fossa. An extraperitoneal pouch is prepared to receive the kidney and the renal vessels are anastomosed to the adjacent external iliac artery and vein.

The ureter is usually implanted into the recipient's bladder. Implantation into the colon or an isolated small bowel loop (an ileal conduit) is rarely used.

Outcome and prognosis
Rejection episodes are uncommon with the newer regimens of immunosuppression, outlined on page 198. Although recipients cope well with common viral illnesses, they are prone to opportunistic infection with *Pneumocystis* sp. or cytomegalovirus (CMV). Cancer is also more common in transplant recipients.

Current long term graft survival rates average 80% for cadaveric transplants and 90% for living related grafts.

Liver transplantation

The first successful liver transplants were carried out in the late 1960s. Before 1980, 1-year survival was less than 40%. The introduction of cyclosporin revolutionised liver transplantation and, worldwide, more than 4000 transplants are performed per year with the 1-year survival rates exceeding 70%.

The main indications for transplantation in adults are:

- cirrhosis secondary to viral hepatitis
- fulminant liver failure.

Transplantation is performed less often for:

- hepatocellular cancer
- alcoholic cirrhosis.

In children, congenital biliary atresias are the most widespread indication for liver transplantation.

Donor sources
Whole organ livers are obtained from brain-dead donors. Because there are technical difficulties encountered in transplanting a large liver into a small recipient (e.g. from an adult to a child) several alternative types of transplant have been developed. These are:

- reduced-size transplants: using part of the left liver lobe only as a graft; this is especially useful in children
- split-liver transplants: dividing the liver into two anatomical halves corresponding to the left and right lobes to enable two transplants from one donor.

Living related transplants are occasionally undertaken, again using part of the left lobe. This form of transplantation is usually undertaken between mother and child.

Transplant surgery
The operative procedure is complex. Essentially the organ is transplanted orthotopically after the recipient liver has been removed. During this procedure, the venous return to the heart is diverted away from the liver bed by an extracorporeal veno-venous bypass.

Outcome and prognosis
Haemorrhage and biliary complications including obstructive jaundice are the most common early postoperative complications. Opportunistic infections related to immunosuppression are also frequent.

Despite these setbacks, patients can expect up to a 70% 1-year survival.

Cardiac transplantation

Successful cardiac transplantation was established as recently as 1970–1980. Currently about 3000 transplants are performed annually worldwide.

The main indication for cardiac transplantation is end-stage cardiac failure, which is most commonly caused by:

- viral cardiomyopathy
- ischaemic heart disease.

Less common indications include:

- valvular heart disease
- congenital heart disease.

There are few contraindications to transplantation other than the presence of active infection (especially HIV or hepatitis) or major liver or renal dysfunction.

Donor sources

Donor hearts are invariably obtained as part of a multiple organ retrieval from a brain-dead donor. In contrast to kidney and liver transplants, a freshly harvested cold perfused heart has a short survival time of only 4–6 hours. Because of this, recipient preparation and organ retrieval, which often take place at different centres, have to be carefully coordinated to minimise any delays.

Transplant surgery

Cardiopulmonary bypass is established and the recipient's heart excised before performing an orthotopic heart transplant.

Outcome and prognosis

Many patients will die in the early postoperative period because of the severity of their pre-existing cardiac illness, despite a technically successful transplant. Sepsis precipitated by immunosuppression is another important cause of mortality. Deaths caused by rejection are less common.

About 80% of all transplant patients will survive at least 1 year after operation.

Pulmonary transplantation

Successful lung transplantation has only been achieved since the late 1980s. The main indications for transplantation are:

- chronic fibrotic lung disease
- chronic obstructive airways disease
- chronic pulmonary sepsis
- pulmonary hypertension.

Transplant surgery

There are three types of operation:

- combined heart and lung transplants
- single lung transplants
- bilateral lung transplants.

The choice of operation depends upon the extent of pulmonary disease and any coexistent cardiac disease.

Outcome and prognosis

Rejection and/or infection are the main causes of graft failure. Lung transplantation is less successful than heart, liver or renal transplantation; approximately 60% of patients will survive 1 year after surgery.

Small bowel transplantation

Small bowel transplantation remains experimental. The main indication is intestinal failure in patients who have had massive small bowel resection who, for whatever reason, can no longer be treated by total parenteral nutrition.

Transplant surgery

Currently, controversy exists regarding the relative merits of small bowel transplantation either alone or in combination with liver transplantation. Various clinical trials are currently underway in the major transplant centres worldwide.

Outcome and prognosis

To date, there have been few long-term survivors.

Self-assessment: questions

Multiple choice questions

1. With regard to transplantation in general:
   a. Currently most human transplants are xenotransplants
   b. A renal transplant is an example of an orthotopic transplant
   c. Allotransplantation means transplantation from a non-identical donor to a recipient of the same species
   d. Heterotopic transplants are rarely performed
   e. Currently renal transplants are the most commonly performed transplant operation

2. The following points concern transplant rejection:
   a. A blood group A graft placed in a blood group O recipient will not be rejected if there is a good HLA system match between donor and recipient
   b. Close HLA class I and II matching is essential if rejection is to be prevented
   c. An acute pattern of rejection usually develops within weeks/months of transplantation
   d. Hyperacute rejection is characterised by severe vascular damage, with thrombosis and endothelial destruction
   e. Cellular and humoral mechanisms are responsible for the phenomenon of acute rejection

3. With regard to renal transplantation:
   a. Most kidneys can be preserved for up to 24 hours between harvesting and transplantation
   b. A 60% survival rate can be expected following cadaveric transplantation
   c. The kidney is usually transplanted into a heterotopic site in either the left or right iliac fossa
   d. Renal transplant patients are prone to infection with *Pneumocystis* sp. or cytomegalovirus
   e. Diabetic nephropathy can recur in a healthy kidney following transplantation

4. With regard to liver transplantation:
   a. Biliary atresia is a common indication for transplantation in adults
   b. Multiple transplants can be provided from a single donor liver
   c. Liver transplantation is an example of an orthotopic transplant
   d. Up to 70% of all transplant patients can expect to live for 1 year after transplantation
   e. Liver transplantation is contraindicated in patients with hepatocellular carcinoma

5. With regard to cardiac and pulmonary transplantation:
   a. A freshly harvested cold perfused heart will survive for up to 12 hours before transplantation
   b. Acute rejection is the most frequent cause of death following cardiac transplantation
   c. Cardiopulmonary bypass is an essential step prior to performing an orthotopic cardiac transplant
   d. Ischaemic heart disease accounts for 40% of all patients requiring cardiac transplantation
   e. Coronary artery disease can develop in a healthy transplanted heart

Self-assessment: answers

Multiple choice answers

1. a. **False.** Xenotransplantation means transplanting between members of different species. Most human transplants are allotransplants, i.e. transplanting between members of the same species.
   b. **False.** Grafts are termed orthotopic if they are transplanted into their 'normal' anatomical site. Renal transplants are usually heterotopic, occupying an ectopic site usually in the right or left iliac fossa.
   c. **True.** Most human transplants are allografts.
   d. **False.** Renal transplants, the most common of all human transplants, are heterotopic.
   e. **True.** Approximately 3000 renal transplants are performed per year in the UK. The usual limiting factor is the availability of suitable donor kidneys.

2. a. **False.** The ABO blood group is one of the key compatibility systems in tissue matching. A blood group A graft will be immediately rejected by a blood group O recipient by circulating anti-group A antibodies in the recipient. This will occur even if there is a good donor/recipient match in the HLA system.
   b. **False.** The HLA class I and II antigen systems are extremely complex and perfect matching is rarely achieved between donor and recipient because of the wide number of antigenic permutations. However, this does not prevent transplantation. Immunosuppressive agents such as cyclosporin are used to overide the recipient immune response to the graft.
   c. **True.** Hyperacute rejection occurs within minutes of transplantation. An acute rejection response occurs within several months of transplantation.
   d. **True.** The transplanted organ becomes acutely swollen and tender and ceases to function. Vascular thrombosis and endothelial damage are the key microscopic features.
   e. **True.** Only hyperacute rejection is mediated predominantly by circulating humoral antibodies.

3. a. **True.** There is a functional deterioration if transplantation is delayed beyond this time.
   b. **False.** Graft survival rates following transplantation average 80%.
   c. **True.** A renal transplant is the most common type of heterotopic transplant.
   d. **True.** Opportunistic infections are more frequent in patients following renal or other types of transplant. This is related to suppression of the patient's own immune system by the immunosuppressive agents used to prevent rejection.
   e. **True.** Diabetic nephropathy and some forms of glomerulonephritis can recur in a transplanted kidney. Occasionally repeat transplantation is required.

4. a. **False.** This is the major indication for transplantation in childhood. Most adult transplants are undertaken for cirrhosis secondary to viral hepatitis or for fulminant liver failure.
   b. **True.** A split liver transplant, dividing the liver into two anatomical halves corresponding to the left and right lobes of the liver, enables two transplants from one donor.
   c. **True.** The liver is transplanted into its normal anatomical site, i.e. it is an orthotopic transplant.
   d. **True.** The immunosuppressive agent cyclosporin has revolutionised the outcome of liver transplantation. Currently 70% of transplanted patients will survive 1 year.

5. a. **False.** A heart has a short survival period after harvesting, usually 4–6 hours. For this reason, recipient preparation and donor harvesting, which often take place at different centres, need to be carefully coordinated.
   b. **False.** Most early deaths are caused by the severity of the patient's pre-existing cardiac illness. These patients will die despite a technically successful transplant.
   c. **True.** Cardiopulmonary bypass enables systemic perfusion to continue during the transplant procedure.
   d. **True.** Ischaemic heart disease and viral myocarditis together account for 80–90% of all transplant patients.
   e. **True.** 'Transplant' coronary artery disease does occur. It is probably a form of chronic rejection rather than a complication of developing atheromatous disease.

Index